NINTH EDITION

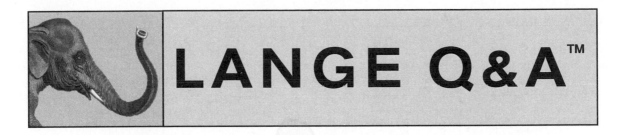

LANGE Q&A™

PSYCHIATRY

Ivan Oransky, MD
Clinical Assistant Professor of Medicine
New York University School of Medicine
New York, New York

Sean Blitzstein, MD
Director, Psychiatry Clerkship
Clinical Professor of Psychiatry
University of Illinois at Chicago School of Medicine
Chicago, Illinois

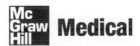

New York Chicago San Francisco Lisbon London Madrid Mexico City Milan
New Delhi San Juan Seoul Singapore Sydney Toronto

Lange Q&A™: Psychiatry, Ninth Edition

Copyright © 2007 by The McGraw-Hill Companies, Inc. All rights reserved. Printed in the United States of America. Except as permitted under the United States Copyright Act of 1976, no part of this publication may be reproduced or distributed in any form or by any means, or stored in a data base or retrieval system, without the prior written permission of the publisher.

Lange Q&A™ is a trademark of The McGraw-Hill Companies, Inc.

2 3 4 5 6 7 8 9 0   QPD/QPD   0 9 8 7

ISBN-13: 978-0-07-147567-9
ISBN-10:   0-07-147567-2

Notice

Medicine is an ever-changing science. As new research and clinical experience broaden our knowledge, changes in treatment and drug therapy are required. The authors and the publisher of this work have checked with sources believed to be reliable in their efforts to provide information that is complete and generally in accord with the standards accepted at the time of publication. However, in view of the possibility of human error or changes in medical sciences, neither the authors nor the publisher nor any other party who has been involved in the preparation or publication of this work warrants that the information contained herein is in every respect accurate or complete, and they disclaim all responsibility for any errors or omissions or for the results obtained from use of the information contained in this work. Readers are encouraged to confirm the information contained herein with other sources. For example and in particular, readers are advised to check the product information sheet included in the package of each drug they plan to administer to be certain that the information contained in this work is accurate and that changes have not been made in the recommended dose or in the contraindications for administration. This recommendation is of particular importance in connection with new or infrequently used drugs.

This book was set in Palatino by International Typesetting and Composition.
The editor was Marsha S. Loeb.
The production supervisor was Phil Galea.
Project management was provided by International Typesetting and Composition.
Quebecor World Dubuque was printer and binder.

This book is printed on acid-free paper.

Library of Congress Cataloging-in-Publication Data

Lange Q & A. Psychiatry / [edited by] Ivan Oransky, Sean Blitzstein. —9th ed.
    p. ; cm.
   Includes bibliographical references and index.
   ISBN-13: 978-0-07-147567-9 (soft cover : alk. paper)
   ISBN-10: 0-07-147567-2 (soft cover : alk. paper)
   1. Psychiatry—Examinations, questions, etc.   I. Oransky, Ivan.   II. Blitzstein, Sean.
III. Title: Q & A.   IV. Title: Psychiatry.
  [DNLM: 1. Mental Disorders—therapy—Examination Questions.   2. Mental Disorders—diagnosis—Examination Questions.   3. Psychiatry—Examination Questions. WM 18.2 L274   2007]
RC457.E18   2007
616.89'0076—dc22

                                                2006035504

Contents

Preface

Welcome to *Lange Q&A: Psychiatry*, 9th edition. It is an exciting time to be studying or practicing psychiatry as sophisticated imaging techniques herald potential changes in how we think about diagnostic criteria and the brain itself. Such methods aren't yet ready for clinical use, and are certainly not part of the fundamentals of psychiatry tested on the USMLE Step 2 examination, but they are worth noting nonetheless because future generations of medical students—users of future editions of this book—will more than likely need to master such material.

As psychiatry begins to change, so too does the format of the United States Medical Licensing Examination (USMLE) Step 2 examination. This edition of the book reflects those changes so that students can use it to prepare for the examination as effectively as possible. The subjects covered in the eighth and previous editions—from psychopathology to psychopharmacology and legal issues—are represented in nine chapters and 800 questions including two final chapters that are practice tests of 100 questions each that simulate the real examination. The "definitions" chapter has been eliminated.

Because so many students rely heavily or solely on books of questions such as this, answers include, in addition to a discussion of the correct answer, a discussion of why the incorrect answers were wrong. That way, learning is not restricted to one term or discussion per question. All diagnostic criteria refer to the American Psychiatric Association's *Diagnostic and Statistical Manual of Mental Disorders, Fourth Edition, Text Revision* (DSM-IV-TR), the most recent edition. A list of references is included for those students who wish to pursue further reading, but is not indexed directly to questions because many students will be using this book, as I did, at the last minute before their examinations.

As much as possible, we have done our best to replicate the format of the examination. That means that in this edition, all of the questions are clinical vignettes and there are no negatively phrased questions (e.g., *except, least likely*). None of the vignettes have more than two questions, and many have just one. Still, because there are many times the number of questions in this book as there are psychiatry questions on the USMLE Step 2, some sets of questions based on a single vignette remain to give you a sense of how a single vignette can raise more than one important (and testable) issue.

There is material in this edition, as in previous editions, that is unlikely to appear on the examination. That's because I recognize that some students use this book to review material during their psychiatry clerkships as well as in direct studying for the examination. The answers to those "non-USMLE-type" questions begin with a note that these are in a format unlikely to be found on that test.

A few words on how best to use this book. If you are first picking it up within a few weeks of Step 2 and don't have time to review the entire book, I'd recommend hitting Chapters 8 and 9, the practice examinations. These best reflect what you'll see on the examination and will point out gaps in your knowledge.

If you have more time—say, a few months—pick some questions from each chapter, other than Chapters 8 and 9 to test your knowledge of each subject, then concentrate on those chapters in which you're weakest.

Finally, if you're using this book during your clerkship, it's probably best to work through all the chapters and save Chapters 8 and 9 for the end of your clerkship review. You'll find basic questions that will help you master the material but that may not appear on Step 2.

Ivan Oransky, MD

Acknowledgments

This book continues to reflect the hard work and dedication of a large group of contributors to past editions of the predecessor book, *Appleton & Lange Review of Psychiatry*. This list reflects the titles and affiliations of those contributors at the time of publication of earlier editions.

R. Andrew Chambers, MD
Resident
Department of Psychiatry
Yale University School of Medicine
New Haven, Connecticut

Joseph R. Check, MD
Assistant Clinical Professor of Psychiatry
Yale University
New Haven, Connecticut

Vladimir Coric, MD
Chief of Inpatient Services
Clinical Neuroscience Research Unit
Assistant Clinical Professor of Psychiatry
Yale University
New Haven, Connecticut

Frank G. Fortunati, MD, JD
Resident
Department of Psychiatry
Yale University School of Medicine
New Haven, Connecticut

Brian Greenlee, MD
Resident
Department of Psychiatry
University of Kentucky
Lexington, Kentucky

Julie E. Peters, MD
Resident
Department of Psychiatry
Yale University School of Medicine
New Haven, Connecticut

Greer Richardson, MD
Resident
Department of Psychiatry
Yale University School of Medicine
New Haven, Connecticut

William Roman, MD
Resident
Department of Psychiatry
Yale University School of Medicine
New Haven, Connecticut

Louis Sanfilippo, MD
Assistant Clinical Professor of Psychiatry
Yale University
New Haven, Connecticut

Raziya Sunderji, MD
Resident
Department of Psychiatry
Yale University
New Haven, Connecticut

Blake Taggart, MD
Resident
Department of Psychiatry
Yale University School of Medicine
New Haven, Connecticut

Elizabeth Walter, MD
Resident
Department of Psychiatry
Yale University School of Medicine
New Haven, Connecticut

Chung-Che Charles Wang, MD
Resident
Department of Psychiatry
Yale University
New Haven, Connecticut

Thanks to medical students Adam Beall, Alvin Kwok, and Mark McDonnell, who made helpful suggestions on how to improve from the eighth edition. Thanks also to the extremely patient Marsha Loeb, our editor at McGraw-Hill. And of course, thanks to the patients and professors who taught me psychiatry.

Ivan Oransky, MD

CHAPTER 1

Psychological Testing
Questions

DIRECTIONS (Questions 1 through 27): Each of the numbered items in this section is followed by answers. Select the ONE lettered answer that is BEST in each case.

Questions 1 and 2

A 34-year-old woman suffering from severe depression and chronic renal failure is a candidate for electroconvulsive therapy (ECT).

1. Which test listed below can be used to monitor the patient's depressive symptoms with the greatest reliability and validity?

    (A) Thematic Apperception Test (TAT)
    (B) Rorschach Test
    (C) Halstead-Reitan Neuropsychological Battery
    (D) Draw-a-Person Test
    (E) Beck Depression Inventory

2. The most useful test to assess for memory impairments in the setting of ECT is which of the following?

    (A) Brown-Peterson Task
    (B) Beck Depression Inventory
    (C) State-Trait Anxiety Inventory
    (D) Bulimia Test—Revised
    (E) Eating Disorder Inventory-2 (EDI-2)

Mr. Brown was the doctor and Peterson was the physician and memory following ECT will be evaluated;

Questions 3 and 4

You admit an 83-year-old widowed White woman for further evaluation because she is no longer able to care for herself at home. She has lost 30 lb in the past year, has poor hygiene, and admits to increasing forgetfulness.

3. A commonly administered screening test to evaluate for dementia is which of the following?

    (A) Geriatric Rating Scale
    (B) Glasgow Coma Scale
    (C) Folstein Mini-Mental Status Examination (MMSE)
    (D) Mental Status Examination (MSE)
    (E) Blessed Rating Scale

4. Another psychiatric diagnosis that may mimic dementia in this patient is which of the following?

    (A) panic disorder
    (B) depression
    (C) posttraumatic stress disorder
    (D) generalized anxiety disorder
    (E) obsessive-compulsive disorder

Questions 5 and 6

A 28-year-old single African American man with a long history of schizophrenia and prominent thought disorganization asks you if there are psychological tests that would demonstrate which part of his brain "isn't working." You explain that no test can indicate exactly which part of his brain is different from those without schizophrenia and suggest a certain test to assess his ability to organize and correctly process information.

Read Ans

5. The neuropsychological test you recommend is which of the following?

    (A) MMSE
    (B) Wisconsin Card Sorting Test (WCST)
    (C) Bender Gestalt Test
    (D) Luria-Nebraska Neuropsychological Battery
    (E) Draw-a-Person Test

    Wisconsin card sorting test → see Frontal Lobe working.

6. This test assesses which of the following?

    (A) executive functions of the brain
    (B) attentional state
    (C) the ability to draw
    (D) orientation
    (E) memory

    executive Functions → Frontal Lobe messed up schizophrenia

Questions 7 and 8

While reading a medical journal, you find an article about a new screening test that predicts a patient's risk for suicide. The authors have shown that high scores on their screening test correlate with an increased risk for completed suicide. Nine months later, another group repeats the study and demonstrates that male patients consistently scored higher on the screening test than female patients. Furthermore, the authors of the second article state that when gender is taken into account, the previously reported correlation between the screening test and increase in suicide rate vanishes. The authors of the second study conclude that this limits the usefulness of the screening test to predict a patient's risk of suicide.

7. The authors of the initial article regarding the screening test suggested that their test was useful because of which of the following?

    (A) internal reliability
    (B) test-retest reliability
    (C) content validity
    (D) predictive validity
    (E) discriminative validity

    screening test can predict who is at high risk suicide. has predictive validity.

8. The authors of the second paper faulted the usefulness of this screening tool because of its lack of which of the following?

    (A) internal reliability
    (B) test-retest reliability
    (C) content validity
    (D) predictive validity
    (E) discriminative validity

    screening test does not take into account sexes has discriminative validity.

Questions 9 and 10

A patient is administered a test that consists of viewing a set of 10 inkblots sequentially. The responses to the inkblots are noted by the examiner in relationship to the content of the perception, the area of the blot that forms the basis of the response, and the aspects of the area that are used to form the response.

9. The test being administered is which of the following?

    (A) TAT
    (B) Rorschach Test
    (C) Sentence Completion Test
    (D) Draw-a-Person Test
    (E) Minnesota Multiphasic Personality Inventory (MMPI)

10. This type of projective test is best classified as which of the following?

    (A) self-expression
    (B) constructions
    (C) completions
    (D) associations
    (E) choice of ordering

11. An 89-year-old married African American woman is admitted to the medical service with a diagnosis of failure to thrive. The team following her has asked you to assess her. In their notes, they observe that the patient is not oriented to time. To evaluate orientation, you perform which of the following?

   (A) Spatial Orientation Memory Test
   (B) Fargo Map Test
   (C) Stroop Test
   (D) WCST
   (E) Temporal Orientation Test

Questions 12 and 13

A 25-year-old single African American woman who carries the diagnosis of dependent personality disorder is referred for psychological testing. Your first consideration is whether to perform a set of projective or objective tests.

12. You decide to perform projective tests because of which of the following reasons?

   (A) They provide numerical scores.
   (B) They ask specific questions with itemized responses.
   (C) They are unstructured and allow for a variety of responses from the examinee.
   (D) Statistical analysis is easily undertaken on the data.
   (E) You want to determine how the patient feels about you.

13. After performing a battery of projective tests, you chose to continue testing with the MMPI-2. You chose this test because of which of the following reasons?

   (A) It is the most widely used test in the evaluation of personality structure.
   (B) It can be scored by nonprofessionals.
   (C) It is a specific type of projective test.
   (D) The patient is single.
   (E) It is designed to evaluate attitudes about test taking at the time the test is administered.

Questions 14 and 15

A 20-year-old college student is referred for testing to evaluate poor academic performance. He reports that he has always "struggled" to pass his classes despite studying for many hours. He attends all of his lectures and is able to pay attention, yet he does not seem to be able to adequately learn the material. While he is very frustrated, he denies significant depression.

14. Which of the following tests would be most appropriate to determine this patient's problem?

   (A) MMPI-2
   (B) Draw-a-Person Test
   (C) Wechsler Adult Intelligence Scale—Revised (WAIS-R)
   (D) Wechsler Intelligence Scale for Children (WISC)
   (E) Wechsler Memory Test (WMT)

15. The IQ is calculated by which of the following formulas?

   (A) performance IQ/verbal IQ × 100
   (B) mental age/full-scale IQ × 100
   (C) chronological age/performance IQ × 100
   (D) mental age/chronological age × 100
   (E) actual IQ/theoretic IQ × 100

Questions 16 and 17

A 72-year-old man is suspected to have suffered a stroke in his right parietal region.

16. The test most likely to show abnormalities is which of the following?

   (A) WMT
   (B) WCST
   (C) MMPI-2
   (D) Rey-Osterrieth Test
   (E) Rorschach Test

mnemonic "MCI° MAImental CA chronological I = IQ"

17. This test assesses which of the following?

   (A) visual nonverbal memory
   (B) verbal memory
   (C) tactile memory
   (D) long-term procedural memory
   (E) long-term implicit memory

18. A 70-year-old man with multiple medical problems is suspected to have had a stroke, affecting his ability to speak. The test most likely to adequately describe the nature of the difficulty is which of the following?

   (A) Stroop Test
   (B) Boston Diagnostic Aphasia Examination
   (C) Folstein MMSE
   (D) Bender Gestalt Test
   (E) Sentence Completion Test

19. A compulsive gambler tells her psychiatrist that once she begins to play the slot machines, she cannot stop, particularly if she wins a few times. Which of the following reinforcement schedules best explains the phenomena?

   (A) continuous
   (B) fixed-interval
   (C) fixed-ratio
   (D) variable-interval
   (E) variable-ratio

20. When an examiner asks a patient to count backward by 7, starting at 100 (referred to as serial sevens), what is principally being tested?

   (A) recent memory
   (B) remote memory
   (C) concentration
   (D) fund of knowledge
   (E) mathematics skills

21. A 39-year-old woman presents to the outpatient mental health clinic at the request of her oncologist 3 weeks after being diagnosed with metastatic breast cancer. The patient denies strong feelings in relation to the diagnosis, but talks a great deal about the epidemiology of breast cancer and the available treatment options. Which of the following defense mechanisms is she using?

   (A) sublimation
   (B) dissociation
   (C) intellectualization
   (D) rationalization
   (E) self-observation

22. A 35-year-old woman presents with episodic anxiety and complains of the occasional feeling that she has heard or perceived things prior to actually hearing them. She expresses her concern that she is "going crazy." You assure her that this can occur in anxiety disorders. What is this phenomenon called?

   (A) déjà vu
   (B) jamais vu
   (C) déjà entendu
   (D) folie à deux
   (E) la belle indifférence

23. After being severely reprimanded by his employer, a man goes home and is extremely nasty to his wife. What is his behavior an example of?

   (A) sublimation
   (B) dissociation
   (C) displacement
   (D) rationalization
   (E) conversion

24. A psychiatrist discovers that she is frustrated and easily angered with one of her patients for no obvious reason. While talking to a colleague, she admits that the patient reminds her of her abusive father. Which of the following best describes the clinician's reaction?

   (A) transference
   (B) countertransference
   (C) reaction formation
   (D) displacement
   (E) projection

25. A 36-year-old woman was placed on alprazo-lam (Xanax) 3 years ago for panic disorder. After watching a news report on television, she became frightened about addiction. She abruptly stopped the medication and during the next 3 days experienced increased anxiety attacks, but claims that she is now doing better. She denies any tremor, sweating, increased heart rate, or uneasiness except in relation to the panic attacks. Which of the following best describes this phenomenon?

   (A) recurrence
   (B) rebound
   (C) withdrawal
   (D) dystonic reaction
   (E) akathisia

26. A 37-year-old patient presents to your office for the first time for long-term psychotherapy. You decide it would be helpful to compile a personality inventory. You place a set of 10 inkblots in front of the patient and note the responses in terms of the content of the per-ception and the use of the various areas of the inkblot. To score and interpret this test using a data based system, one would rely on which of the following?

   (A) Exner Comprehensive System
   (B) Five-Factor Model
   (C) Eysenck Personality Questionnaire
   (D) California Personality Inventory
   (E) MMPI-2

27. You are asked to evaluate a 68-year-old man on the inpatient medicine service for increasing confusion. The patient was admitted 2 days earlier for pneumonia. After performing a mental status evaluation, you suspect delirium. The patient dropped out of school in the sev-enth grade. The best test to assess this patient's ability to maintain and focus attention is which of the following?

   (A) serial sevens
   (B) counting by two's to 20
   (C) serial threes

   (D) Random Letter Test
   (E) simple calculations

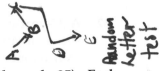

DIRECTIONS (Questions 28 through 35): Each group of items in this section consists of lettered headings followed by a set of numbered words or phrases. For each numbered word or phrase, select the ONE lettered heading that is most closely asso-ciated with it. Each lettered heading may be selected once, more than once, or not at all.

Questions 28 through 35

Match the clinical presentation with the appropriate neuropsychological test.

   (A) MMPI-2
   (B) WISC
   (C) Rey-Osterrieth Test
   (D) Beck Depression Inventory
   (E) Blessed Rating Scale
   (F) WAIS-R
   (G) Boston Diagnostic Aphasia Examin
   (H) Rorschach Test
   (I) Folstein MMSE
   (J) Bender Gestalt Test
   (K) WCST
   (L) Wada Test

28. A 40-year-old woman who scores the Folstein MMSE gave many a don't know, I'm too tired to answ to assess for the possibility of de

29. A 65-year-old man has diffici sequencing, and planning a impairment in memory.

30. The family of an 80-year-c dementia has asked you to to continue to live in his c You would like to ask h their assessment of how

31. A 16-year-old boy w mental retardation pre poor school perfo behavior toward pe

21.

u

18. **(B)** The *Boston Diagnostic Aphasia Examination* is a comprehensive set of tests given by a skilled interviewer to evaluate aphasic disorders and to help define further interventions to improve speech. The Stroop Test aids in the evaluation of concentration. The Folstein MMSE is used for rapid assessment of dementia and delirium. The Bender Gestalt Test is a constructional test for evaluation of brain damage and has some ability to differentiate the location of the lesion. The Sentence Completion Test is a projective test used to describe personality structure.

19. **(E)** Behavior is most difficult to extinguish when reinforced on a partial rather than continuous schedule. Gambling on a slot machine is even more likely to continue because it is reinforced on a variable-ratio schedule, that is, money is given based on a random (but unknown) number of times.

20. **(C)** *Concentration* refers to the ability to sustain focus on a cognitive task. Performing serial sevens and spelling *world* backward are tests of concentration. Although a certain facility with the remaining choices is necessary to perform each task (no cognitive function is tested in absolute isolation), the serial sevens test provides a window on a patient's concentration. *Remote memory* involves the recall of events long past, for example, information from a patient's childhood. *Recent memory* is recall of events occurring in the last several minutes. *Fund of knowledge* is a test of information the patient readily has available to him or her; knowledge of current events is often used to assess this. The *MSE* often contains tests of mathematics skills, but testing mathematics skills is not the purpose of the serial sevens test. Any test of cognitive function must take into account the patient's cultural, educational, and social background.

(C) *Intellectualization* is the utilization of abstract thinking to deal with or cover internal or external stressors; in this case, the unacceptable feelings of having cancer. *Sublimation* is a defense mechanism employed to deal with unacceptable feelings or desires by channeling them into socially acceptable behaviors. Like sublimation, *rationalization* is a defense against undesired motivations, but in this case, the motivations are concealed by elaborate and reassuring explanations that avoid the actual underlying motives. *Dissociation* is a defense mechanism that deals with stressors with a breakdown of the usual integration of memory, behavior, and perception. *Self-observation* is a defense mechanism involving the reflection of one's own thoughts and behavior with appropriate responses.

22. **(C)** *Déjà entendu* is the feeling that one is hearing something one has heard before. It is usually associated with anxiety states or fatigue. *Déjà vu* is a similar experience, but refers to the sensation that something has been seen before. *Jamais vu* is the opposite of déjà vu in that it refers to something that should be familiar but seems quite unfamiliar. *Folie à deux* is a shared delusion aroused in one person by the influence of another. *La belle indifférence* is the indifference shown toward a deficit or loss of function classically seen in a conversion disorder.

23. **(C)** The man is naturally angry, anxious, and sensitive at being reprimanded by his employer. He has found it difficult to express his feelings toward the disturbing person, the employer. Instead of suppressing or repressing the anger, or sublimating his tension in more forceful work, he displaces his anger onto a safer target, his wife. This is an example of displacement.

24. **(B)** *Transference*, in strict terms, is the patient's reexperiencing of past experiences in the setting of psychoanalytic psychotherapy. *Countertransference* is the analyst's (or therapist's) response to this. These terms have come to mean the transferring of emotions and feelings that one has from one's past to the other person; in the case of transference, the feelings are experienced in the patient and relate to how he or she feels about the therapist. In the case of countertransference, the feelings are experienced in the analyst or therapist and reflect how he or she feels about the patient. Reaction

formation, displacement, and projection are all defense mechanisms used by the ego to keep potentially anxiety-provoking feelings out of awareness. *Reaction formation* is the formation of thoughts that are opposite to the anxiety-provoking feelings. *Displacement* is the transferring of a feeling toward an object that is less threatening, as in the family pet or one's spouse or children. *Projection* is the false attribution of one's own unacceptable feelings to another.

25. **(B)** *Rebound* is a return of symptoms that are brief and transient and is frequently associated with the abrupt discontinuation of benzodiazepines. *Recurrence* is the long-term return of the original symptoms. Withdrawal is characterized by a specific set of signs and symptoms specific to a particular substance. These are not necessarily similar to the original symptoms that were being treated by the medication. *Akathisia* is the subjective sensation of motor and mental restlessness. A *dystonic reaction* is an increase in muscle rigidity and spasticity that is usually associated with the use of neuroleptics.

26. **(A)** The test that is being described here is the Rorschach Test. One data-based system used to score and interpret the Rorschach Test is the *Exner Comprehensive System*. It is limited in its validity and requires highly trained examiners. All of the other choices are types of personality assessment not associated with the Rorschach Test. The *Eysenck Personality Questionnaire* constructs questions designed to assess aspects of personality predicted to exist by theoretical constructs. The *MMPI-2* is the most widely used and highly standardized test of personality. The *California Personality Inventory* is similar to the MMPI but is used in counseling situations, rather than with pathologic populations.

27. **(D)** In this instance, the *Random Letter Test*, which relies on concentration, cooperation, and the ability to hear, is the test of choice. The other tests rely not only on attention but also on calculation abilities and educational level. The Random Letter Test consists of telling a patient a letter and then in a monotone listing a random string of letters. The patient responds by raising a finger to indicate when he or she hears the key letter.

28. **(D)** The Beck Depression Inventory is a 21-item test with 3 responses per item that is an easily used screening tool to evaluate for depression. Because it would be unusual for an individual so young to have dementia and because many of the answers reflect a lack of interest, the Beck Depression Inventory, in conjunction with the Folstein MMSE, may help distinguish depression from dementia.

29. **(K)** The WCST assesses executive functions of the brain such as organizational abilities, mental flexibility, and the ability to abstract and reason. These capacities are believed to be located in the frontal lobes. Damage to the frontal lobes can lead to abnormalities on this test.

30. **(E)** The Blessed Rating Scale is a tool that asks friends or family of the patient to assess the ability of the patient to function in his or her usual environment.

31. **(F)** An assessment of IQ is indicated to rule out mental retardation and help better understand the individual's level of intellectual level of functioning. IQ assessment will also aid the school in developing an individualized study program for this student. Because the patient is older than 15, the WAIS-R would be used.

32. **(H)** The Rorschach Test is a projective test that may be used to assess personality structure. The patient has characteristics of schizoid personality disorder, which may be better elucidated with further skilled assessment in the context of his clinical history.

33. **(I)** The Folstein MMSE is a quick, easily administered test that allows for immediate assessment of dementia. Scores of less than 24 are suggestive of a dementia.

34. **(A)** The MMPI-2 is an objective test consisting of several hundred true/false questions used to assess an individual's personality. It is the most widely used and highly standardized test of personality.

35. **(L)** The Wada Test is used to evaluate hemispheric language dominance prior to surgical amelioration of seizure focus. Whereas most right-handed individuals show left hemispheric dominance for language, left-handed individuals may be either right or left dominant. The test consists of injecting sodium amytal into the carotid artery and observing the transient effects on speech. Injection into the left carotid artery anesthetizes the left side of the brain, and those with left hemispheric language dominance show interrupted speech.

The Rey-Osterreith figure is sensitive to deficits in copying and lack of attention to detail in people with right-sided parietal lobe lesions. The appropriate test to evaluate IQ would be the WISC. The Boston Diagnostic Aphasia Examination is a series of tests given by an experienced clinician to evaluate and make treatment recommendations for individuals with aphasia. The Bender Gestalt Test involves copying figures, which helps to determine if organic brain disease is present.

CHAPTER 2

Child and Adolescent Psychiatry
Questions

DIRECTIONS (Questions 1 through 73): Each of the numbered items in this section is followed by answers. Select the ONE lettered answer that is BEST in each case.

Questions 1 and 2

A 17-year-old boy with a history of major depressive disorder (MDD) comes to your office for a routine visit. When you walk into the examining room, you notice that the boy is sitting slumped forward with his head bent down. He does not make eye contact and says nothing. You suspect that he is having a recurrence of depressive symptoms and are concerned about his risk for suicide.

1. Which of the following statements regarding depression and suicide in adolescents is true?

   (A) Rates of suicidal behavior are similar in adolescent girls and boys.
   (B) More girls than boys commit suicide.
   (C) Suicide is a considerable risk in depressed adolescents and should be specifically addressed during an interview.
   (D) A prior suicide attempt does not increase an adolescent's risk of a subsequent one.
   (E) The adolescent suicide rate has remained stable over the past few decades.

   adol suicide is ↑;

2. Which of the following is the most common method by which adolescents commit suicide?

   (A) drug overdose
   (B) stabbing or cutting

   (C) jumping from buildings
   (D) hanging
   (E) firearms

Questions 3 and 4

A mother brings her 7-year-old son to you because she is worried about him. She tells you that he sits up in bed in the middle of the night and screams. She says he is inconsolable but eventually falls back to sleep. She starts crying as she tells you she cannot sleep after these episodes and is exhausted at work during the day.

3. Which of the following initial responses is most appropriate?

   (A) "I can see this is very upsetting for you."
   (B) "I know you're upset, but this problem will get better."
   (C) "I can see you're upset, but you're really overreacting."
   (D) "Tell me why you can't fall back to sleep after your son does."
   (E) "Are you worried that this is your fault?"

   Not "D" since Does Not console;

4. During what stage of sleep do these episodes most likely occur?

   (A) stage 1
   (B) stage 2
   (C) stages 3–4
   (D) rapid eye movement (REM) stage
   (E) any stage

Sleep terror and sleepwalking
Stage 3-4 thats why NOT remembered;

Questions 5 and 6

A 17-year-old girl with a history of asthma presents for a physical examination prior to entering college. You note that she appears sad. Upon further questioning, you learn that she has felt depressed for the past 6 months since breaking up with her boyfriend of 2 years. She says she feels tired all the time and comes home from school every day, lies on the couch, and sleeps or watches television. She reports that she quit the senior celebration committee, no longer "hangs out" with her friends, cannot imagine things will improve, and is considering not going to college. In addition, she has been binge eating and abusing laxatives. Her physical and laboratory examinations are normal. You diagnose her with MDD, single episode and bulimia nervosa, purging type.

5. Which of the following is the most appropriate pharmacologic agent to use to treat this girl's MDD?

    (A) carbamazepine (Tegretol)

    (B) imipramine (Tofranil)
    (C) lithium
    (D) olanzapine (Zyprexa)
    (E) sertraline (Zoloft)

6. Which of the following types of psychotherapy is most effective for the treatment of bulimia nervosa in adolescents?

    (A) cognitive-behavioral therapy
    (B) family therapy
    (C) psychoanalytic psychotherapy
    (D) psychodynamic psychotherapy
    (E) group therapy

Questions 7 and 8

A 6-year-old boy is brought to the clinic by his parents at the request of the boy's teachers. The teachers report that he is quiet in class. When he does talk, he frequently makes errors with verb tense. His parents recall that his speech was delayed. On examination, the boy is friendly and cooperative. His speech is clear, but he uses simple sentences with a limited vocabulary. Otherwise, he has a normal physical and laboratory examinations are normal.

7. Which of the following *Diagnostic and Statistical Manual of Mental Disorders, Fourth Edition, Text Revision* (DSM-IV-TR) diagnoses is most appropriate?

    (A) disorder of written expression
    (B) expressive language disorder
    (C) phonological disorder
    (D) stuttering
    (E) developmental coordination disorder

8. Which of the following would be most helpful in confirming the diagnosis?

    (A) Intelligence quotient (IQ) test
    (B) Children's Assessment Scale (CAS)
    (C) Diagnostic Interview for Children and Adolescents (DICA)
    (D) Diagnostic Interview Schedule for Children (DISC)
    (E) Schedule for Affective Disorders and Schizophrenia for School-Age Children (K-SADS)

Questions 9 and 10

A 6-month-old girl is brought in by her grandmother for a routine visit. The physical examination is normal except that the baby has not gained weight as expected. As of earlier visits, the baby had been gaining weight appropriately. The grandmother reports that the baby likes to eat and is generally happy and playful. On further questioning, the grandmother describes chaotic mealtimes at home and says that the baby drools more than usual.

9. Which of the following DSM-IV-TR eating disorders is the most likely diagnosis?

    (A) anorexia nervosa
    (B) bulimia nervosa
    (C) pica
    (D) rumination disorder
    (E) feeding disorder of infancy or early childhood

10. Which of the following tests would be most helpful in making the diagnosis?

(A) serum lead level
(B) calculation of the percentage of expected weight that the child's weight is
(C) 24-hour video monitoring
(D) complete blood count (CBC)
(E) esophageal pH measurement

Questions 11 and 12

An 8-year-old boy is referred to you by a school nurse because he has been complaining of stomachaches every morning in school. On interviewing the boy's mother, you learn that he does not like to go to school, insists on coming home immediately after school each day, and sleeps in his parents' bed at night. The mother denies other complaints.

11. Which of the following is the most likely diagnosis?

(A) social phobia
(B) posttraumatic stress disorder (PTSD)
(C) separation anxiety disorder
(D) reactive attachment disorder of early childhood
(E) specific phobia

12. This boy's stomachaches are an example of which of the following?

(A) coprolalia
(B) anhedonia
(C) reaction formation
(D) coprophagia
(E) somatization

Questions 13 and 14

A 5-year-old boy is brought to the pediatric emergency department because he is frantically trying to run away from lions that he says are chasing him. He says that when he sees the lions he has to jump out of their way or else they will attack him.

13. Which of the following disorders is the most likely diagnosis?

(A) schizophrenia
(B) panic disorder
(C) autistic disorder
(D) moderate mental retardation
(E) substance-induced psychotic disorder

pH measurement can Dx the gastric reflux causing the rumination D/o

14. Which of the following is the most common psychiatric emergency in the child and adolescent population?

(A) psychotic behavior
(B) assaultive behavior
(C) suicidal behavior
(D) homicidal behavior
(E) sexually inappropriate behavior

suicide is the second most common cause of Death in adolescents

Questions 15 and 16

A 15-year-old girl with a history of separation anxiety disorder presents complaining of distress over her habit of biting her fingernails. Since starting high school 6 months earlier, the girl says that her nail-biting has been "out of control" and that she is extremely embarrassed about how her fingers look. All her fingers bleed every day, and they throb constantly. The girl reports that high school is stressful and that her grades are suffering because her nail-biting interferes with her ability to do her homework. She denies obsessional thoughts or compulsions. Physical and laboratory examinations are normal, with the exception of the girl's hands. Her fingers show signs of extreme nail-biting and there are abrasions on the back of her right hand.

15. Which of the following is true of the girl's academic difficulties related to her nail-biting?

(A) They are part of the diagnostic criteria for her Axis I diagnosis and therefore do not need to be coded elsewhere.
(B) They should be coded on Axis II.
(C) They should be coded on Axis III.
(D) They should be coded on Axis IV.
(E) They should be coded on Axis V.

16. Which of the following responses is most appropriate to use to determine the etiology of the abrasions on the dorsum of the girl's right hand?

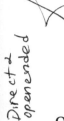

(A) "Tell me about the scratches on your hand."
(B) "Do you scratch yourself in addition to biting your nails?"
(C) "How did the scratches happen?"
(D) "I see you have scratches on your hand. Do you have a cat?"
(E) "Sometimes I see girls who make themselves throw up. Have you ever done that?"

Questions 17 and 18

An 8-year-old boy with a history of MDD treated with fluoxetine (Prozac) is brought to the pediatric emergency department after running into the street in front of a car on the way home from school. The boy says that he wants to be dead and refuses to say more. The boy was not hit by the car, and physical and laboratory examinations are normal.

17. Which of the following symptoms of MDD is seen more commonly in children than in adolescents?

(A) hypersomnia
(B) hopelessness
(C) psychomotor agitation
(D) weight change
(E) drug abuse

18. Which of the following is the most common method by which children attempt suicide?

(A) substance ingestion
(B) stabbing or cutting
(C) jumping from buildings
(D) hanging
(E) firearms

Questions 19 and 20

An 11-year-old boy with enuresis presents to the clinic for routine follow-up. His bed-wetting has not responded to behavioral interventions, so you had previously initiated treatment with intranasal desmopressin (DDAVP). You complete a full physical and laboratory examination.

19. During this visit, you would be most likely to identify which of the following signs and symptoms as an adverse effect of DDAVP?

(A) sedation
(B) hypotension
(C) liver toxicity
(D) tremor
(E) headache

20. Which of the following laboratory abnormalities are you most likely to identify in association with DDAVP?

(A) hyponatremia
(B) hypocalcemia
(C) hypokalemia
(D) hypomagnesemia
(E) hypophosphatemia

Desmopressin can lead to fluid retention so it causes headache and hyponatremia;

Questions 21 and 22

A 9-year-old boy with a history of panic disorder treated with cognitive-behavioral therapy is brought to your office by his mother because he has been irritable and depressed. On physical examination, the boy appears depressed but otherwise normal. Laboratory examination is normal. After a thorough history and mental status examination, you diagnose the boy with MDD and decide to initiate treatment with fluoxetine.

21. What is the approximate comorbidity of childhood anxiety disorders and MDD?

(A) 10%
(B) 25%
(C) 33%
(D) 50%
(E) 75%

22. You inform the boy and his mother of possible adverse effects of fluoxetine. Which of the following is the most common adverse effect of fluoxetine?

(A) hypotension
(B) nausea
(C) liver toxicity
(D) weight gain
(E) sedation

I HE DCTE mnemonic

Questions 23 and 24

A 3-year-old girl with moderate mental retardation is brought to the clinic by her mother because she has been complaining that her arm hurts. On physical examination, the girl has several bruises on her thorax and a tender right forearm. On laboratory examination, you discover a normocytic, normochromic anemia and basophilic stippling. On x-ray, you find signs of multiple fractures of different ages and increased density at the metaphyseal plate of the growing long bones.

23. Which of the following is the most appropriate treatment?

    (A) edetate calcium disodium (CaEDTA)
    (B) flumazenil (Romazicon)
    (C) naloxone (Narcan)
    (D) deferoxamine (Desferal)
    (E) acetylcysteine (Mucomyst)

    EDTA lead; Deferoxamine - Ferc - iron tox;

24. Which of the following is the most likely cause of this girl's bruises?

    (A) thrombocytopenia
    (B) developmental coordination disorder
    (C) malnutrition
    (D) physical abuse
    (E) hepatic failure

Questions 25 and 26

A 24-month-old girl is brought to the clinic by her mother for a routine visit. The mother tells you that the girl has not spoken her first clear word yet, at times seems not to understand what people say to her, and does not play with her 3-year-old brother. The mother also tells you that her daughter seems clumsy and has started to make odd repetitive movements with her hands. According to the girl's chart,

she had a normal head circumference at birth, at 6 months, and at 12 months, and had seemed to be developing normally. On physical examination, you note that the rate of head growth has slowed.

25. Which of the following pervasive developmental disorders is the most appropriate diagnosis?

    (A) autistic disorder
    (B) Rett disorder
    (C) childhood disintegrative disorder
    (D) Asperger disorder
    (E) pervasive developmental disorder not otherwise specified

26. Which of the following statements best describes this girl's disorder?

    (A) It is seen exclusively in girls.
    (B) There is never an Axis II diagnosis.
    (C) There are no clear characteristic chromosomal abnormalities associated with the disorder.
    (D) There are familial clusters of the disorder.
    (E) It is the most common of the pervasive developmental disorders.

Autism most common; Retts is only girls and its an X chromosome defect;

Questions 27 and 28

A 12-year-old boy is referred by the court for evaluation. He skips school, stays out late at night, and verbally abuses his parents. He has run away from home on three separate occasions prompting his parents to call the police.

27. This adolescent is most likely to have an additional Axis I diagnosis from which of the following DSM-IV-TR diagnostic categories?

    (A) substance-related disorders
    (B) schizophrenia and other psychotic disorders
    (C) anxiety disorders
    (D) eating disorders
    (E) somatoform disorders

28. Which of the following personality disorders is this boy most likely to develop?

    (A) antisocial personality disorder
    (B) paranoid personality disorder
    (C) schizoid personality disorder
    (D) schizotypal personality disorder
    (E) avoidant personality disorder

Antisocial PD. → *psychopathy*

Questions 29 and 30

A 10-year-old girl who has recently been diagnosed with diabetes mellitus Type I is referred to you by her pediatrician for an evaluation. You notice that she seems sad. After interviewing the girl and her parents, you determine that she meets DSM-IV-TR criteria for adjustment disorder with depressed mood.

29. Which of the following criteria for the diagnosis of adjustment disorder distinguishes it from MDD?

    (A) Symptoms develop following an identifiable stressor.
    (B) Symptoms develop within 3 months of the onset of the stressor.
    (C) Symptoms do not persist for more than 6 months following termination of the stressor.
    (D) Symptoms cause marked distress or significant impairment in functioning.
    (E) Symptoms do not represent bereavement.

30. Approximately what percentage of children who are diagnosed with diabetes mellitus Type I develop adjustment disorder following their medical diagnosis?

    (A) 1%
    (B) 5%
    (C) 10%
    (D) 33%
    (E) 75%

like 1 in 3

31. A 9-month-old girl is brought to the clinic by her foster mother for a routine examination. The girl's biological mother was infected with human immunodeficiency virus (HIV), was enrolled in a methadone maintenance program, and was using cocaine. The baby girl's HIV

test is negative but you are concerned about the possibility of developmental delays due to the mother's cocaine use. You learn that this girl has a 2-year-old brother who is infected with HIV. Which of the following is the best place for HIV-infected children under the age of 3 who cannot be cared for by their family?

    (A) a hospital
    (B) a group home
    (C) a foster home
    (D) a nursing home
    (E) a hospice

Questions 32 and 33

A 9-year-old boy is referred to you for evaluation after increasingly disruptive behavior in school. The teachers report that at any time, without warning, the boy will make a disruptive sound or shout out in class. They describe him as polite and neat but restless and jumpy.

32. Which of the following is the most likely diagnosis?

    (A) oppositional defiant disorder
    (B) conduct disorder
    (C) separation anxiety disorder
    (D) panic disorder
    (E) Tourette disorder

33. Which of the following medications is most appropriate?

    (A) bupropion (Wellbutrin)
    (B) paroxetine (Paxil)
    (C) venlafaxine (Effexor)
    (D) haloperidol (Haldol)
    (E) clonidine (Catapres)

clonidine—alpha agonist and first line for Tourette's

Questions 34 and 35

A 7-year-old boy with leukemia is referred to you because of concerns for his mood. His parents report that he fluctuates between appearing depressed and acting angry. At times he plays quietly in his room, but at other times he displays angry outbursts, often hitting his 4-year-old brother.

34. Which of the following methods would be the most useful way to interview this child?

   (A) Sit quietly and allow the child to talk.
   (B) Encourage the child to talk about whatever is on his mind.
   (C) Provide toys and allow the child to play.
   (D) Use the DISC.
   (E) Ask the child specific questions about how he feels about his disease.

35. Which of the following is true for children with a medical illness and a psychiatric illness?

   (A) The psychiatric illness does not need to be treated until the medical illness is resolved.
   (B) The psychiatric illness should not be treated pharmacologically in the setting of a medical illness.
   (C) The psychiatric illness should be treated by the same physician who is treating the medical illness.
   (D) The psychiatric illness should be treated aggressively in the setting of a medical illness.
   (E) Psychotherapy is unlikely to be effective in the setting of a medical illness.

Questions 36 and 37

An 8-year-old boy presents to your office for a routine visit. One month earlier, you diagnosed him with Tourette disorder and prescribed medication. He and his parents report that the medication has been helpful.

36. Which of the following is the most common initial symptom of Tourette disorder?

   (A) eye tics such as blinking
   (B) facial tics such as grimacing or licking
   (C) vocal tics, such as throat clearing or grunting
   (D) whole-body tics, such as body rocking or pelvic thrusting
   (E) self-abusive tics such as hitting

eye blinking tics are the most common tics of Tourettes but than vocal tics come before motor tics;

37. Which of the following is true regarding the DSM-IV-TR diagnosis of Tourette disorder?

   (A) Motor and vocal tics must occur concurrently.
   (B) Onset must be before the age of 21.
   (C) Tics must be present every day consecutively for at least 1 year.
   (D) Vocal tics must improve production of words.
   (E) Multiple motor tics must occur.

Tourette Dx age 7-18; Tourette s pt needs multiple tics for the DX but its Not concurrent;

Questions 38 and 39

After you complete a routine physical examination of a healthy 11-year-old girl, the girl's mother asks to talk with you in private. She tells you that her daughter was given an IQ test in school and that she scored a 68. The mother is extremely upset and wonders if it is her fault that her daughter is "dumb." She says she lies awake at night worrying and wonders why her daughter would have done so poorly on the test.

38. Which of the following is the most common predisposing factor for mental retardation?

   (A) heredity
   (B) pregnancy and perinatal problems
   (C) early alterations in embryonic development
   (D) general medical conditions acquired during infancy and childhood
   (E) environmental influences and mental disorders other than mental retardation

super

39. According to DSM-IV-TR, mental retardation is coded on which of the following axes?

   (A) Axis I
   (B) Axis II
   (C) Axis III
   (D) Axis IV
   (E) Axis V

Questions 40 and 41

An 8-year-old boy with a family history of tic disorders is referred to you for an evaluation of behavioral difficulties in school. His teachers report that he is unable to sit still, constantly fidgets, and is unable to complete class work because he is so easily distracted. The boy's mother reports that he has always had a lot of energy. She says that preparing to leave for school in the morning is extremely difficult because of her son's disorganization and forgetfulness. Otherwise, she has no complaints. She denies that her son produces any repetitive movements or sounds.

40. Which of the following is the most likely diagnosis?

    (A) dementia
    (B) conduct disorder
    (C) oppositional defiant disorder
    (D) attention deficit hyperactivity disorder (ADHD)
    (E) disruptive behavior disorder not otherwise specified

41. Which of the following classes of medications is most likely to unmask an underlying predisposition to developing tics?

    (A) stimulants
    (B) selective serotonin reuptake inhibitors (SSRIs)
    (C) monoamine oxidase inhibitors (MAOIs)
    (D) D$_2$ antagonists
    (E) benzodiazepines

Questions 42 and 43

A 6-year-old boy is referred to you by his school to evaluate his difficulty with reading. It is suspected that he suffers from a reading disorder, but a subtle impairment in vision or hearing must be ruled out as a causative or contributing factor.

42. Learning disorders are most commonly associated with which of the following disorders?

    (A) ADHD
    (B) bipolar disorder
    (C) Tourette disorder
    (D) Asperger disorder
    (E) schizophrenia

43. Which of the following percentages approximates those children and adolescents with learning disorders who drop out of school?

    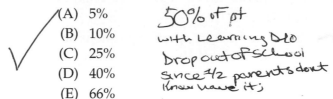

    (A) 5%
    (B) 10%
    (C) 25%
    (D) 40%
    (E) 66%

(handwritten note: 50% of pt with Learning D/O Drop out of School since 1/2 parents dont know have it;)

Questions 44 and 45

An 8-year-old child is referred to you for an evaluation of bed-wetting. Several behavioral interventions have been attempted, including eliminating fluid intake in the evening, scheduled awakenings at night to use the bathroom, and a urine alarm (a bell and pad). These techniques have been unsuccessful, and the child continues to urinate in bed every night.

44. A child with enuresis is most likely to be which of the following?

    (A) an otherwise normal boy
    (B) an otherwise normal girl
    (C) a child with mental retardation
    (D) a child with autistic disorder
    (E) a child with obsessive-compulsive disorder (OCD)

45. Which of the following medications is most appropriate for you to prescribe to treat the enuresis?

    (A) methylphenidate (Ritalin)
    (B) paroxetine
    (C) trazodone (Desyrel)
    (D) imipramine
    (E) benztropine (Cogentin)

Questions 46 and 47

A 10-year-old boy is referred to you because his pediatrician suspects that he may have ADHD. After a thorough history, physical examination, and laboratory investigation you make the diagnosis of ADHD.

After discussing the adverse effects of medications, you prescribe methylphenidate to be taken in the morning and at lunch on school days.

46. Which of the following is a common adverse effect of methylphenidate?

    (A) tremor
    (B) hypotension
    (C) weight gain
    (D) insomnia
    (E) liver toxicity

Also stimulants suppress appetite
Stimulants cause insomnia so not after 12pm)

47. Stimulants such as methylphenidate effectively treat symptoms of ADHD in what percentage of patients?

    (A) 10%
    (B) 25%
    (C) 33%
    (D) 50%
    (E) 70%

Questions 48 and 49

During a routine office visit, the mother of a 22-month-old girl tells you that she is concerned about her daughter's behavior. Since the birth of her son 4 months earlier, the mother states that her daughter is more irritable and angry. The mother is especially concerned that her daughter is aggressive and violent toward the baby.

48. Which of the following statements is the most appropriate response to this mother?

    (A) "If you simply ignore your daughter's behavior, it will pass."
    (B) "Your daughter's behavior is normal for her age."
    (C) "Every day, schedule some time for you and your daughter to spend together without the baby."
    (D) "Explain to your daughter that the baby needs more attention that she does right now."
    (E) "Your daughter must be precocious since the terrible twos are starting early."

49. At 22 months of age, this girl should be able to do which of the following?

    (A) copy a circle
    (B) copy a square
    (C) identify her left hand
    (D) tell her age and gender
    (E) ride a tricycle

Questions 50 and 51

A 4-year-old boy is referred to you for evaluation because he has not started walking. He appears healthy and well-cared for. He readily comes with you to the examining room. In your office, he notices a windup toy and immediately becomes engrossed in winding it up, watching it move around until it winds down, and winding it up again. After about 10 minutes, you attempt to take the toy from him and he becomes extremely upset, making an insistent, piercing cry.

50. Which of the following is the most likely diagnosis?

    (A) oppositional defiant disorder
    (B) conduct disorder
    (C) separation anxiety disorder
    (D) autistic disorder
    (E) selective mutism

51. Which of the following qualities is associated with a more favorable prognosis for children similar to this boy?

    (A) easily toilet trained
    (B) organized in play
    (C) interested in mechanical toys
    (D) able to converse
    (E) able to dance to a beat

Questions 52 and 53

A 17-year-old girl comes to your office for a routine visit. She states that she feels fine and offers no complaints. On physical examination, you find that her weight is 92 lb and her height is 5 ft 5 in. One year earlier, her weight had been 126 lb, and her height was 5 ft 5 in. After further discussion, you learn that this girl is terrified of gaining weight and thinks that she looks fat and needs to lose more weight. She reports that she has not menstruated in the past 6 months.

52. Which of the following laboratory abnormalities are you most likely to discover?

    (A) hypercholesterolemia
    (B) increased thyroid-stimulating hormone (TSH)
    (C) hypocarotenemia
    (D) leukocytosis
    (E) hyperkalemia

53. Which of the following findings is most consistent with this girl's disorder?

    (A) sinus tachycardia
    (B) increased resting energy expenditure
    (C) elevated serum estrogen levels in girls
    (D) elevated serum testosterone levels in boys
    (E) increased ventricular-brain ratio on brain imaging

Questions 54 and 55

An 8-month-old boy is brought to the clinic by his mother. She complains that her son has been experiencing screaming and crying fits when she leaves him with a babysitter. She says that in the past he did not object to being left with a babysitter and asks you why he becomes so upset now and what she can do about it.

54. Which of the following statements is the most appropriate response?

    (A) "This behavior is characteristic of autistic children."
    (B) "It is possible that your son has separation anxiety disorder."
    (C) "This behavior suggests that you're not spending enough time with your son."
    (D) "It sounds as though your son is overly attached to you."
    (E) "This behavior is normal at your son's age and will pass with time."

55. Which of the following statements is true regarding attachment by an infant to a caretaker?

    (A) Attachment is prevented by mental illness in the caretaker.
    (B) Attachment requires consistent interaction with the caretaker.
    (C) Attachment is prevented by physical abuse from the caretaker.
    (D) Attachment usually does not occur if the infant is blind.
    (E) Attachment requires contact beginning in the perinatal period.

Side Note attachment can also occur during physical abuse butits reactive attachment

Questions 56 and 57

A 14-year-old boy is referred to you due to extreme difficulties in school. He has been held back a grade and is still not passing. During the course of your evaluation, you learn that the boy hears voices telling him that he is stupid and to leave the classroom. Afraid to disobey, he goes to the bathroom frequently. He has difficulty falling asleep at night because the voices keep him awake. In addition, you learn that the boy believes others can read his thoughts. Physical and laboratory examinations are normal.

56. You suspect that the boy may be suffering from schizophrenia. Which of the following subtypes of schizophrenia is most probable?

    (A) paranoid type
    (B) disorganized type
    (C) catatonic type
    (D) undifferentiated type
    (E) residual type

57. Which of the following is the worst prognostic feature of schizophrenia with onset in childhood?

(A) affective symptoms
(B) acute onset
(C) onset before the age of 10
(D) good premorbid adjustment
(E) well-differentiated symptoms

Questions 58 and 59

A 9-year-old girl with a family history of bipolar disorder is referred to you by her school because of disruptive behavior in class that has been worsening over the past 3 months. Her teachers report that her energy level is high.

58. Which of the following would be most helpful in distinguishing between mania and ADHD in children?

(A) pressured speech
(B) distractibility
(C) motoric overactivity
(D) low self-esteem
(E) impulsivity

ADHD children have anxiety and low selfesteem

59. Which of the following disorders is more common among girls than among boys?

(A) ADHD
(B) conduct disorder
(C) Rett disorder
(D) Tourette disorder
(E) Asperger disorder

Questions 60 and 61

A 6-year-old boy is brought to your office by his mother for evaluation of an upper respiratory infection. The mother mentions that her son has started sucking on his thumb again. In addition, she mentions that the boy's grandmother died recently and asks how children view death.

60. At what age can a child normally appreciate that death is irreversible?

(A) 2 years
(B) 3 years
(C) 5 years
(D) 7 years
(E) 12 years

Age 9 children understand death is irreversince understand time;

61. Which of the following defense mechanisms is the boy employing when he starts sucking his thumb?

(A) repression
(B) acting out
(C) denial
(D) regression
(E) blocking

Questions 62 and 63

A 12-year-old boy with Tourette disorder comes to your office for a routine visit. Two weeks earlier, you had prescribed clonidine for his illness. The boy reports that his tics have subsided slightly since starting the clonidine, but complains about the medicine.

62. This boy is likely experiencing which of the following as an adverse effect of clonidine?

(A) sedation
(B) light-headedness due to hypotension
(C) dry mouth
(D) tremor
(E) nausea

clonidine is centrally acting so more likely lead to sedation than hypotension

63. If this boy's 7-year-old brother were to have ADHD, which of the following classes of medications would be the most appropriate choice for him?

(A) a stimulant such as methylphenidate
(B) a tricyclic antidepressant (TCA) such as desipramine (Norpramin)
(C) an SSRI such as fluoxetine
(D) an MAOI such as phenelzine (Nardil)
(E) a neuroleptic such as haloperidol (Haldol)

✓ **64.** A 6-year-old boy is brought to the emergency department by his mother, who reports that he was playing on some steps in front of the house when he slipped and fell. She tells you that she is concerned that he might have broken his arm. An x-ray of the boy's arm shows a fracture of the ulna, as well as signs of several old fractures of varying ages. Which of the following is the most appropriate action?

(A) Refer the boy to an orthopedist for further evaluation.

(B) Tell the mother that you notice that the boy has had multiple broken bones and recommend that she limit the boy's sports activities.

(C) Set the current broken bone in a cast and recommend that the boy see his pediatrician for follow-up care.

(D) Recommend calcium supplements and a multiple vitamin daily.

(E) Tell the boy that you notice that he has had multiple broken bones and ask him how each of these fractures happened.

65. The mother of one of your 4-year-old patients calls and asks you for advice. She says that her son has been stealing toys from other children at school and bringing them home with him. Which of the following suggestions is most appropriate?

(A) The mother should return the toys herself and buy her son similar toys.

(B) The mother should tell her son that if he stops stealing, she will give him a reward each week.

(C) The mother should point out to her son that he is stealing and punish him for it.

(D) The mother should help her son return the toys.

(E) The mother should ignore the entire situation because her son's behavior is part of a developmental phase that will pass.

66. A 14-year-old girl presents to her pediatrician complaining that she has been freaking out. The girl describes episodes of palpitations, shaking, gasping for air, and feeling like she is going to die. These feelings intensify for a few minutes and resolve spontaneously. These episodes have occurred at various times, in various situations, and the girl is worried that she is going crazy. Which of the following is the most appropriate treatment?

(A) valproate (Depakote)

✓ (B) risperidone

(C) clozapine (Clozaril)

(D) sertraline

(E) carbamazepine

67. A 5-year-old girl with asthma is seen by her pediatrician for a routine visit. After returning home from the clinic, the girl asks her friend to "play doctor." This behavior is a manifestation of which of the following phenomena?

(A) reaction formation

(B) identification

(C) displacement

(D) rationalization

(E) dissociation

68. A 4-year-old boy whose mother had rubella during her pregnancy is brought to the clinic for a routine visit. The physical and laboratory examinations are normal. The highest risk of physical and/or mental defects in the fetus as a result of maternal rubella infection occurs during which month of the pregnancy?

(A) first

(B) third

(C) fifth

(D) seventh

(E) ninth

Rubella → MR, → woman in psych out pt daughter

69. A 10-year-old girl with a history of asthma is brought to the clinic after a recent increase in asthma symptoms. During the visit, you learn that she is being beaten by her mother's boyfriend. Under which of the following circumstances, does the law require mandatory reporting of suspected child abuse by a physician who evaluates a child?

(A) in all cases

(B) only when the physician believes it is in a child's best interests

(C) only when consent of a parent or guardian is obtained

(D) only in cases in which the child shows behavioral manifestations of abuse

(E) only when the physician has examined all children in the family

70. A 4-year-old boy is referred to you because he will not speak in preschool. Over the course of about 2 months, he gradually stops talking. Initially his mother reports that he objected to going to preschool, but no longer complains. She states that at times, her son is quiet and stays in his room, but that she has not noticed a significant change in his speech or behavior. Which of the following is the most likely diagnosis?

(A) selective mutism

(B) MDD

(C) separation anxiety disorder

(D) social phobia

(E) dysthymic disorder

71. A 2-year-old boy is referred to you for evaluation due to the suspicion that the child is the victim of physical abuse secondary to Munchausen syndrome by proxy. Which of the following family members is most frequently the perpetrator who fabricates the presenting illness?

(A) brother

(B) sister

(C) father

(D) mother

(E) uncle

72. A frustrated mother brings her 14-year-old son to a child psychiatrist after he is expelled from three high schools in 1 year. She reports the boy has tried twice to set his school on fire, has slashed school bus tires, and has broken into the principal's office to steal athletic trophies. In addition, he has been suspended numerous times for getting into fights with other students. She shudders and tearfully relates that she recently caught him singeing one of the family cats with a cigarette butt. The diagnosis of the above disorder is required for which of the following disorders?

(A) schizotypal

(B) borderline

(C) obsessive-compulsive

(D) antisocial

(E) histrionic

73. A 15-year-old girl is brought into the pediatrician's office by her mother, who is concerned about her lack of apparent appetite. The patient is wearing baggy clothes, but her weight is in the 70th percentile for her height. She admits that she "does not eat much," but she claims to have a voracious appetite. She is active in the school musical productions, and she is very worried about "getting fat" and not getting the lead part. Her past medical history is unremarkable, and although she started menstruating at age 13, she has not had her period for at least 5 months. Which of the following laboratory abnormalities would be most likely found in this patient?

(A) decreased corticotropin-releasing hormone (CRH)

(B) hypercholesterolemia

(C) hyperglycemia

(D) hyperthyroidism

(E) leukocytosis

DIRECTIONS (Questions 74 through 83): Each set of items in this section consists of a list of lettered headings followed by several numbered words or phrases. For each numbered word or phrase, select the ONE lettered option that is most closely associated with it. Each lettered option may be selected once, more than once, or not at all.

74. A 13-year-old girl is seen by her psychiatrist 1 year after an automobile accident. She demonstrates intact language ability and complex motor skills. She has no abnormalities in the perception of stimuli that are identifiable, but she has lost the ability to read since the accident. What deficit is she demonstrating?

    (A) anomia
    (B) aphasia
    (C) alexia
    (D) apraxia
    (E) agnosia

anomia
↓
recognize object but cannot Name!
(a-nomia means No Name)

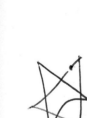

75. Britney is a 10-year-old girl without significant medical history brought to the pediatrician by her father for evaluation. Over the past school year, she has been having increasing difficulties going to sleep. Although she has "always had bedtime rituals," they have extended in complexity and length. Most of her time in the evening is now spent going around the house numerous times, locking and unlocking the doors and windows. While she knows the chances of a burglary are slim, she is extremely anxious about her safety, and she "can't stop" the urges to perform these behaviors. As a result, she only obtains 5 hours of sleep, and she has been falling asleep in class with diminishing grades. Infection with which of the following organisms might have contributed to her current illness?

    (A) herpes simplex virus
    (B) HIV
    (C) prion proteins
    (D) streptococcus
    (E) treponema

Questions 76 through 79

    (A) Rett disorder
    (B) bulimia nervosa
    (C) stereotypic movement disorder
    (D) social phobia
    (E) separation anxiety
    (F) pica
    (G) enuresis
    (H) conduct disorder
    (I) panic disorder
    (J) Asperger disorder

76. A 7-year-old boy with *Toxocara* and visceral larva migrans

77. A 17-year-old girl with hypokalemia

78. A 6-year-old boy with rectal bleeding and anemia

79. A 15-year-old boy with a urine toxicology screen positive for cocaine

Questions 80 through 84

    (A) OCD
    (B) pica
    (C) hypochondriasis
    (D) Tourette disorder
    (E) panic disorder
    (F) bulimia nervosa
    (G) anorexia nervosa
    (H) Asperger disorder
    (I) pyromania
    (J) trichotillomania

80. A 14-year-old girl with episodes of palpitations, chest pain, shortness of breath, and diaphoresis who has a normal physical and laboratory examination

81. A 10-year-old girl with physical findings that include hypotension, bradycardia, and lanugo hair

82. An 8-year-old boy with erythematous, chapped hands, and an otherwise normal physical and laboratory examination

83. A 13-year-old girl with a bald patch on the back of her head and an otherwise normal physical and laboratory examination

DIRECTIONS (Questions 84 and 85): Each of the numbered items in this section is followed by answers. Select the ONE lettered answer that is BEST in each case.

Questions 84 and 85

84. An 8-year-old boy is brought to your office by his anxious mother who says that he cannot read at grade level. She says he was doing well until last year in second grade when he began falling behind. He has become somewhat of a behavioral problem in school since his troubles with reading began. His mother insists that he is "at least as smart as every other kid in that school" but says she would be relieved to hear that he has a learning disorder "so he can get the help he needs." You read with the child and confirm that he is having difficulty. You should do which of the following?

(A) Tell the mother to schedule some sessions with a reading specialist.

(B) Ask the child if he likes to read.

(C) Test the child's vision.

(D) Prescribe methylphenidate for ADHD.

(E) Reassure the mother that her son is doing fine.

85. As the school psychologist, you are asked to see a fourth grader who has been consistently acting out in class. He often lies about things he has done in class, such as trying to cheat on tests. You learn that at home he sprays water on the family dog and sometimes barks at him. After he does so, he is seen cackling to himself. The most likely diagnosis is which of the following?

(A) autistic disorder

(B) Tourette disorder

(C) conduct disorder

(D) oppositional defiant disorder

(E) childhood schizophrenia

DIRECTIONS (Questions 86 through 95): Each set of items in this section consists of a list of lettered headings followed by several numbered words or phrases. For each numbered word or phrase, select the ONE lettered option that is most closely associated with it. Each lettered option may be selected once, more than once, or not at all.

Questions 86 through 89

(A) autism

(B) selective mutism

(C) childhood schizophrenia

(D) Rett disorder

(E) Asperger disorder

(F) ADHD

86. A 6-year-old girl whose parents are going through a divorce will not speak during school.

87. A 6-year-old girl who had reached normal early development milestones now does not speak in school or at home.

88. A 6-year-old boy who performs well in school but does not seem to talk when other children approach him and generally avoids other children.

89. A 6-year-old boy who is having difficulty in school and avoids interactions with his classmates and others, who notice him making odd repetitive movements with his hands.

Questions 90 through 95

(A) mild mental retardation

(B) moderate mental retardation

(C) severe mental retardation

(D) profound mental retardation

(E) average intelligence

90. A 14-year-old boy with an IQ of 34

91. A 14-year-old boy with an IQ of 96

92. A 14-year-old boy with an IQ of 68

93. A 14-year-old boy with an IQ of 52

94. A 14-year-old boy with an IQ of 24

95. A 14-year-old boy with an IQ of 56

Answers and Explanations

1. **(C)** Suicide is a considerable risk in depressed adolescents, and should be specifically addressed during an interview with a patient who appears depressed or agitated or has a history of a suicide attempt. Surveys of adolescents in the general community have estimated that approximately 9% of adolescents have attempted suicide at least once in their lives. Among adolescents with known psychiatric disorders, the rate is much higher. More girls than boys demonstrate suicidal behavior, but nearly five times more teenage boys successfully commit suicide than do teenage girls, because boys more frequently use guns and violent methods to attempt suicide. History of a prior suicide attempt is an important risk factor for suicide in all age groups; the majority of those who successfully complete suicide have attempted suicide in the past. The adolescent suicide rate has increased substantially during the past few decades.

2. **(E)** The use of firearms is the most common method by which adolescents die by suicide. Drug overdose is the most common method of suicide attempts, but accounts for fewer completed suicides. Stabbing, cutting, jumping from buildings, and hanging are other methods frequently employed.

3. **(A)** A simple, nonjudgmental statement, such as "I can see this is very upsetting for you," conveys to the mother that you are concerned about her and that, at least on some level, you understand her and sympathize with her suffering. This form of sentence also acts as an open-ended question that is most likely to elicit the most important information most efficiently. The mother may be most troubled by something other than her son's episodes and her daytime sleepiness. Specifically directed statements, such as "Tell me why you can't fall back to sleep after your son does," or leading questions, such as "Are you worried that this is your fault?" are less likely to be helpful in gaining this information than an open-ended statement or question. Usually, any statement containing "but" is inappropriate as the initial response to a person who is describing a problem to you. Statements such as "I know you're upset, but this problem will get better" or "I can see you're upset, but you're really overreacting" may indicate that you do not take the problem seriously or that you are minimizing how the person feels. Such an approach may prevent you from obtaining further important ation.

4. **(C)** Episodes of sleep terror, as well as of sleepwalking, occur during deep sleep (stages 3–4). Sleep terror does not occur during stage 1 or 2 of sleep or during REM sleep.

5. **(E)** An SSRI, such as sertraline, is the first-line agent for MDD in children and adolescents. TCAs such as imipramine cause more adverse effects than SSRIs typically do, and an overdose is much more likely to be lethal. Mood stabilizers such as carbamazapine and lithium are used for bipolar disorder and as adjuncts to the treatment of MDD refractory to antidepressant medications alone. Antipsychotics such as olanzapine are usually reserved for use as adjuncts when psychosis develops.

6. **(A)** Bulimia nervosa is most effectively treated with cognitive-behavioral therapy. Family

therapy, psychoanalytic psychotherapy, and group therapy may be used as adjuncts to cognitive-behavioral therapy, but are not as effective in changing the behaviors associated with bulimia nervosa.

7. **(B)** This boy most likely suffers from expressive language disorder. Typical symptoms include having a markedly limited vocabulary, making errors in tense, and having difficulty recalling words or producing sentences with developmentally appropriate length or complexity. In addition, the boy's difficulties are interfering with academic functioning. There is no indication that this boy has difficulty with written expression, so a diagnosis of disorder of written expression is inappropriate. This boy does not suffer from a phonological disorder because his speech is clear and he has not failed to develop expected speech sounds. Similarly, he is not suffering from stuttering, a DSM-IV-TR communications disorder diagnosis, because there is no disturbance in the fluency and time patterning of his speech. There is no indication that he has difficulty with motor coordination, so a diagnosis of developmental coordination disorder would be inappropriate.

8. **(A)** An IQ test would be most helpful in confirming the diagnosis of expressive language disorder because a diagnosis of mental retardation must be ruled out. The CAS, DICA, DISC, and K-SADS are semistructured interviews that aid primarily in the assessment of mood disorders, anxiety disorders, disruptive behavior disorders, and eating disorders.

9. **(D)** The most likely diagnosis is rumination disorder, in which there is repeated regurgitation and rechewing of food for a period of at least 1 month following a period of normal functioning. Rumination disorder is often seen in infants who have a variety of caretakers in an unstable environment. The drooling exhibited by this baby is most likely the milk or food that has been regurgitated. Lack of appropriate weight gain is typical when the baby does not reswallow the food. This baby is not suffering from anorexia nervosa because she likes to eat and does not display fears of becoming

overweight. Similarly, she is not suffering from bulimia nervosa because she does not display episodes of binge eating with compensatory behavior, such as self-induced vomiting or misuse of laxatives. A diagnosis of pica would require that the baby persistently eat nonnutritive substances such as dirt, plaster, hair, bugs, or pebbles. A diagnosis of feeding disorder of infancy or early childhood is not appropriate because the baby's disturbance is better accounted for by a diagnosis of rumination disorder.

10. **(E)** To confirm the diagnosis of rumination disorder, an associated gastrointestinal or other general medical condition, such as esophageal reflux, must be ruled out. Esophageal pH measurement indicates if acidic gastric contents move into the esophagus during periods when the infant is not eating or actively regurgitating, as occurs in esophageal reflux. Measurement of the serum lead level is appropriate when pica is suspected, because old paints may contain lead, which can cause significant neurologic problems when ingested. Calculating the percentage of expected weight represented by the infant's current weight would be required for a diagnosis of anorexia nervosa (85% or less) but is not a criterion for rumination disorder. Twenty-four-hour video monitoring would greatly aid in assessing the baby's behavior and the context in which the disturbance occurs, but would not rule out a gastrointestinal condition as the cause of this problem. Results of a CBC would not be helpful in determining the diagnosis.

11. **(C)** This boy's behavior and symptoms are most consistent with separation anxiety disorder, characterized by developmentally inappropriate and excessive anxiety concerning separation from the home or from those to whom the individual is attached. Consistent with this diagnosis, the boy does not like to go to school, comes home immediately after school, sleeps in his parents' bed at night, and has repeated physical symptoms when at school. The boy does not suffer from social phobia disorder because he does not have a marked and persistent fear of a social or performance

situation with exposure causing intense anxiety, expressed as a tantrum or a panic attack. The boy is not suffering from PTSD because there is no evidence of a traumatic event that is persistently reexperienced and has caused symptoms of increased arousal and avoidance of associated stimuli. For a diagnosis of reactive attachment disorder of infancy or early childhood, the boy would need to have suffered markedly disturbed social relatedness, in most contexts, beginning before the age of 5. Finally, a diagnosis of specific phobia would require the display of marked and persistent fear cued by the presence of anticipation of a specific object or situation, expressed as a tantrum or panic attack.

12. **(E)** *Somatization* is a defense mechanism in which emotional concerns are manifested as physical symptoms. *Coprolalia* is the repetitive speaking of obscene words, seen in severe cases of Tourette disorder. *Anhedonia* is the lack of interest or pleasure in activities that were once enjoyable, seen in MDD. *Reaction formation* is a defense mechanism in which an unacceptable impulse is transformed into its opposite. *Coprophagia* is the eating of feces.

13. **(E)** Substance-induced psychotic disorder is the most common cause of florid visual hallucinations in a child. The child may have ingested prescription drugs, illicit drugs, over-the-counter medications, or a household agent. Schizophrenia rarely presents in young children. When it does, it is much more likely to present with auditory hallucinations than with visual hallucinations. Hallucinations do not occur in panic disorder, autistic disorder, or mental retardation.

14. **(C)** Suicidal behavior is the most common psychiatric emergency in children and adolescents. Psychotic behavior, particularly assaultive behavior, and homicidal behavior are less common emergencies. Sexually inappropriate behavior alone is rarely an emergency.

15. **(D)** This girl's academic difficulties related to her nail-biting should be coded on Axis IV along with any other psychological and environmental problems that may affect the diagnosis, treatment, and prognosis of her Axis I disorder (or are a significantly distressing effect of her Axis I disorder). The fact that the girl's behavior is interfering with normal activities (e.g., homework) is part of the diagnostic criteria for her Axis I diagnosis, but the stress of falling grades requires coding on Axis IV. Mental retardation and personality disorders are coded on Axis II. Medical (physical) disorders are coded on Axis III. The Global Assessment of Functioning (GAF), the clinician's judgment of the individual's overall level of functioning, is coded on Axis V.

16. **(A)** A direct but open-ended statement, such as "Tell me about the scratches on your hand," is most likely to be helpful in this situation. It is not a secret that the abrasions are there, but the patient has not mentioned them. Usually, a patient appreciates a direct question rather than wonder if you ignored or did not notice something obvious. Questions such as "Do you scratch yourself in addition to biting your nails?" or "Do you have a cat?" are not open-ended; they require "yes" or "no" answers and are unlikely to yield new information. "How did the scratches happen?" may sound accusatory; patients are more likely to offer information if you seem nonjudgmental. Signs of bulimia nervosa include erosion of tooth enamel caused by acidic vomitus and abrasions on the dorsum of the hand due to scraping by the upper teeth as the individual pushes the hand to the back of the throat to induce vomiting. If this girl does not volunteer information that confirms to you that she is not inducing vomiting, you should use a reassuring statement such as "Sometimes I see girls who make themselves throw up. Have you ever done that?"

17. **(C)** Psychomotor agitation is more commonly seen in children with MDD compared to adolescents with MDD. Children with MDD may appear more anxious and irritable than sad and depressed. Hypersomnia, hopelessness, weight change, and drug abuse are more commonly seen in adolescents with MDD compared to children with MDD.

18. **(A)** Substance ingestion is the most common method children use when attempting suicide. Other methods frequently used by children include stabbing, cutting, jumping from buildings, hanging, running in front of vehicles, and gas inhalation. Firearms are used less frequently than substance ingestion but are more often lethal. It is important to note that some suicide attempts may be mistaken for accidents, so it is important to directly ask children if they intended to hurt or kill themselves.

19. **(E)** Headaches and nausea are common adverse effects associated with the synthetic antidiuretic hormone DDAVP. Sedation, hypotension, liver toxicity, and tremor are not associated with desmopressin.

20. **(A)** DDAVP is effective in treating enuresis because it suppresses urine production for 7–10 hours following administration by an intranasal spray. It lacks the pressor effects of an antidiuretic hormone, but can cause a mild hyponatremia. Hypocalcemia, hypokalemia, hypomagnesemia, and hypophosphatemia are not side effects of the drug.

21. **(D)** The approximate comorbidity of childhood anxiety disorders (overanxious disorder, separation anxiety disorder, panic disorder) and MDD is 50%. The approximate comorbidity of childhood anxiety disorders and ADHD is 30%.

22. **(B)** The most common adverse effects of fluoxetine include gastrointestinal symptoms, insomnia, agitation, and headaches. In general, hypotension, liver toxicity, weight gain, and sedation are not side effects associated with fluoxetine.

23. **(A)** CaEDTA is a chelating agent used to treat lead toxicity. Flumazenil is used to reverse the sedating effects of excess benzodiazepines, and naloxone is used to reverse the effects of excess opiates. Deferoxamine is a chelating agent used to treat iron toxicity. Acetylcysteine is used to treat acetaminophen toxicity.

24. **(D)** The girl's bruises are most likely the result of physical abuse, which is strongly suggested by the presence of multiple fractures of different ages. Thrombocytopenia and malnutrition are rare in the United States. In developmental coordination disorder, there is a delay in achieving major milestones and clumsiness, but there is not typically a pattern of repeated injury. Hepatic failure is extremely rare in a 3-year-old child.

25. **(B)** This girl's history and presentation are consistent with Rett disorder, which is characterized by normal prenatal and perinatal development, normal head circumference at birth, and normal psychomotor development through the first 5 months of life. Between the ages of 5 and 48 months, there is deceleration of head growth, loss of hand skills with development of stereotyped hand movements such as hand wringing, loss of social interaction (which may improve later), appearance of poorly coordinated gait or trunk movements, and severely impaired expressive and receptive language development with severe psychomotor retardation. Autistic disorder and pervasive developmental disorder, not otherwise specified, are not appropriate diagnoses because this girl's presentation is better accounted for by Rett disorder. Children with childhood disintegrative disorder do not develop normally for at least 2 years after birth. Children with Asperger disorder do not show delay in language development (e.g., single words are used by the age of 2).

26. **(A)** Rett disorder is the only DSM-IV-TR disorder that is seen only in girls. Children with Rett disorder commonly suffer from mental retardation, which is coded on Axis II. Although there are no clear characteristic laboratory findings associated with the disorder, there is a genetic test available. There are no known familial clusters of the disorder. Autistic disorder is the most common of the pervasive developmental disorders.

27. **(A)** This boy is most likely to have a substance-related disorder in addition to conduct disorder. Children and adolescents with conduct disorder often have a substance-related disorder and/or ADHD. Schizophrenia and other psychotic

disorders, anxiety disorders, eating disorders, and somatoform disorders are less frequently associated with conduct disorder.

28. **(A)** Children and adolescents who are diagnosed with conduct disorder are at increased risk for antisocial personality disorder as adults. Antisocial personality disorder is not diagnosed until after the age of 18, and one of the criteria is evidence of conduct disorder prior to the age of 15. Earlier onset of conduct disorder is associated with an increased risk of developing antisocial personality disorder. Conduct disorder is not as closely associated with paranoid personality disorder, schizoid personality disorder, schizotypal personality disorder, or avoidant personality disorder.

29. **(C)** By definition, symptoms of adjustment disorder do not last longer than 6 months after a stressor or the termination of its consequences. If depressive symptoms persist, MDD may be diagnosed. In both adjustment disorder and MDD, symptoms may develop following a stressor, may develop within 3 months of the onset of a stressor, must cause marked distress or significant impairment in functioning, and must not represent bereavement.

30. **(D)** Following a diagnosis of diabetes mellitus Type I, approximately 33% of children develop symptoms of adjustment disorder.

31. **(C)** A foster home is the optimal place for young children with HIV. In a foster home, a child has the psychological benefit of belonging to a family and is more likely to receive adequate emotional support than in a group setting. In addition, the risk of opportunistic infections is higher in group settings, such as hospitals, group homes, nursing homes, and hospices, than in private home environments.

32. **(E)** Tourette disorder is the most likely diagnosis because the boy's outbursts are consistent with vocal tics, and the report of "restless and jumpy" behavior is consistent with misinterpretation of motor tics. Tourette disorder most commonly develops in grade school-age boys, and the involuntary tics may be misinterpreted

as purposefully disruptive behavior. Of note, there is frequent comorbidity with ADHD. This boy does not suffer from oppositional defiant disorder or conduct disorder because he is polite and neat and does not display hostile, destructive, or angry behaviors. There is no evidence that this boy experiences distress and worry when separated from an important attachment figure as in separation anxiety disorder. The outbursts are not typical of panic disorder, in which there are discrete panic attacks, periods of intense fear, or discomfort with physical manifestations such as palpitations and subjective difficulty breathing.

33. **(E)** Clonidine has become the first-line treatment for Tourette disorder. It has a limited side effect profile and helps control symptoms of the two frequently associated comorbid disorders: ADHD and OCD. TCAs have been shown to be effective in the treatment of Tourette disorder, but other antidepressants such as bupropion, paroxetine, and venlafaxine are not known to be effective. High-potency antipsychotics such as haloperidol and pimozide were traditionally the first-line agents for Tourette disorder. The newer atypical antipsychotics, such as risperidone, are not known to be effective in treating the disorder.

34. **(C)** A play interview in which a child is provided with toys and allowed to play is an effective and efficient way to interview a child. Even with encouragement, a child is unlikely to produce much spontaneous talk in the uncomfortable setting of sitting with a stranger evaluating him or her. Likewise, asking specific questions is not as helpful as observing the child's play. Semistructured interviews are useful tools in combination with play interviews. The DISC is unreliable in 6–9-year-old children.

35. **(D)** A psychiatric illness in a child or adolescent with a medical illness should be treated aggressively using the type of treatment most effective for the specific psychiatric illness. Effective treatment of a mental illness may positively affect a medical illness if improvement of psychiatric symptoms enables the child to more

fully participate in treatment of the medical illness. In addition, emotional state is related to immune response. Appropriate pharmacologic treatment should be avoided only if there are specific contraindications based on the medical treatment the child is receiving. There is no need for the psychiatric illness to be treated by the same physician who is treating the medical illness. In general, the effectiveness of psychotherapy is related to the specific mental illness, not to the existence of, or lack of, a medical illness.

36. **(A)** Eye tics such as blinking and eye rolling are the most common initial symptoms in Tourette disorder. Facial tics such as grimacing or licking movements and vocal tics such as throat clearing or grunting are the next most common initial symptoms. Whole-body tics, such as body rocking or pelvic thrusting, and self-abusive tics, such as hitting, may develop later.

37. **(E)** In Tourette disorder, multiple motor tics and one or more vocal tics must be present at sometime during the illness. The motor and vocal tics do not need to occur concurrently. Onset is before the age of 18. The average age of onset is 7. Tics must be present nearly every day or intermittently for at least 1 year, with no tic-free period longer than 3 consecutive months. Vocal tics include various sounds such as grunts, yelps, coughs, and throat clearing, as well as words.

38. **(C)** Early alterations in embryonic development, such as chromosomal changes (e.g., Down syndrome) and prenatal damage due to toxins (e.g., maternal alcohol consumption), are the most common predisposing factors for mental retardation, accounting for approximately 30% of cases. Heredity accounts for about 5%. Pregnancy and perinatal problems account for approximately 10%. General medical conditions acquired during infancy and childhood account for approximately 5%. Environmental influences and mental disorders, other than mental retardation, account for approximately 15–20%. There is no clear etiology in 30–40% of cases.

39. **(B)** Mental retardation is coded on Axis II. All psychiatric disorders except mental retardation and personality disorders are coded on Axis I. Medical (physical) disorders are coded on Axis III. Psychosocial and environmental problems of clinical significance are coded on Axis IV. The GAF, the clinician's judgment of the individual's overall level of functioning, is coded on Axis V.

40. **(D)** This boy's history is typical of ADHD, combined type. He is fidgety and distractible in school as well as at home, and this is interfering with his ability to function. Forgetfulness due to distractibility is commonly seen in ADHD and is not a sign of dementia. This boy does not display excessive aggression, destruction of property, deceitfulness, theft, or serious violations of rules, as seen in conduct disorder. His behaviors are not negativistic, hostile, or defiant, so he does not suffer from oppositional defiant disorder. Disruptive behavior disorder not otherwise specified is a diagnosis reserved for cases in which there are conduct or oppositional defiant behaviors that do not meet the full criteria for conduct disorder or oppositional defiant disorder but cause significant impairment.

41. **(A)** Stimulant medications have been associated with an increased risk of developing tics. In general, if a child suffers from tics or has a family history of tics, stimulant medications should be avoided and a TCA should be used to treat ADHD if necessary. SSRIs, MAOIs, D_2 antagonists, and benzodiazepines are not known to exacerbate tics.

42. **(A)** Learning disorders are commonly associated with ADHD. Children with conduct disorder, oppositional defiant disorder, MDD, and dysthymic disorder are also at increased risk for learning disorders. Bipolar disorder, Tourette disorder, Asperger disorder, and schizophrenia are not commonly associated with learning disorders.

43. **(D)** Approximately 5% of students in public schools are identified as suffering from a learning disorder. Nearly 40% of those students drop out of school.

44. **(A)** Most commonly, enuresis occurs in otherwise normal boys. Enuresis is more common in boys than in girls. There is no increased prevalence of enuresis in children with mental retardation, autistic disorder, or OCD.

45. **(D)** Imipramine, a TCA, is the standard agent used in the pharmacologic treatment of enuresis. Methylphenidate is commonly used in the treatment of attention deficit disorder, paroxetine is an SSRI, trazodone is an antidepressant most often used for insomnia, and benztropine is used to prevent extrapyramidal symptoms caused by neuroleptic use.

46. **(D)** The most common adverse effects of methylphenidate and other stimulant medications include insomnia, decreased appetite, weight loss, dysphoria, and irritability. Tremor, hypotension, weight gain, and liver toxicity are not common.

47. **(E)** Stimulant medications, such as methylphenidate, are effective in diminishing symptoms of ADHD in approximately 70% of patients.

48. **(C)** Since the birth of the baby, the parents have probably spent a lot of time tending to the new baby's needs and paying less attention to their daughter. The girl may feel rejected, jealous, and angry. The most helpful approach is for the mother to spend time alone with her daughter every day, giving her undivided attention, and showing her that she is still loved and wanted. The girl is unlikely to be reassured by a single discussion about how the baby needs more attention than she does. Being consistently irritable, angry, and violent is not normal behavior at 20 months or at 24 months. The girl's behavior should not be ignored.

49. **(A)** A developmentally normal child can copy a circle at the age of 2. She can tell her age and gender and ride a tricycle at age 3. She can copy a square and can identify her left hand at age 5.

50. **(D)** This boy's behavior is characteristic of autistic disorder. He suffers from impaired social interactions and attachments, restricted interests and behaviors, and impaired communication. He does not object to going with a stranger to the examining room, does not interact with the physician, becomes preoccupied with a toy to an abnormal degree, and screams when the toy is taken away. He is not primarily negativistic and hostile as in oppositional defiant disorder. He is not aggressive, destructive, deceitful, or in violation of rules, as in conduct disorder. He does not become upset when separated from his mother, as in separation anxiety disorder.

51. **(D)** Children with autistic disorder have more favorable prognoses if they are able to converse meaningfully rather than unable to interact positively with others. They are often easily toilet trained, often enjoy mechanical toys, are rigidly organized in their play, and may become preoccupied with the rhythm or beat of music. These latter characteristics are not associated with a good prognosis.

52. **(A)** Hypercholesterolemia is common in anorexia nervosa. Other findings associated with the starvation state are mild normocytic normochromic anemia and leukopenia. Hypercarotenemia, causing yellowing of the skin, may be seen if many carrots are eaten in an attempt to satisfy the appetite with a low-calorie food. TSH is not typically altered. If vomiting is induced, hypokalemia, hypochloremia, and metabolic alkalosis may be seen.

53. **(E)** During anorexia nervosa, the body is in a state of starvation and, as a result, most bodily functions are suppressed. The resting energy expenditure is decreased, there is a sinus bradycardia, serum estrogen levels are low in girls, and serum testosterone levels are low in boys. Brain imaging may show an increase in ventricular-brain ratios secondary to starvation.

54. **(E)** Stranger anxiety occurs as part of normal child development and is evidence of the development of a strong bond of attachment. It does not suggest that a parent is inattentive; it usually appears by 7–8 months and generally resolves with time. Typically, stranger anxiety

is stronger toward completely unknown persons than toward those who are more familiar. Autistic children lack this developmental marker. Because stranger anxiety at this age is developmentally appropriate, this boy cannot be diagnosed with separation anxiety disorder and is not overly attached to his mother.

55. **(B)** Bonding is believed to begin in the immediate postdelivery period. However, the slow-growing attachment between an infant and his or her caretakers occurs with ongoing interaction over time and does not require contact in the perinatal period. Attachment occurs in the face of many obstacles, including sensory deficit, maltreatment, and physical disabilities on both sides.

56. **(A)** Schizophrenia, paranoid type, is the most likely diagnosis because of the frequency of the auditory hallucinations without prominent disorganization or inappropriate affect, as seen in disorganized type, or motor abnormalities, as seen in catatonic type. Criteria for paranoid type are met, so this is not an undifferentiated type. Hallucinations are not present in residual type.

57. **(C)** Very early onset of schizophrenia, before the age of 10, is rare and associated with a poor outcome. A better outcome is associated with more affective symptoms, acute onset, older age at onset, good premorbid functioning, well-differentiated symptoms, and lack of a family history of schizophrenia.

58. **(D)** Children with ADHD often suffer from low self-esteem, while children with mania are more likely to be euphoric. Pressured speech, distractibility, motoric overactivity, and impulsivity are seen in children with both disorders.

59. **(C)** Rett disorder occurs exclusively in girls. ADHD, conduct disorder, Tourette disorder, and Asperger disorder are seen more commonly in boys.

60. **(D)** Typically, children are 7 or 8 years old when they begin to understand the irreversibility of death. To understand that death is irreversible, a child must be aware of the continuity of time,

be able to fantasize, and have a solid sense of his or her own individuality. Usually, this level of maturity is achieved between the ages of 6 and 10.

61. **(D)** This boy is displaying *regression*, a defense mechanism in which there is an attempt to return to an earlier developmental phase to avoid the tension and conflict at the present level of development (e.g., distress over the grandmother's death). *Repression* is a defense mechanism in which an idea or feeling is expelled or withheld from consciousness. *Acting out* is a defense mechanism in which an unconscious wish or impulse is expressed through action to avoid an accompanying affect. *Denial* is a defense mechanism in which the awareness of a painful aspect of reality is avoided by negating sensory data. *Blocking* is a defense mechanism in which a thought, impulse, or effect is transiently inhibited, causing tension or distress.

62. **(A)** Sedation is a frequent adverse effect of clonidine upon initiating treatment. With continued treatment, the sedation usually subsides. Dry mouth is a less common adverse effect. Hypotension is a rare adverse affect. In general, tremor and nausea are not seen.

63. **(A)** Stimulants are the most commonly used medication in the treatment of ADHD, and although they can unmask tic disorders, ADHD treatment guidelines state that stimulants can still be used with tics. A recent study found that stimulants did not worsen tics in those with tic disorders. Although TCAs are as effective as stimulants, there have been reports of sudden death using the medications, and they are not used. SSRIs may be used to augment treatment in some cases, but not as a first-line treatment. MAOIs and neuroleptics are not used for ADHD.

64. **(E)** The finding of multiple fractures especially when they are of different ages is a red flag for physical abuse. Even though the boy may be scared to report what happened for fear of punishment, it is important to try to talk with him alone and find out as much as possible. It is not

appropriate to refer the boy to an orthopedist or his pediatrician prior to investigating the possibility of physical abuse. Recommending limited sports or extra vitamins does not address the question of whether the boy is safe at home.

65. **(D)** The most appropriate advice is that the mother should help her son return the toys. The boy is in a developmental period when his conscience is being established, and the parental model is important. The parent can show the child how to act responsibly by helping him return the toys himself. At the age of 4, a child cannot adequately grasp the abstract concept of stealing, so punishment is not helpful. His sense of time is limited, so he cannot integrate the idea of a reward after a week.

66. **(D)** SSRIs such as sertraline are effective in the treatment of panic disorder. Mood stabilizers, such as valproate and carbamazepine, and antipsychotics, such as risperidone and clozapine, are not indicated for the treatment of panic disorder.

67. **(B)** *Identification* is the process of adopting other people's characteristics. Identification with a parent is important in personality formation. This girl's behavior may occur as an attempt to imitate the doctor because she admires her, or it may represent an effort to cope with anxiety about the doctor because she fears her. *Reaction formation* is a defense mechanism in which an unacceptable impulse is transformed into its opposite. *Displacement* is a defense mechanism in which emotions are shifted from one idea or object to another that resembles the original but evokes less distress. *Rationalization* is a defense mechanism in which rational explanations are offered in an attempt to justify unacceptable attitudes, beliefs, or behaviors. *Dissociation* is a defense mechanism in which a person's character or sense of identity is temporarily but drastically modified in order to avoid emotional distress.

68. **(A)** When the mother is infected with rubella during the first month of the pregnancy, the risk of congenital defects is 50%. The risk of defects decreases inversely with the duration of pregnancy at the time of disease.

69. **(A)** In all jurisdictions in the United States, clinicians are required to report all cases of suspected child abuse. The law does not leave the issue to the clinician's discretion.

70. **(A)** This boy's history is most consistent with selective mutism. He does not speak at school but continues to talk at home. Consistent failure to speak in a specific social situation despite speaking in other situations is not characteristic of MDD, separation anxiety disorder, social phobia, or dysthymic disorder.

71. **(D)** The mother is most commonly the perpetrator of intentionally producing physical or psychological symptoms in her child in order to assume the sick role by proxy. The victim is usually a preschool child, and an Axis I diagnosis of physical abuse of a child may be appropriate.

72. **(D)** DSM-IV-TR criteria for antisocial personality disorder requires evidence of a conduct disorder before the age of 15. No other personality disorder requires a previous diagnosis of conduct disorder. In addition, there is no evidence of a reduced capacity for close relationships or eccentric behavior, making a diagnosis of schizotypal personality disorder unlikely. Recurrent suicidal behavior or an identity disturbance is a common finding in borderline personality disorder, and there is no evidence of excessive attention-seeking behavior, thus making histrionic personality disorder unlikely.

73. **(B)** This patient meets the criteria for anorexia nervosa, a serious and potentially life-threatening eating disorder, characterized by intense fear of gaining weight, distortion of body image, and weight <85% of normal. The purposeful starvation can lead to numerous physiological abnormalities, including amenorrhea and anemia. It can also lead to elevated cholesterol, increased secretion of corticotropin-releasing hormone, hypoglycemia, hypothyroidism, and leukopenia.

74. **(C)** *Alexia* is the inability to read. *Anomia* is the specific inability to name objects even though the object is recognizable and can be described by the patient. *Aphasia* is more global and is an abnormality in either the expression or the comprehension of language. *Agnosia* is the inability to recognize objects, but as in anomia, the object can be perceived by the patient's intact senses. *Apraxia* is an inability to perform learned motor skills despite normal strength and coordination.

75. **(D)** This patient is suffering from OCD. Although all of the other listed organisms may cause psychiatric symptoms, prior infection with Group-A beta-hemolytic *Streptococcus* has been associated with several psychiatric illnesses, such as OCD and Tourette disorder.

76. **(F)** When children with pica eat soil or feces, eggs of *Toxocara canis* or *cati* may be ingested causing visceral larva migrans. The other disorders are not associated with behavior likely to include ingestion of parasite eggs.

77. **(B)** Bulimia nervosa is seen in 1–3% of adolescent girls and young women. In the purging type of disorder, repeated vomiting can produce fluid and electrolyte abnormalities, most frequently hypokalemia, hyponatremia, and hypochloremia. Metabolic alkalosis may occur as well. The other disorders are not associated with hypokalemia.

78. **(C)** One of the presentations of stereotypic movement disorder is self-inflicted bodily injury that is severe enough to require medical attention. An individual's repetitive motor behavior may cause chronic rectal bleeding severe enough to lead to anemia. The other disorders are not associated with rectal bleeding.

79. **(H)** Adolescents with conduct disorder often abuse substances including alcohol, marijuana, and cocaine. The other disorders are not as often associated with substance abuse.

Rett disorder **(A)** is characterized by normal prenatal and perinatal development, normal head circumference at birth, and normal psychomotor development through the first 5 months of life. Between the ages of 5 months and 48 months, there is deceleration of head growth, loss of hand skills with development of stereotyped hand movements such as hand wringing, loss of social interaction (which may improve later), appearance of poorly coordinated gait or trunk movements, and severely impaired expressive and receptive language development with severe psychomotor retardation. To date, Rett disorder has been observed only in girls. Patients suffering from social phobia **(D)** demonstrate a marked and persistent fear of a social or performance situation with exposure causing intense anxiety expressed as a tantrum or a panic attack. Separation anxiety disorder **(E)** is characterized by developmentally inappropriate and excessive anxiety concerning separation from the home or from those to whom the individual is attached. Enuresis **(G)** refers to bedwetting. In panic disorder **(I)**, there are discrete panic attacks, periods of intense fear or discomfort with physical manifestations such as palpitations, and subjective difficulty breathing. Asperger disorder **(J)** is a particular type of autism most commonly seen in boys.

80. **(E)** Palpitations, chest pain, shortness of breath, and diaphoresis commonly occur during panic attacks. These symptoms do not occur routinely in any of the other disorders.

81. **(G)** Hypotension, bradycardia, and lanugo hair are classic sequelae of starvation seen in anorexia nervosa. These signs are not associated with any of the other disorders.

82. **(A)** Chapped hands and other dermatologic problems are often present in OCD due to excessive washing with water or caustic cleaning agents. Chapped hands are not specifically associated with any of the other disorders.

83. **(J)** Trichotillomania usually occurs around ages 5–8 or age 13. The repeated pulling out of hair results in decreased or complete loss of hair in a specific area. The scalp, eyebrows, and eyelashes are the sites most commonly involved. Patches of baldness are not associated with any of the other disorders. Pica **(B)** is the eating of

nonnutritional substances such as dirt or paint. Hypochondriasis **(C)** is the preoccupation that one has a serious disease based on misinterpretation of symptoms, despite appropriate medical evaluation and reassurance. Eye tics such as blinking and eye rolling are the most common initial symptoms in Tourette disorder **(D)**. Facial tics such as grimacing or licking movements and vocal tics such as throat clearing or grunting are the next most common initial symptoms. Whole-body tics, such as body rocking or pelvic thrusting, and self-abusive tics, such as hitting, may develop later. Bulimia nervosa, seen in 1–3% of adolescent girls and young women, is a purging type of eating disorder. Asperger disorder **(H)** is a pervasive developmental disorder characterized by impairments in social interactions and the development of stereotyped or repetitive patterns of behaviors without significant delay in language skills or cognitive function. Asperger occurs more commonly in males and is commonly referred to as a *high-functioning autism*. A DSM-IV-TR diagnosis of pyromania **(I)** requires several criteria, including deliberate and purposeful fire setting and tension or affective arousal before the act, which is not better accounted for by conduct disorder, a manic episode, or antisocial personality disorder.

84. **(C)** Although it is possible that this child has a learning disorder such as dyslexia that is keeping his reading skills from progressing, it is important to rule out a vision problem that could be easily fixed with glasses and that would in fact impair other parts of his life. The child may need a reading specialist, or even have ADHD, but all the interventions for these conditions will be for naught if you miss a simple vision problem.

85. **(C)** This child is fulfilling the DSM-TR criteria for conduct disorder, namely, three of the four following acts: aggression toward people and animals, destruction of property, deceitfulness, and serious violations of rules. There is nothing to suggest an autistic spectrum disorder, particularly because it would probably have been diagnosed much earlier; his actions seem willful and not repetitive or stereotyped. Similarly, although one manifestation of Tourette syndrome might be a bark-like noise, it would not occur only at will and be directed only at the dog. Oppositional defiant disorder requires 6 months of negativistic, hostile, and defiant behavior directed mostly at authority figures. Finally, there is no evidence of the psychosis, such as hallucinations, that would characterize childhood schizophrenia.

86–89. **(86–B, 87–D, 88–E, 89–A)** The purpose of these questions is to differentiate some of the autistic spectrum disorders by symptom and epidemiology. Selective mutism is rare, and children who suffer from it are only mute in certain situations (e.g., school). It often involves a stressful life event such as parents' divorce. The 6-year-old girl in question 85 who had reached normal early development milestones but now does not speak in school or at home is most likely to have Rett disorder **(D)**, which is also rare and seen only in girls. The boy in question 86 who performs well in school but avoids social interactions is most likely to have Asperger disorder, because those with autism, as in question 87, are likely to have other symptoms such as repetitive movements and to have difficulty in school. There is no evidence in any of the cases for the psychosis that would suggest childhood schizophrenia.

90–95. **(90–C, 91–E, 92–A, 93–B, 94–D, 95–A)** Although these are not "board-style" questions, it is worth reminding yourself of the definitions of the severity of mental retardation: mild (IQ of 55–70), moderate (IQ of 40–54), severe (IQ of 25–39), and profound (IQ below 25).

CHAPTER 3

Adult Psychopathology
Questions

DIRECTIONS (Questions 1 through 116): Each of the numbered items in this section is followed by answers. Select the ONE lettered answer that is BEST in each case.

Questions 1 and 2

A 22-year-old single White man is referred to you for a 1-year history of strange behavior characterized by talking to the television, accusing local police of bugging his room, and carrying on conversations with himself. His mother also describes a 3- to 4-year history of progressive withdrawal from social activities. The patient dropped out of college in his final year and since then has been living in his room at home. Attempts to hold a job as a busboy at a local restaurant and as a night janitor have abruptly ended after disputes with the employers.

1. How prevalent is this patient's illness in the general population?

   (A) 0.1%
   (B) 0.5%
   (C) 1%
   (D) 3%
   (E) 5%

2. The monozygotic (identical) twin concordance for this patient's illness is which of the following?

   (A) 10%
   (B) 25%
   (C) 50%

(D) 100%
(E) the same incidence as in the general population

Questions 3 and 4

A patient reports to you that for the past week or two he has had the belief that his intestines and his heart have been removed. When asked about his lack of getting out in the world, he responds "What world? There is no world!"

3. This aspect of the patient's illness would best be referred to as which of the following?

   (A) schizoaffective disorder
   (B) Capgras syndrome
   (C) folie à deux
   (D) Cotard syndrome
   (E) major depression

4. If this patient consistently reported to you the belief that his mother and father have been replaced by "cyborg alien robots" that look identical to his parents, this would be most indicative of which of the following?

   (A) delusional disorder
   (B) Capgras syndrome
   (C) folie à deux
   (D) Cotard syndrome
   (E) simple schizophrenia (simple deteriorative disorder)

[handwritten margin note, left side, rotated: "postpartum psychosis is often associated with Bipolar D/o which is 80% horrible)"]

5. A 32-year-old woman 6 days postpartum is brought into the emergency room at the encouragement of her husband. She is a poor historian, not believing that anything is wrong. He states that his wife has no past psychiatric history, although she does have an unknown family history of "some sort of mental illness." He is very worried as over the last several days his wife has not been sleeping even while the newborn is. He has noticed her walking around their apartment in the middle of the night weeping while talking to no one in particular. She has begun ignoring their baby, but he brought her in today because earlier she volunteered that their child "is the Antichrist and must be destroyed." Which of the following is her most likely diagnosis?

(A) bipolar disorder

(B) delusional disorder

(C) major depressive disorder (MDD) with psychotic features

(D) schizoaffective disorder

(E) schizophrenia

[handwritten: "Not 'C' since need 2 wks of depression B4 get MDD"]

6. An 18-year-old woman, without a history of psychiatric illness, has recently started her freshman year of college. The woman is brought to the psychiatric emergency department after being found on the roof of her dormitory dressed only in her underwear despite below freezing temperatures. The campus police who brought her in report that she appeared to be dancing in a disorganized and agitated fashion, speaking angrily to someone that was not apparent to them, and accused the policemen of being "Satan's horsemen" and "adulterers from the Court of King Herod." On psychiatric examination, she reports to you that "Lucifer is telling me I'm an angel of death. He told me to flap my wings and soar to my death." A careful history is obtained. Her roommates report that for the past 5 weeks the patient has been delusional, mostly with religious or persecutory content, and her thoughts seem disorganized. In talking with this patient's family, you would be most likely to gather a history of which of the following?

(A) low intelligence

(B) head trauma

(C) progressive social withdrawal

(D) a neglectful mother

(E) physical or sexual abuse

7. A 42-year-old woman presents to a therapist with a history since early adolescence of dramatic mood swings, quickly becoming deeply depressed for hours to days, usually in response to separation from a loved one. She also admits to "rage attacks," where she will break items, scream, or scratch herself superficially on her arms. She claims to drink in "binges," up to 1–2 pints of hard liquor at a time. She has had over 30 sexual partners, many times without using contraception. Which of the following defense mechanisms is most likely employed by this patient?

(A) altruism

(B) intellectualization

(C) splitting

(D) sublimation

(E) undoing

8. In performing a Mental Status Examination (MSE) on a 26-year-old male graduate student, you make the following notes: The patient is poorly oriented to time and place, is dressed in pink bathroom slippers, and is wearing only a trench coat. He reports auditory hallucinations and fears that his classmates are conspiring to embarrass him in front of his teachers. If, in the course of this patient's chronic mental illness, he becomes jobless, homeless, and destitute, the history would exemplify which concept?

(A) stress-diathesis model

(B) downward drift hypothesis

(C) sometimes intolerable side effects of antipsychotic drugs

(D) socioeconomic burden of schizophrenia

(E) Bleuler's classical model of schizophrenia

9. A 36-year-old patient you have seen twice is brought to your walk-in department by family members. On previous occasions, he presented with delusions, hallucinations, and prominent negative symptoms. During the visit, he exhibits motoric, waxy flexibility and resistance to all instructions. He methodically repeats words and phrases and appears to crudely mimic your movements. The most likely diagnosis is which of the following?

(A) elective mutism

(B) malingering

(C) schizophrenia, disorganized type

(D) schizophrenia, catatonic type

(E) drug-induced psychosis

Ryan - schizophrenia catatonic type

10. A 49-year-old bank teller without a psychiatric history is referred to your office for the first time by her internist for an evaluation. For the past 2 months, she has been increasingly convinced that a well-known pop music star is in love with her and that they have had an ongoing affair. She is well-groomed, and there is no evidence of thought disorder or hallucinations. Her husband reveals that she has been functioning well at work and in other social relationships. Which of the following is the most likely diagnosis?

(A) delusional disorder

(B) acute reactive psychosis

(C) prodromal schizophrenia

(D) paranoid personality disorder

(E) schizophreniform disorder

Questions 11 and 12

A 46-year-old divorced, middle-class, African American woman is admitted to your inpatient psychiatric ward after a suicide attempt by overdosing on acetaminophen (Tylenol). She has a history of multiple psychiatric hospitalizations with similar presentations. She has been unable to work because of her depression and has lost interest in activities she once enjoyed. Additionally, the patient reports a 2-week history of decreased sleep, difficulty concentrating, low energy, hopelessness, and a decreased appetite.

11. Which of the following factors would influence you to recommend electroconvulsive therapy (ECT)?

(A) severe, melancholic depression and history of poor response to medications

(B) severe, adverse reactions to all selective serotonin reuptake inhibitors (SSRIs), tricyclic antidepressants (TCAs), and continued suicidal ideation

(C) known history of psychotic symptoms in the context of her depressive symptoms

(D) known history of bipolar illness

(E) poor compliance with medications

12. The most important diagnosis to rule out in this patient before administering an antidepressant medication would be which of the following?

(A) panic disorder

(B) bipolar disorder

(C) obsessive-compulsive disorder (OCD)

(D) drug-induced depressive disorder

(E) malingering

Questions 13 and 14

A 34-year-old White man complains of feeling blue at his first visit to you. An MSE reveals a disheveled appearance, a depressed mood, psychomotor retardation, and suicidal thoughts. Thought processes are significant for thought blocking and some slowing. Deficits with remote and short-term memory are noted. Judgment and insight are also impaired. Your diagnosis is a major depressive episode.

13. The type of sleep disturbance you would most expect to see in this patient is which of the following?

(A) sleeping too deeply (difficulty being awakened)

(B) early morning awakening

(C) increased rapid eye movement (REM) stage latency

(D) decreased response to sedative drugs

(E) sleeping too lightly (awakened too easily)

14. You would expect the biochemical/hormonal profile of this patient to be significant for which of the following?

    (A) increased catecholamine activity
    (B) increased cortisol secretion
    (C) increased sex hormones
    (D) increased immune functions
    (E) decreased monoamine oxidase (MAO) activity

Dep ↑ MAO consuming all the Biogenic amines; think about how the drug works;

Questions 15 and 16

A 52-year-old man with a history of major depression is treated with paroxetine (Paxil). He has been your patient for 2 years and has recently missed his last two appointments reporting to you that "I've been spectacular!" You have documented two calls from his wife since his last visit. She initially reported that her husband has been "very different." You learn that he has spent more money on frivolous items than he ever has. In addition, when she went to the bank to withdraw money for groceries, she was told that the account was overdrawn. Recently, his wife called again to make an appointment for her husband. She reports that one moment her husband is giddy and without notice he quickly becomes agitated and angry. During the interview, the patient questions your credentials and accuses you of being more loyal to his wife than to him. Most of the interview is spent interrupting the patient as you try to decipher his rapid speech.

15. Which of the following statements is true?

    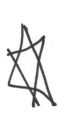

    (A) Patients with bipolar disorder usually have a more favorable course than depressive patients.
    (B) A lower percentage of patients with bipolar disorder eventually get treatment as compared to patients with unipolar depression.
    (C) Bipolar disorder has a stronger genetic link than depression.
    (D) More women are diagnosed with bipolar disorder than with major depression.
    (E) Bipolar disorder is more common than major depression in the northern hemisphere.

The patient returns for a follow-up visit 4 weeks after you initiate treatment with divalproex sodium. He presents looking irritable and demonstrates pressured speech and grandiose delusions. He reports that he is the lost son of a famed millionaire. He exhibits symptoms of depression characterized by decreased sleep, poor appetite and concentration, and thoughts of suicide. He admits to drinking alcohol every day since his last visit. His wife reports that his moods seem to change with the seasons.

16. In addition to starting valproic acid, the other pharmacologic management change indicated at the prior visit would have been to which of the following?

    (A) Check the patient's serum paroxetine level.
    (B) Select a more effective antidepressant.
    (C) Stop the antidepressant.
    (D) Select a medication as needed for insomnia.
    (E) Start lithium.

Questions 17 and 18

17. A patient places a call after hours to the practice you are covering. You do not have access to the patient's chart but learn that the history suggests the patient experiences dysthymia followed by episodes of hypomania. In making a decision about the patient's medication, you quickly recognize the diagnosis. Which of the following choices best categorizes the patient's diagnosis?

    (A) bipolar II disorder
    (B) bipolar I disorder
    (C) cyclothymia
    (D) bipolar III disorder
    (E) double depression

18. On a subsequent visit, the patient brings his brother to your office. His brother asks what his risk of developing a mood disorder is. What do you answer?

    (A) the same as anyone in the general population
    (B) 25%

mnemonic
Bipolar → 2 poles → risk 20-25%

(C) 10%

(D) 1%

(E) the answer is unknown

Questions 19 and 20

A 26-year-old White woman presents to the psychiatric emergency department in an acutely distressed, nervous state. The emergency department staff are unable to calm her down or gain an adequate history from the patient. She complains of terrible anxiety. She is slightly diaphoretic, tachycardic, and the pupils are mildly dilated. She is on no medications.

19. The cause of anxiety important to rule out in this patient is which of the following?

(A) cocaine induced

(B) hypochondriasis

(C) serotonin syndrome

(D) specific phobia

(E) lysergic acid diethylamide (LSD) induced

20. Abdominal pain in this patient might cause you to investigate which of the following?

(A) blood alcohol level

(B) acetaminophen level

(C) urinary porphobilinogen

(D) urine toxicology screen

(E) serum catecholamine metabolites

21. A 46-year-old man is admitted to the emergency department acutely diaphoretic, tachycardic, hypertensive, tremulous, and agitated. He refuses to give a urine sample for toxicology studies. He is apparently hallucinating, judging from his insistence that he be allowed to "squash those bugs on the wall" (there are none). One would expect to most likely see this

patient's type of hallucinations in the context of which of the following?

(A) delirium

(B) delusional disorders

(C) schizophrenia

(D) conversion disorder

(E) brief psychotic disorder

Questions 22 and 23

A 62-year-old woman presents to the nursing home where you work as a consulting psychiatrist. She has had a history of bilateral temporal lobectomy for an intractable seizure disorder. After a few weeks at the new facility, the staff report the following observations about the patient in addition to her short-term memory difficulties: She is extremely docile and displays very little emotion. She has a large appetite and compulsively puts both food and nonfood items in her mouth. She also displays sexual disinhibition, often walking out of her room without her pants on.

22. This patient's clinical condition is most consistent with which of the following?

(A) Pick disease

(B) Klüver-Bucy syndrome

(C) Arnold-Chiari syndrome

(D) punchdrunk syndrome

(E) Möbius syndrome

23. The loss of what temporal lobe structure is most closely associated with this condition?

(A) hippocampus

(B) insula

(C) superior temporal gyri

(D) amygdala

(E) inferior horn of the lateral ventricle

Questions 24 and 25

A 22-year-old woman is referred by her gynecologist for the treatment of a possible eating disorder. The gynecologist informs you that the patient presented with a chief complaint of amenorrhea that had been present for 4 months. In addition, the patient is at 83% of her expected body weight. Upon evaluation, the patient describes a repeated pattern of bingeing on large meals followed by forced vomiting. She also uses laxatives every night before she goes to bed "to prevent constipation." The patient reports that she had been running 3 miles every day, but in the last few weeks she has become too tired to run.

24. The most accurate diagnosis for this patient is which of the following?

(A) exercise-induced amenorrhea
(B) OCD
(C) psychogenic gastritis
(D) anorexia nervosa
(E) bulimia nervosa

25. Laboratory findings associated with severe cases of this disorder include which of the following?

(A) decreased serum cortisol levels
(B) blunted thyroid-stimulating hormone (TSH) response to thyrotropin-releasing hormone (TRH)
(C) polycythemia
(D) low serum growth hormone
(E) high serum blood urea nitrogen (BUN)

26. A 23-year-old college student has experienced frequent episodes of feeling utter doom for the past 3 months. During these episodes, he also experiences tremulousness, sweating, dizziness, and tingling in his extremities. He reports experiencing these episodes at least once a week and is now becoming fearful of attending classes lest he have an episode. The medication of choice for this condition is which of the following?

(A) alprazolam (Xanax)
(B) fluoxetine (Prozac)

(C) chlordiazepoxide (Librium)
(D) phenelzine (Nardil)
(E) divalproex sodium

Questions 27 and 28

A 34-year-old woman complains of a 3-month history of "feeling down" that has steadily worsened. After losing her job as a sales representative 1 month ago, she has been living with her parents and has not looked for work. The patient reports that she is unmotivated to do anything even the things she used to enjoy. She says that "nothing really matters...I don't matter." She has been sleeping 10–14 hours a night and has no appetite. More than once, she has pondered suicide as a possible escape route.

27. Given this patient's diagnosis, what is the likelihood that she would fail to suppress her cortisol levels in a dexamethasone suppression test?

(A) 10%
(B) 30%
(C) 50%
(D) 70%
(E) 90%

28. What is the likelihood that she would have a blunted response of TSH to an administration of TRH?

(A) 10%
(B) 30%
(C) 50%
(D) 70%
(E) 90%

29. A 37-year-old woman, who works the night shift at a local grocery store taking inventory, reports that her childhood and college years were uneventful but happy. She spends most of her time alone when she is not at work. She does not venture out of her house and her social contacts are limited to work-related interactions with coworkers. She is an avid plant lover and she spends most of her free time taking care of her indoor plants. She

reports that she is quite content with her life. The most accurate diagnosis for this patient is which of the following?

(A) agoraphobia
(B) avoidant personality disorder
(C) schizoid personality disorder
(D) schizotypal personality disorder
(E) autistic disorder

30. An 18-year-old, pregnant, human immunodeficiency virus (HIV)-positive White woman presents for the treatment of heroin addiction. She reports using heroin for the last 8 months with substantial efforts to quit for the last 4 months. She is now homeless and has recently been arrested for shoplifting. Which of the following is important to discuss with the patient when considering methadone maintenance?

(A) Methadone may cause bone decay.
(B) Methadone substantially reduces libido.
(C) Methadone worsens dependence on heroin.
(D) Effective treatment is likely to require more than 60 mg/day of methadone.
(E) Methadone may cause Cushing syndrome.

31. Following the birth of her first child, a 29-year-old woman is diagnosed with postpartum psychosis. Which of the following would be the most important first step in the management of this patient?

(A) Admit her to the hospital.
(B) Begin a mood stabilizer.
(C) Begin an antidepressant.
(D) Begin an atypical antipsychotic.
(E) Begin ECT.

32. A 42-year-old business executive presents for his first contact with a mental health provider. He reports that for the last 4 months he has been feeling depressed. His low energy level and poor motivation are affecting his job performance and the CEO of his company advised him to "take a couple of weeks off." The patient reports that he started feeling down when his wife discovered that he was involved in his third extramarital affair. Since then he has moved into a small apartment by himself. He is sleeping almost 12 hours every night, has a poor appetite, and is experiencing financial difficulty due to indiscriminate purchases. He laments the loss of his former self. He reports that he used to need only 4–5 hours of sleep and once was able to "party all night and work all day." This case best illustrates an Axis I diagnosis of which of the following?

(A) bipolar I disorder
(B) bipolar II disorder
(C) MDD
(D) narcissistic personality disorder
(E) impulse control disorder not otherwise specified

33. A 52-year-old woman who has been treated with medication for 3 years for a chronic mood disorder reports that although she feels well, she wonders if her medication is causing side effects. She complains of dry mouth, trouble urinating, and occasional dizziness when she gets out of bed. Which of the following medications is she most likely being prescribed?

(A) fluoxetine
(B) imipramine (Tofranil)
(C) phenelzine
(D) lithium
(E) divalproex sodium

Questions 34 and 35

A 72-year-old man is brought in by his wife to your geriatric psychiatry clinic. The patient's wife is concerned about his progressive confusion over the last year. She is particularly distressed that he repeatedly asks the same questions throughout the day. She also notes that her husband has become increasingly unsteady on his feet and needs to use a walker when they go out. She wonders if these symptoms may be related to the meningitis he suffered from 3 years ago.

34. For you to make a diagnosis of normal pressure hydrocephalus (NPH), further investigation in this case would have to reveal which of the following?

    (A) elevated opening pressure upon lumbar puncture
    (B) a history of incontinence
    (C) oculomotor difficulties
    (D) frontal release signs
    (E) perseveration

35. Neuroimaging with noncontrast computed tomography (CT) in this case of NPH is most likely to reveal which of the following?

    (A) dilated lateral ventricles
    (B) normal ventricles
    (C) frontal sulcal widening
    (D) focal subcortical hypointensities
    (E) cerebellar atrophy

Questions 36 and 37

A 48-year-old man has been drinking up to 6 beers per night during the week and up to 12 beers a night on the weekend. A year ago, he had his driver's license suspended for drunk driving. His marriage is failing. Last month, he was diagnosed with a gastric ulcer as a result of alcohol consumption. He admits to an alcohol problem and has tried to stop on numerous occasions. He finds that he experiences insomnia if he does not drink for more than 2 days.

36. The feature of this case that suggests alcohol dependence rather than alcohol abuse is which of the following?

    (A) the patient's inability to stop drinking despite knowledge of its harmful effects and his desire to quit
    (B) the high quantity of alcohol consumed on a regular basis
    (C) the patient's history of drunk driving
    (D) the fact that the patient cannot sleep if he does not drink
    (E) a medical complication due to drinking

37. On laboratory examination, this patient is likely to have which of the following?

    (A) increased alanine aminotransferase (ALT) and aspartate aminotransferase (AST), with increased ALT/AST ratio
    (B) decreased uric acid
    (C) increased gamma-glutamyl transpeptidase (GGT)
    (D) microcytic anemia
    (E) decreased serum triglycerides

38. A 26-year-old computer programmer without a past psychiatric history has been married for 4 years. His wife is expecting their first child. She reports that 3 months ago the patient became preoccupied with the idea that she became pregnant by another man. During this time, he began missing work and isolated himself in his bedroom. His affect has progressively become more blunted. Recently, he believes that his wife is carrying a child conceived by "extraterrestrial forces." He urged her to have an abortion and she refused. The patient denies any history of substance abuse and his recent medical evaluation was within normal limits. Which of the following is the most appropriate diagnosis?

    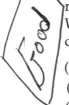

    (A) brief psychotic disorder
    (B) delusional disorder
    (C) psychosis not otherwise specified
    (D) schizophreniform disorder
    (E) schizophrenia

39. A 27-year-old woman was involved in a major automobile accident 2 weeks ago in which a friend sitting next to her in the passenger

seat was killed. Since the accident, she has experienced recurrent thoughts of the accident and has recurrent nightmares each night. Lately, she is reluctant to drive and has chosen to ride a bus to work. When she does ride in the car as a passenger, she feels nervous and is overly concerned about the safety of her companion's driving. The most appropriate diagnosis for this patient is which of the following?

(A) acute stress disorder

(B) adjustment disorder

✓ (C) posttraumatic stress disorder (PTSD)

(D) generalized anxiety disorder (GAD)

(E) MDD

Questions 40 and 41

An 18-year-old woman diagnosed with schizophrenia presents to the psychiatric emergency department after a suicide attempt by carbon monoxide poisoning. Medical evaluation was noncontributory and a urine toxicology screen was negative. The patient reports that she sat in her mother's car with a glove stuck into the exhaust pipe and eventually fell asleep awaiting death. She relates that she believes that she was personally responsible for the Holocaust and that she should therefore die in a similar way. The patient's mother reports that she has been refusing to take haloperidol (Haldol) for the past 3 weeks.

40. The lifetime risk of death by suicide in patients with schizophrenia is closest to which of the following?

(A) 1%

(B) 5%

 (C) 10%

(D) 30%

(E) 50%

Death in schizophrenia is the same as the relative risk in relatives 10%.

41. A 27-year-old internal medicine resident is working in an outpatient clinic. He prefers the inpatient service and is unhappy most of the time he is there. Today, however, he is looking forward to his clinical work because one of his appointments is a follow-up visit for a single, attractive 31-year-old woman who is finishing her antibiotic regimen for treatment of pneumonia. The best psychodynamic term for this doctor's response to his patient is which of the following?

(A) countertransference

 (B) empathy

(C) identification

(D) projection

(E) transference

Questions 42 and 43

A 31-year-old woman was admitted to a psychiatric hospital after a failed suicide attempt by medication ingestion. Recently, she broke up with her boyfriend whom she met in a bar 4 months ago. She is noted for episodes of mood lability, marked by feelings of depression, and anger directed toward the psychiatric resident who completed the rotation 5 days after her admission. When the resident left, she reported that she was having urges to cut her wrists. As the patient was nearing her discharge date, she reported that "all the staff hates me except for Dr Johnson." Dr Johnson, a medical student, had a recent difference of opinion with the nursing staff regarding the patient's discharge.

42. The single most appropriate diagnosis for this patient is which of the following?

(A) psychotic disorder not otherwise specified

✓ (B) MDD

(C) histrionic personality disorder

(D) cyclothymic disorder

(E) borderline personality disorder

43. The outpatient treatment of choice for patients with the diagnosis illustrated in this case is which of the following?

(A) antidepressant medications

(B) benzodiazepine medications

(C) mood stabilizer medications

(D) neuroleptics

(E) psychotherapy

Questions 44 and 45

A 34-year-old woman presents for the treatment of her severe, medication-refractory, major depression. She is referred to you by her outpatient psychiatrist because of your expertise in ECT. After reviewing her past psychiatric history and interviewing the patient, you conclude that she should indeed undergo ECT.

44. In discussing the effects of ECT with the patient, you should relate that the most likely side effect may be which of the following?

    (A) amnesia
    (B) anesthesia-related respiratory complications
    (C) fractures from convulsions
    (D) abnormal cardiac arrhythmias
    (E) psychosis

45. You tell the patient to expect the best possible outcome, she is likely to require how many treatments?

    (A) 2
    (B) 4
    (C) 10
    (D) 20
    (E) 40

Dr. Stable said ECT tx is 10 months

Questions 46 and 47

A 38-year-old woman presents to your clinic telling you that she has had disturbing, recurrent thoughts about harming her 7-month-old infant. She imagines using a knife to stab her child. Since having these distressing thoughts, she has removed all sharp objects from her kitchen. Because of this, she has not been able to prepare meals at home and has chosen to buy fast food or take-out food for the family meals. She has not shared these thoughts with her husband.

46. The most accurate diagnosis for this condition is which of the following?

    (A) impulse control disorder not otherwise specified
    (B) OCD
    (C) obsessive-compulsive personality disorder
    (D) psychosis not otherwise specified
    (E) schizotypal personality disorder

47. The first-line pharmacotherapy for this condition is which of the following?

    (A) lorazepam (Ativan)
    (B) benztropine (Cogentin)
    (C) nortriptyline (Pamelor)
    (D) haloperidol
    (E) fluvoxamine (Luvox)

48. A 72-year-old woman presents to the emergency department from a nursing home. On physical examination, she appears malnourished and dehydrated. The medical service initiates intravenous fluid replacement. On MSE, she is alert and oriented to person only. She reports that the president is Lyndon B. Johnson. During the interview, the patient is easily distracted. She often forgets things shortly after she learns them. One hour later, her MSE has improved, reporting the correct day, time, and place. However, she cannot remember why she is there. When asked about the current president, she cannot remember his name but describes his appearance. She is able to perform serial sevens slowly but accurately without distraction. Based on the information in this case, the most appropriate diagnosis for this patient's presenting symptoms is which of the following?

    (A) amnestic disorder not otherwise specified
    (B) cognitive disorder not otherwise specified
    (C) delirium
    (D) dementia not otherwise specified
    (E) major depression

Questions 49 and 50

You are a research psychiatrist conducting a double-blind, placebo-controlled trial of a new antidepressant. You have enrolled 200 patients in the study, all of whom meet the criteria for uncomplicated major depression. You plan to randomize 100 patients to a placebo medication and the other 100 patients to the experimental antidepressant.

49. Of the 100 patients taking the placebo, approximately how many patients would be expected to improve after 4–6 weeks?

(A) 5
(B) 10
(C) 30
(D) 50
(E) 70

50. Of the 100 patients taking the experimental antidepressant (assuming this drug is as efficacious as standard antidepressants), approximately how many patients would be expected to improve after 4–6 weeks?

(A) 10
(B) 30
(C) 50
(D) 70
(E) 90

Questions 51 and 52

A 24-year-old man is brought to the psychiatric emergency department by his parents. They report that he has been living with them since he dropped out of college a year ago. In the last few months, he has spent an increasing amount of time by himself in his room. Rather than look for employment, he is absorbed in doing crossword puzzles. The parents also report that in the last 2 months, their son's behavior has become increasingly bizarre. His sleep schedule has become disorganized and he has started wearing his clothes inside out. They note that he makes strange gestures while at the dinner table. In addition, he has begun smiling for very long periods of time although there is nothing to laugh at. At times, the patient does not respond to questions asked of him, and at other times, he simply repeats the questions.

51. The type of schizophrenia that best describes the presentation is which of the following?

(A) catatonic type
(B) disorganized type
(C) paranoid type
(D) residual type
(E) undifferentiated

52. Recent epidemiologic trends concerning this type of schizophrenia are notable for which of the following?

(A) increased prevalence compared to 35 years ago
(B) about the same prevalence compared to 35 years ago

(C) its being the most common subtype of schizophrenia
(D) decreased prevalence compared to 35 years ago
(E) its having an association with history of LSD use

53. A 32-year-old single successful Wall Street executive tells you that on weekends he likes to visit a dominatrix. His regular, paid appointment with this person is described as humiliating and somewhat painful but also very sexually arousing. He describes his life as otherwise normal. The best way to describe this case by *Diagnostic and Statistical Manual of Mental Disorders, Fourth Edition, Text Revision* (DSM-IV-TR) diagnostic criteria is which of the following?

(A) fetishism
(B) frotteurism
(C) no diagnosis
(D) sexual masochism
(E) sexual sadism

Questions 54 and 55

A 28-year-old woman presents complaining of falling asleep during the day. She says this problem has been ongoing for 3 months. It has been interfering with her work as a telephone operator because she falls asleep two or three times a day while speaking with customers. At times, she finds herself falling asleep at her desk and she is awakened when her head hits the computer console in front of her. Oddly enough, she reports, this can happen when she becomes particularly stressed out as she is managing many calls. The patient also reports that this disturbance has not improved even though she is sure she sleeps 8 hours each night.

54. The most appropriate diagnosis for this case is which of the following?

   (A) circadian rhythm sleep disorder
   (B) dyssomnia not otherwise specified
   (C) narcolepsy
   (D) nightmare disorder
   (E) primary hypersomnia

55. The most useful pharmacotherapy for this condition is which of the following?

   (A) lorazepam at bedtime
   (B) bupropion (Wellbutrin)
   (C) phenelzine
   (D) methylphenidate (Ritalin)
   (E) fluoxetine

Questions 56 and 57

A 27-year-old woman is brought into the psychiatric emergency department by her distraught husband because she has been acting strangely. She reports that for about 1 year the neighborhood children have been watching and following her sometimes even breaking into her home. She adds that for the last 6 months she has been hearing a conversation between two voices typically when she is alone. Her husband says that she has been increasingly withdrawn and rarely talks anymore with her family and friends. She now spends most of the day in their bedroom. He reports that he often hears her talk to herself and has seen her checking the telephone for "bugs."

56. As you begin to discuss the possible diagnosis and treatment options with the patient, she tells you that she is 6 months pregnant. Which of the following psychiatric medications is considered safest in pregnancy?

   (A) lithium
   (B) divalproex sodium
   (C) haloperidol
   (D) chlorpromazine
   (E) fluoxetine

57. The patient's husband tells you that he does not believe the patient needs medication. He is a spiritual man and wants to take her to a healer from his community. What can you tell him about the prognosis of this disorder?

   (A) The majority of people spontaneously recover.
   (B) If she does not take medication, the patient will suffer a chronic deteriorating course.
   (C) Prognostic factors may be taken into account, but the actual course of the illness for this patient cannot be predicted.
   (D) If the patient does not take medication, she will require permanent commitment in a psychiatric facility.
   (E) There is no risk to the medication you've prescribed.

58. A 28-year-old woman presents for her annual gynecology appointment. She complains that in the week before her period, she often experiences marked anger and irritability and argues more with her boyfriend. She also reports diminished energy and concentration and sleeping more than is usual for her. These symptoms, in addition to breast tenderness and headaches, always remit in the week after her menses is finished. The most likely diagnosis is which of the following?

   (A) MDD
   (B) normal female behavior
   (C) premenstrual dysphoric disorder (PMDD)
   (D) GAD
   (E) dysthymic disorder

59. Mr P is a 37-year-old accountant who presents to the primary care clinic with complaints of insomnia. Upon further questioning, he admits that he has felt "blue" for 6 weeks since getting passed over for promotion. Since that time, he has had poor sleep often awakening early in the morning. He also has had a decreased appetite with a 10–15-lb weight loss, poor energy, guilt over "not being good enough," and he has been distracted at work. For the past 3 days, he has had thoughts of "ending my life." What is this patient's most likely risk of completed suicide?

(A) 0–10%
(B) 10–20%
(C) 20–30%
(D) 30–40%
(E) 40–50%

Questions 60 and 61

A 36-year-old man is brought to the emergency department in respiratory arrest. On examination, he is unresponsive, and the medical student rotating through the emergency department observes pinpoint pupils and antecubital track marks. There is suspicion that the patient's condition may be the result of a drug overdose.

60. The patient most likely has overdosed on which of the following drugs?

(A) cocaine
(B) phencyclidine (PCP)
(C) heroin
(D) alcohol
(E) inhalants

61. Which of the following would reverse the effects of the suspected drug?

(A) acetylcysteine
(B) naloxone
(C) deferoxamine
(D) methylene blue
(E) methadone

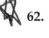

62. A 38-year-old male veteran from the Gulf War presents to the mental health clinic at the urging of his family members. While stationed in the Middle East, he had witnessed a friend killed during an explosion. Since that time, he has had chronic insomnia with ongoing nightmares of the event as well as occasional flashbacks. He describes always being "on edge," avoiding crowds, and becoming easily startled with loud noises. He admits to regular alcohol use, especially when his symptoms are worse, up to 12 beers at a time. Which of the following is the most appropriate treatment to begin for this patient?

(A) atypical antipsychotic
(B) benzodiazepine
(C) lithium
(D) serotonin-specific reuptake inhibitor
(E) valproic acid

SSRI are used for PTSD but anticonvulsants may be added adjuvantly if pt needs something specifically for flashback

63. A 40-year-old married woman is referred by her internist to a psychologist for further treatment. She presents an 8-month history of recurrent bouts of "terror," associated with chest pain, tachypnea, tremors, flushing, nausea, and fears that "I'm going to die." These episodes last for approximately 15 minutes and do not have a particular stressor. As a result, she has had increasing difficulty traveling far from her home due to concerns over having further attacks. Despite adequate treatment with sertraline, she remains symptomatic and in significant distress. Which of the following psychotherapies would be the most appropriate for her condition?

(A) cognitive-behavioral therapy (CBT)
(B) eye movement desensitization and reprocessing
(C) insight-oriented therapy
(D) interpersonal psychotherapy
(E) supportive psychotherapy

64. You are treating a 48-year-old housewife on an inpatient medical unit for exacerbation of asthma. On the day that you inform her of her pending discharge, she complains of feeling feverish and achy and has a nonproductive cough. The nursing staff reports that she has a sudden fever of 103°F. You treat the fever with acetaminophen and perform a physical examination, order chest x-rays, draw blood, and order a urinalysis. While you are awaiting these results, the nurse informs you that she witnessed the patient dipping her thermometer into a hot cup of tea before another nurse went back into the patient's room to read the thermometer. The most likely diagnosis to account for this woman's behavior is which of the following?

    (A) conversion disorder
    (B) factitious disorder
    (C) hypochondriasis
    (D) malingering
    (E) somatoform disorder

Questions 65 and 66

A 32-year-old man is brought to the psychiatric emergency department by the police after having been arrested for public nudity. Laboratory tests show a negative drug screen and alcohol levels. On MSE, you find that the patient cannot sit down and is only partly cooperative. He interrupts the interview several times demanding to be allowed to contact his lawyer "because my rights given to me by God and ordained by the Jeffersonians and Washingtonians and Lincolnians have been infringed...and you, sir, are committing illegalities of the highest order." His speech is pressured.

Examination of the patient's psychiatric records indicate that he has a history of a major depressive episode treated successfully with an SSRI for 1 year when he was age 23. The patient's parents arrive in the emergency department and tell you that the patient is a college graduate and a computer programmer. Lately, his job has been rather stressful as he has been overlooked for promotion, and his girlfriend left him 1 month ago. He is also in a great deal of credit card debt.

65. The most likely diagnosis for this patient is which of the following?

    (A) adjustment disorder
    (B) bipolar disorder
    (C) MDD
    (D) PTSD
    (E) schizophrenia

66. The mean age of onset for this disorder is closest to which of the following ages?

    (A) 10
    (B) 20
    (C) 30
    (D) 40
    (E) 50

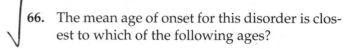 *Bipolar D/O is on average age 30 since when you really make money*

67. A 68-year-old man has a history of a left middle cerebral artery stroke. Which of the following psychiatric disturbances is most common following such a neurologic event?

    (A) anxiety
    (B) OCD
    (C) depression
    (D) mania
    (E) panic symptoms

 super

68. A 25-year-old man presents to your office asking for help stopping smoking. He has tried quitting cold turkey and using nicotine replacement therapy but neither has worked. He wants to know about hypnosis. Which of the following best describes this technique?

    (A) a state in which critical judgment is suspended and a person experiences alterations in perception, memory, or mood in response to suggestions
    (B) an individual psychotherapy directed at changing behavior
    (C) a group psychotherapy directed at changing maladaptive thoughts
    (D) a procedure that directly accesses repressed memories
    (E) an altered brain state that can be mapped by electroencephalogram (EEG)

69. A 48-year-old man presents with a chief complaint of impotence that has troubled him for the last year. Based on epidemiology of known causes of this disorder in this patient's age group, the chance that his problem is due to a psychological cause rather than a medical cause is closest to which of the following?

(A) 10%
(B) 30%
(C) 50%
(D) 70%
(E) 90%

[handwritten, vertical: Almost all of the impotence age 30–60 is psychological. (90%)]

70. Postmortem studies and cerebrospinal fluid (CSF) sampling from living patients have revealed a correlation between aggression, impulsivity, and suicide and a decrease in the metabolites of which of the following neurotransmitters compared to control subjects?

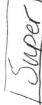

[handwritten: Super]

(A) dopamine
(B) gamma-aminobutyric acid (GABA)
(C) glutamate
(D) norepinephrine
(E) serotonin

71. A 38-year-old woman diagnosed with multiple sclerosis of moderate severity has had symptoms of depression and memory loss increasing over the last year. On MSE, you notice blunted affect and decreased speed of mental processing. A magnetic resonance imaging (MRI) examination is likely to reveal which of the following?

(A) normal brain
(B) global cerebral atrophy
(C) ventricular enlargement
(D) multiple plaques of frontal white matter
(E) rare periventricular plaques

72. The patient is an 80-year-old widowed woman admitted to the hospital under the medical service who is "confused." Her primary medicine

team has consulted a psychiatrist to help with the evaluation and management of her condition. On examination, she is somnolent at times, fluctuating with alert. She is not cooperative, hostile, and clearly hallucinating. Her insight and memory are poor. The primary team wishes to know if she is "delirious or demented." Which of the following signs/symptoms in this patient is the most specific for delirium?

(A) aggressivity
✓(B) fluctuating consciousness
(C) poor memory
(D) psychosis
(E) uncooperativeness

73. A 45-year-old married woman, formerly employed as an accountant, had onset of severe anhedonia, amotivation, anergia, and flattened affect when she was 40 years old. Initially, her psychiatrist thought she might be suffering from major depression because of her prominent family history of depression on her father's side. At age 41, she had the sudden onset of auditory hallucinations and a fixed false belief that the government was harassing her. Her psychiatrist then diagnosed her with schizophrenia and placed her on neuroleptics. After starting these medications, her auditory hallucinations disappeared and she no longer believed in her delusions. However, she continued to have amotivation, anhedonia, and flattened affect, and was unable to return to her employment as an accountant. Which prognostic indicator suggests a poorer prognosis in this case?

(A) the onset of symptoms relatively late in the patient's life
(B) the fact that the patient is married
(C) a positive family history of depression
(D) the sudden onset of psychotic symptoms
(E) the predominance of negative symptoms

[handwritten: Late onset Schiz Do Better since already know how to function and can just return to baseline;]

Questions 74 and 75

A 34-year-old woman with schizophrenia has been stable on her psychiatric medications for 3 years and has become pregnant for the first time. Her family psychiatric history is not known because she was adopted. The father of the unborn child does not have schizophrenia.

74. What percentage most closely approximates the likelihood that this patient's child will have schizophrenia?

    (A) 1%
    (B) 5%
    (C) 10%
    (D) 20%
    (E) 30%

75. Suppose adoption records indicate that the patient has an identical twin that was adopted into another family. Which percentage most closely represents the likelihood that her twin sister has schizophrenia?

    (A) 10%
    (B) 30%
    (C) 50%
    (D) 70%
    (E) 90%

76. You are a research psychiatrist who is studying signs and symptoms associated with certain psychiatric disorders that are not mentioned in the DSM-IV-TR for those disorders. Your spreadsheet contains a category of patients who have sensory gating deficits, short-term memory difficulties, and abnormalities in smooth-pursuit eye movements. The most frequent DSM-IV-TR diagnosis you are likely to find in this category is which of the following?

    (A) attention deficit hyperactivity disorder (ADHD)
    (B) major depression
    (C) OCD
    (D) PTSD
    (E) schizophrenia

77. A 23-year-old single White medical student comes to your office complaining of difficulty sleeping. During the past year, he has been worrying excessively about a number of things, including his studies, his relationship with his parents, and that his girlfriend of 2 years is going to break up with him, despite being happy with their relationship. He admits that he has difficulty controlling the time he spends worrying. He notes feeling irritable at times and has been experiencing muscle tension. Because of these symptoms, he has trouble with schoolwork and his grades have suffered. He does not endorse a depressed mood and asks, "Can you help me with my problems?" You diagnose him with GAD, and prescribe a combination of psychotherapy and benzodiazepines. Three months later, the patient comes back to your office reporting that his mood has been down in the dumps, and he feels like he may never feel better. Recently, he has been thinking that life was not worth living anymore and has passive thoughts of suicide. When asked about specific suicidal plans, he reports recent thoughts of taking an overdose of pills. The most appropriate next step would be which of the following?

    (A) Tell the patient he is going to get better and schedule weekly outpatient visits.
    (B) Prescribe lorazepam for his excessive worries.
    (C) Refer the patient to the psychiatric emergency department.
    (D) Prescribe an antidepressant and instruct him to follow up with you in 1 month.
    (E) Call his parents to pick him up and arrange for a family meeting.

78. The patient is a 36-year-old married White female who presents to the emergency room with a 2-month history of depression, terminal insomnia, fatigue, decreased appetite, anhedonia, and excessive guilt. When pressed, she admits to suicidal ideation for the past week, with thoughts of "taking all of my medicines." After further questioning, she states that "I would

never do it" as she is a devout Catholic who attends church regularly. Which of the following characteristics increases this patient's risk of suicide?

(A) age
(B) gender
(C) marital status
(D) race
(E) religion

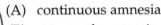

protestants and Jews have a high suicide rate since religion is strict and suicide is not discussed

Questions 79 and 80

A 29-year-old married White woman is brought into the psychiatric emergency department by her husband who reports that despite feeling depressed 1 month ago, she now has been acting bizarre for the past week. On initial interview, the patient states, "I feel superbly supreme, and you have no idea what an amazing person I am! I am a direct descendant of Queen Elizabeth!" The patient is talking so fast you cannot interrupt her. Her husband reports that the patient has not slept in over a week and that she has recently been adjusting her own medication(s) since her last appointment over a month ago. In addition, her husband reports that this past week alone she has bought a new car, a diamond tennis bracelet, and her third designer handbag.

79. The most likely diagnosis is which of the following?

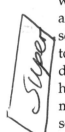

(A) a mood disorder
(B) a psychotic disorder
(C) a personality disorder
(D) an anxiety disorder
(E) a factitious disorder

80. Which of the following medications was most likely to be the one adjusted by the patient?

(A) buspirone
(B) ranitidine (Zantac)
(C) divalproex sodium
(D) propranolol
(E) zolpidem (Ambien)

81. A patient in the emergency department tells the physician that over the past 3 weeks his television has been talking directly to him. From what specific type of delusion is this patient suffering?

(A) thought insertion
(B) somatic
(C) thought broadcasting
(D) paranoid
(E) idea of reference

82. A 45-year-old patient tells her doctor that after hearing that her husband died, she could not remember leaving her office and going home. In every other respect, her memory is intact. Which of the following types of amnesia is this an example of?

(A) continuous amnesia
(B) retrograde amnesia
(C) localized amnesia
(D) generalized amnesia
(E) selective amnesia

83. Mr V is a 26-year-old single male brought into the emergency room for acute paranoia. He admits to smoking "pot laced with something," and soon after, he quickly became fearful that other individuals were going to harm him. He was unable to be calmed down by his friends and he developed palpitations and started screaming that he was going to die. He claims to only smoke cannabis on weekends and he denies any prior psychiatric history. Although he was adopted, he was informed his birth mother had been schizophrenic and he himself is now afraid of developing it. What are his chances of developing schizophrenia?

(A) 0–10%
(B) 10–20%
(C) 20–30%
(D) 30–40%
(E) 40–50%

84. When asked about his level of education, a 48-year-old man with a history of schizophrenia describes his high school grounds, friends he had at the time, clubs he joined, and his high school graduation. He concludes by saying, "And that was the end of my schooling." Which of the following does this answer demonstrate?

    (A) loosening of associations
    (B) circumstantiality
    (C) tangentiality
    (D) pressured speech
    (E) perseveration

85. In her psychiatrist's office, a patient suddenly lowers herself to the floor, begins flailing about wildly, then flings a garbage pail against the wall, and runs out of the office. Immediately afterward, she returns. She is alert and oriented, yet does not remember the incident. What is the most likely diagnosis?

    (A) temporal lobe epilepsy
    (B) jacksonian seizure
    (C) tonic-clonic seizure
    (D) complex partial seizure
    (E) pseudoseizure

86. In a 29-year-old man being treated for depression, which of the following statements would most likely characterize his sleep patterns?

    (A) His sleep patterns are unaffected.
    (B) He has less sleep latency.
    (C) He has few if any episodes of early morning awakening.
    (D) He experiences less REM latency.
    (E) His REM sleep tends to be distributed to the latter half of the night.

87. A 26-year-old man with narcolepsy explains that he has episodes of brief paralysis without any loss of consciousness or other deficits. These attacks are usually precipitated by laughter or anger. What is this phenomenon known as?

    (A) hypersomnia
    (B) cataplexy
    (C) hypnagogic hallucinations

    (D) hypnopompic hallucinations
    (E) catalepsy

88. A 22-year-old man is brought to the emergency department 2 weeks after a motor vehicle accident in which he suffered significant head trauma. His parents are concerned because, although the patient recognizes them on the telephone and responds appropriately, when he sees them face-to-face, he believes them to be imposters who have replaced his real parents. He agrees that these people look like his real parents but is convinced that they are indeed imposters. What delusion is this known as?

    (A) cacodemonomania
    (B) doppelganger
    (C) folie à deux
    (D) Capgras syndrome
    (E) delusion of reference

89. A 50-year-old woman is admitted to the hospital after complaining that she is dead. She believes that her flesh is rotting and that she is able to smell the rancid odor. What delusion is this known as?

    (A) Cotard syndrome
    (B) Capgras syndrome
    (C) Fregoli syndrome
    (D) cacodemonomania
    (E) koro

90. A 36-year-old man presents to the emergency department after being found without clothing in the street. He has multiple excoriations all over his body and states that bugs are crawling all over him. His toxicology screen is positive for cocaine. What is this particular tactile hallucination known as?

    (A) hypnagogia
    (B) hypnopompia
    (C) haptia
    (D) formication
    (E) synesthesia

91. A 21-year-old man is noted to be restless and constantly moving. He states that he feels as if

he has to be moving all the time and is uncomfortable if he sits still. Which of the following is this sensation known as?

(A) akathisia
(B) akinesia
(C) tardive dyskinesia
✓ (D) dystonia
(E) rabbit syndrome

92. A 21-year-old woman diagnosed with panic disorder comes to the outpatient mental health clinic with increased frequency of panic attacks and complains of feeling as if her surrounding environment is unreal and strange. As a result of the increasing frequency of her attacks and this new symptom, she has been unwilling to leave her apartment for several weeks. How is the feeling of a surreal environment best described?

(A) depersonalization
✓ (B) derealization
(C) hypermnesia
(D) dereism
(E) paresthesia

Questions 93 and 94

A 60-year-old man with alcoholism is brought to the emergency department by his family after they notice a decline in memory. On evaluation, the patient's remote memory is intact as verified by the family, but his recent recall is severely impaired. The patient provides verbose but erroneous answers in response to questions testing recent recall.

93. This patient's memory distortion is most likely which form of memory disorder?

(A) anterograde amnesia
(B) retrograde amnesia
✓ (C) dissociative amnesia
(D) prosopagnosia
(E) astereognosis

94. Which of the following best describes the patient's answers in response to recent memory testing?

(A) clang associations
(B) flight of ideas
(C) hypermnesia
✓ (D) logorrhea
(E) confabulation

Questions 95 and 96

A 66-year-old college professor is being seen for a regular checkup. On examination, the patient is noted to demonstrate flat speech with no melodic intonation. In addition, although demonstrating proper word choice and grammar, the patient's answers are extensive with unnecessary detail but do reach a point.

95. When describing the lack of emotional component of this patient's speech, which of the following terms should be used?

(A) aprosody
(B) stuttering
✓ (C) scanning
(D) aphasia
(E) dysphagia

96. To describe the patient's thought process in relation to the verbose, highly detailed answer, which of the following terms should be used?

✓ (A) flight of ideas
(B) tangential
(C) circumstantial
(D) loosening of associations
(E) derailment

97. An 86-year-old woman in the intensive care unit awakes at night and mistakes her intravenous (IV) pole for a family member coming for a visit. She calls the nurses to ask them to ✓ have the visitor leave until morning. Which term best describes the perceptual problem?

(A) illusion
(B) gustatory hallucination
(C) micropsia
(D) macropsia
(E) palinopsia

98. A 24-year-old graduate student in philosophy is referred by his student health center for a psychiatric evaluation. Although he claims to have had similar but attenuated symptoms since childhood, since beginning his thesis, he describes an acute worsening of fears that he will contract HIV. While he understands the modes and risks of contraction and practices safe sex, he is unable to "get rid of these thoughts." As a result, he feels compelled to wash his hands many times per day, even to the point of their becoming raw and bleeding. Despite his insight that his concerns are irrational, he is not able to stop the behaviors. A positron emission tomography (PET) scan of this patient's brain would most likely demonstrate increased activity in which of the following structures?

    (A) amygdala
    (B) caudate nucleus
    (C) cerebellum
    (D) hippocampus
    (E) parietal lobes

Questions 99 and 100

While interviewing a 78-year-old woman, you discover that, although she is able to recognize objects, she fails to provide an accurate name for many of them. When the patient is shown a pen, the response given is "that thing that you write with," and when shown a watch she replies "the time teller."

99. The patient's answers are examples of which of the following?

    (A) clang association
    (B) circumlocution
    (C) neologism
    (D) confabulation
    (E) apraxia

100. Which of the following best describes this particular type of language disorder?

    (A) alexia
    (B) apraxia
    (C) anomia

    (D) paralinguistic components of speech
    (E) prosopagnosia

101. A 36-year-old woman complains of depression. She reports a decrease in sleep, weight, and libido. She also complains of recent constipation. The changes in the patient's sleep, weight, libido, and bowel habits are all which of the following?

    (A) neurovegetative signs
    (B) word salad
    (C) conversion
    (D) catatonia
    (E) neologisms

102. A 35-year-old man complains that his partner enjoys sexual activity only when inflicting pain on him. This disturbs and frustrates him. This type of paraphilia exhibited by his partner is known as which of the following?

    (A) sexual masochism
    (B) sexual sadism
    (C) exhibitionism
    (D) frotteurism
    (E) transvestic fetishism

103. A 34-year-old man reveals to his doctor that he derives sexual satisfaction from rubbing up against women he doesn't know while on crowded subway trains. Which of the paraphilias is this an example of?

    (A) exhibitionism
    (B) fetishism
    (C) pedophilia
    (D) voyeurism
    (E) frotteurism

104. An anxious 23-year-old Asian male university student presents to student health services claiming that his penis is shrinking into his abdomen. Despite reassurances from the staff and the physician, he remains convinced of this belief. This patient is likely demonstrating a specific delusion known as which of the following?

(A) koro

(B) kuru

✓ (C) taijin kyofusho

(D) zar

(E) Capgras syndrome

105. A 21-year-old man was arrested after being found outside of a window masturbating. He admitted to having been watching the young girl inside over a period of several months. This patient demonstrates which paraphilia?

(A) transsexualism

✓ (B) hermaphroditism

(C) voyeurism

(D) exhibitionism

(E) transvestic fetishism

106. A 23-year-old single White man is seen in the psychiatric emergency room after he was found running naked through the streets and telling police that he was Jesus Christ. You are able to elicit a history of paranoid ideation from the patient. His parents report a history of progressive withdrawal from social activities. Based on this patient's likely diagnosis, in which brain region is he most likely to have abnormal findings on MRI?

(A) hippocampus

✓ (B) occipital lobe

(C) parietal lobe

(D) cingulate gyrus

(E) basal ganglia

107. You are seeing a 28-year-old unemployed man with a history of auditory hallucinations and recurrent fears that his parents are trying to kill him. He does not know what year it is and is dressed poorly. He makes poor eye contact with you as you interview him. His fears about his parents represent what phenomenon?

(A) formication

(B) trichotillomania

✓ (C) ideas of reference

(D) reaction formation

(E) hallucinations

108. During a shift in the psychiatric emergency room, you are asked to see a 75-year-old man whose family is concerned that he is unable to live by himself. You suspect dementia in the patient who smiles and is pleasant but does not know who the president is or where he lives. If, while you are performing an MSE, the patient stands uncomfortably close to you as you talk to him, this would most likely be an example of which of the following?

(A) formication

(B) flight of ideas

✓ (C) circumstantiality

(D) ideas of reference

(E) loss of ego boundaries

109. You are seeing a 26-year-old single White man who began to experience auditory hallucinations and delusions in college. Since then, he has been hospitalized a number of times, and has not been able to hold a job. His effect is bizarre. What are the negative symptoms of the condition this patient most likely suffers from?

(A) include affective lability

(B) are more prominent than positive symptoms in the prodromal phase of the illness

(C) do not include autistic features

✓ (D) usually become milder over the course of the illness

(E) are easily distinguished from depressive illness

Questions 110 and 111

You are asked to see a 32-year-old man who was diagnosed with major depression 2 weeks ago and prescribed fluoxetine (Prozac). Once you enter the room and introduce yourself, you cannot get a question in as the man speaks rapidly about how terrific a doctor you are and how wonderful his life is. He tells you about the three cars he recently purchased. When you try to interrupt him, he says angrily, "You're just like my skinflint wife."

110. This patient's affect is best described as which of the following?

    (A) expansive and irritable
    (B) guarded and suspicious
    (C) labile and dysphoric
    (D) euphoric and bizarre
    (E) euthymic

111. His speech is best described as which of the following?

    (A) uninterruptible
    (B) pressured
    (C) hypermotoric
    (D) agitated
    (E) tangential

112. A 23-year-old White graduate student comes to the psychiatric emergency room complaining of great anxiety. She has never been seen by a psychiatrist before and is taking no medications. Her vital signs are taken, and are notable for a heart rate of 100 beats/min. She is also slightly diaphoretic and has mildly dilated pupils. Given her present state, one would expect which area of this patient's brain to be hyperactive at this time?

    (A) locus ceruleus
    (B) hippocampus
    (C) thalamus
    (D) amygdala
    (E) basal ganglia

113. One of your regular patients, a 75-year-old man, presents for a regular checkup with his wife. You notice that since his last visit a year ago, the man is more confused and does not seem to know who you are. There is no history of head trauma. The patient is unsteady on his feet, having brought a walker and, his wife notes, embarrassed that he has become incontinent. Neuroimaging with noncontrast CT in this case is most likely to reveal which of the following?

    (A) dilated lateral ventricles
    (B) normal ventricles
    (C) frontal sulcal widening
    (D) focal subcortical hypointensities
    (E) cerebellar atrophy

114. You are asked to give a psychiatric consultation on a 28-year-old woman with systemic lupus erythematosus who was admitted to the medical service. After you see her, one of your medical colleagues tells you that she will no longer speak to any of them because she hates all of them and insists on seeing you because you are the best doctor in the hospital. The psychodynamic term best used to describe the patient's conflict is which of the following?

    (A) acting out
    (B) externalization
    (C) regression
    (D) splitting
    (E) sublimation

115. A 26-year-old woman who recently gave birth to twins presents complaining of falling asleep without warning. Sometimes, she only awakens when one of the twins begins crying loudly. She often finds that she has collapsed ungracefully on the floor. She notes that the episodes tend to occur when she is trying to juggle several tasks at once and feeling overwhelmed. The term used to describe the phenomenon of sudden loss of muscle tone associated with stressful situations is which of the following?

    (A) cataplexy
    (B) catalepsy
    (C) catatonia
    (D) sleep jerks
    (E) primary atonia

116. A 42-year-old woman is admitted to a medical unit after a car accident that rendered her unconscious. A neighbor reports that she was taking an antidepressant but does not know which one. The patient regains consciousness after 3 days and corroborates that she was on an antidepressant but says she cannot remember which one. She is started on paroxetine (Paxil) for her depression. However, 2 days after this medication is started, she develops tachycardia, diaphoresis, and myoclonic jerks. In the central nervous system (CNS), the neurotransmitter associated with the above reaction is mostly synthesized in which of the following?

(A) nucleus accumbens
(B) locus ceruleus
(C) raphe nucleus
(D) caudate nucleus
(E) substantia nigra

DIRECTIONS (Questions 117 through 123): Each group of items in this section consists of lettered headings followed by a set of numbered words or phrases. For each numbered word or phrase, select the ONE lettered heading that is most closely associated with it. Each lettered heading may be selected once, more than once, or not at all.

Questions 117 through 123

Choose the diagnosis that best fits the scenario given.

(A) borderline personality disorder
(B) somatization disorder
(C) conversion disorder
(D) antisocial personality disorder
(E) schizoid personality disorder
(F) schizotypal personality disorder
(G) factitious disorder (Munchausen syndrome)
(H) hypochondriasis
(I) agoraphobia

117. A 46-year-old married White woman is referred to you by a neurologist. She has had an extensive neurologic workup, which was entirely negative, for the sudden onset of right arm paralysis 1 month ago. She says her husband was initially worried she had a stroke. When describing the onset of the paralysis, she relates that she was just about to punish her 15-year-old daughter who has been involved in heavy drug use and increasingly difficult to discipline lately.

118. A 33-year-old divorced White woman is admitted to the inpatient psychiatric ward for apparently attempting suicide by cutting her wrists. When asked why she did it, she describes that "the physical pain makes my emotional pain go away, for a little while, anyway." She vacillates about whether this was a suicide attempt. She relates multiple complaints about various levels of strife with roommates and family members. She is known from previous admissions to the ward for labeling certain staff as her favorites and others as people "I hate." On MSE, you note significant emotional lability. Her father committed suicide when she was 9 years old.

119. A 35-year-old man who has spent much of the past decade in jail or on parole for various misdemeanors and felonies initially presents to your substance abuse unit under a <u>false name</u>. He gives you his history in extensive detail, but it nonetheless seems implausible. You talk to his sister, who tells you, "He's the biggest con artist there is—don't believe a thing he says!" She then relates that the patient stole his mother's car last weekend. She believes he sold it for drugs, which he's done in the past, she says.

120. A 36-year-old woman is referred to you by her gynecologist, who reports a long history of sexual and other nonspecific complaints that have apparently shown no evidence of verifiable disease. The gynecologist further relates that she believes this patient has a long history of doctor shopping. On interview, the patient demands your attention to multiple physical complaints: her back, belly, and chest pain; her dyspareunia and excessive menstrual bleeding; and her constipation and lactose intolerance. She points out additionally that "nobody's been able to figure out why I can't feel anything on the back side of my arm." She has had multiple surgeries for abdominal complaints in the past, all with no significant findings or findings inconsistent with her complaints. She relates that "I've always been sickly, most of my life."

121. A 41-year-old woman claims she is "certain I have breast cancer." Workup by her internist, including physical examination and mammogram, is negative.

122. A 26-year-old woman is admitted for sepsis. Her roommate reports that a few days before admission she found the patient with a needle and syringe full of what the patient admitted was toilet water. The patient's physical examination reveals intravenous needle marks not made by any hospital staff. Records reveal she was admitted a year ago for gastrointestinal distress and later admitted drinking drain cleaner.

123. A 44-year-old stockbroker has discovered over the last few months that he experiences intense anxiety while taking the subway to work. He relates that "I can't go to the supermarket or any large store anymore, especially when they're crowded. I'm afraid my heart's going to jump out of my chest!"

DIRECTIONS (Questions 124 through 126): Each of the numbered items in this section is followed by answers. Select the ONE lettered answer that is BEST in each case.

124. You are seeing a 66-year-old man who was recently treated with thiamine for Wernicke encephalopathy including a sixth nerve palsy. After appropriate treatment and admission to the hospital, the patient's sixth nerve palsy almost completely resolves. However, he has nystagmus and an improved but wide-based gait. He accurately describes his wife, who died 10 years ago, and can name the last five presidents. Immediate memory and attention are normal. Each morning, he is alert and engages in conversation with the medical team, although careful examination reveals he has no memory of them from the day before. How can these symptoms be explained?

(A) alcoholic dementia
(B) Korsakoff syndrome
(C) stroke
(D) delirium
(E) Alzheimer disease

125. You are seeing a 45-year-old man with no psychiatric history who tells you that his parents are conspiring to destroy his privacy. He says they have planted a bug in his refrigerator to see what he eats. He is seeing you on his lunch break from his job of 5 years, and appears well-dressed. He denies illicit drug use, and says that he has a number of close friends who have tried to convince him his refrigerator is not bugged. What is the most likely diagnosis?

(A) schizophrenia
(B) brief psychotic disorder
(C) delusional disorder
(D) paranoid personality disorder
(E) MDD with psychotic features

126. You are asked by the surgical service at your hospital to see a 34-year-old woman well known to them from previous admissions with a number of vague complaints that have no obvious physical cause: abdominal pain, headache, and lower back pain. She appears tearful and says that although she does not think she has anything serious tells you she just wants to figure it all out so she can get home. What is the most likely psychiatric diagnosis?

(A) somatization disorder

(B) conversion disorder

(C) hypochondriasis

(D) malingering

(E) factitious disorder

Questions 127 and 128

A 42-year-old woman who lives alone is brought into the emergency room unconscious after an apparent suicide attempt. She has left a note for her on-again, off-again boyfriend and has taken a bottle of sleeping pills and drunk a bottle of wine. Her neighbor does not know her psychiatric history but says she has been admitted to the hospital for previous suicide attempts.

127. Which of the following disorders is most closely associated with suicide?

(A) alcohol dependence

(B) schizophrenia

(C) mood disorder

(D) multiple sclerosis

(E) cancer

128. Which of the following predictive factors is most associated with suicide risk?

(A) depression

(B) unemployment

(C) age 45 and older

(D) male gender

(E) divorce

DIRECTIONS (Questions 129 through 136): Each of the numbered items or incomplete statements in this section is followed by answers or by completions of the statement. Select the ONE lettered answer or completion that is BEST in each case.

Questions 129 through 136

(A) heroin

(B) Rorschach

(C) alprazolam

(D) Alzheimer disease

(E) Hamilton

(F) schizophrenia

(G) glucocorticoids

(H) shared psychosis

(I) PCP

(J) Korsakoff syndrome

129. Most common diagnosis among psychiatric hospitalized patients in the United States

130. Folie à deux

131. Often causes psychotic and/or depressive symptoms

132. Amyloid plaques

133. Most dangerous withdrawal syndrome

134. Depression rating scale

135. Dementia praecox

136. Confabulation

Questions 137 through 140

Use the list below to identify the proper term for each question.

(A) lability

(B) irritability

(C) dyscalculia

(D) verbigeration

(E) dysarthria

(F) gustation

(G) glossolalia

(H) hypochondriasis

137. A 24-year-old man whom you have been seeing for 2 years in psychotherapy tells you that he was startled to learn that he could speak Spanish, which he never could before.

✓ **138.** A 32-year-old man with schizophrenia repeats the words "wong, wong, wong," followed by "raizon, raizon, raizon."

✓ **139.** A 79-year-old woman who has suffered a stroke is frustrated by her difficulty to form words.

✓ **140.** A 23-year-old man is alarmed that he cannot taste chocolate. What sensation has he lost?

Questions 141 through 145

Five responses to the question "Why did you go to medical school?" are given. Match the response with the appropriate disorder of thought process or component of thought process disorder.

- (A) circumstantiality
- (B) tangentiality
- (C) flight of ideas
- (D) loosening of associations
- (E) clanging
- (F) derailment

141. I don't even need to make money. Money makes the world go 'round, 'round the mulberry bush the monkey chased the weasel. Weasels make good politicians you know.

142. People are in need wherever you go, and I've been to a lot of places. It is amazing how much traveling I have actually done. I do suffer a bad case of wanderlust.

✓ **143.** Medical school in pools with spools of thread till you're dead, Fred.

144. Religions are the most important of all thought. Why do you bleed your school colors? I just wanted some publicity for my movie.

145. Well, medical school was actually something my parents...I am so worried about the state of the world today.

Answers and Explanations

1. **(C)** The patient's 3- to 4-year history of bizarre behavior, delusions, and decline in social functioning strongly suggest that his illness is schizophrenia. Its prevalence is 1%.

2. **(C)** In twin studies, schizophrenia's monozygotic concordance is 50% suggesting that there is a strong genetic component to the illness.

3. **(D)** Nihilistic delusion content is classic for Cotard syndrome, a psychotic/delusional theme seen potentially in multiple psychotic illnesses. The belief that people have been replaced by imposters is the hallmark of Capgras syndrome. Folie à deux is a shared delusion aroused in one person by the influence of another. Although nihilism and negativism can be observed in patients with MDD, the predominance of psychosis in this patient makes that diagnosis unlikely. Similarly, this patient does not meet the criteria for delusional disorder, which is characterized by nonbizarre delusions.

4. **(B)** The belief that people have been replaced by imposters is the hallmark of Capgras syndrome. Simple schizophrenia is a disorder consisting entirely of negative symptoms with no positive symptoms. See the answer to question 3 for definitions of the other choices.

5. **(A)** This case demonstrates an episode of postpartum psychosis characterized by depression, mood lability, delusions, and hallucinations. Although there can be different etiologies, most cases are a result of bipolar disorder. A less frequent underlying etiology is MDD. Primary psychotic illnesses, such as delusional disorder,

schizoaffective disorder, and schizophrenia, are rarer.

6. **(C)** Progressive social withdrawal is commonly seen as part of the prodrome of schizophrenia; at this point the patient's diagnosis must be schizophreniform disorder because her symptoms have lasted longer than 1 month but less than 6 months. All other choices—low intelligence, head trauma, a neglectful mother, and abuse—have not been proven in any conclusive way to be significantly linked to the disease, although early theories held that a history of one or more was a predisposing factor.

7. **(C)** The patient meets the criteria for borderline personality disorder characterized by rapid mood swings, efforts to avoid abandonment, chronic feelings of emptiness, intense anger outbursts, impulsivity, fluctuations between idealization and devaluation, and recurrent self-mutilation or suicidality. Persons with this personality disorder commonly employ primitive defense mechanisms, such as denial, projective identification, and splitting. Splitting is dividing up individuals into "all good" or "all bad" categories. Intellectualization and undoing are considered neurotic defenses, while altruism and sublimation are mature defenses.

8. **(B)** The downward drift hypothesis points out chronic mental illness's tendency to cause its sufferers to move downward through the social strata. This downward movement has to do with the effects of the illness itself, not the side effects of medications or the stress-diathesis model, which addresses an entirely different issue of susceptibility to illness. The socioeconomic

cost of schizophrenia is the result of drift, not its cause. Bleuler is known for his four *As*—association, affect, autism, and ambivalence—used to describe schizophrenia.

9. **(D)** Clearly, on previous occasions, this patient's presentation has strongly suggested schizophrenia and now he is presenting with classic catatonic features: negativism, hypomotorism, and echolalia with echopraxia. The diagnosis of schizophrenia makes elective mutism very unlikely. There is no evidence of secondary gain, making a diagnosis of malingering similarly unlikely. Drug-induced psychosis is unlikely to result in the classical symptoms of catatonic schizophrenia.

10. **(A)** This patient is likely suffering from a delusional disorder. This woman's age, lack of prior psychiatric illness, and high level of social and occupational functioning are not consistent with a schizophrenia-spectrum diagnosis. Although she is delusional, her delusion is not bizarre (i.e., it could possibly happen) and there is no associated hallucinations or disorganization.

11. **(A)** Depression severity, history of poor response to many medications (many clinicians believe that all medication options should be exhausted), and the need for quick antidepressant action are really the only universally accepted criteria that encourage the clinician to use ECT in major depression. Poor compliance would push a clinician toward ECT only if all other methods of encouraging compliance had failed. The other options all describe diagnoses that would likely respond to ECT but would not necessarily move the clinician to ECT over medications.

12. **(B)** It is always essential to rule out bipolar disorder before administering antidepressants, because all antidepressants can induce mania in susceptible patients. However, antidepressants are sometimes carefully administered to bipolar patients who are predominantly depressed. All the other diagnoses mentioned would likely respond favorably to antidepressants, with the exception of drug-induced depression, for which the treatment is removal of the inciting agent.

13. **(B)** Although many sleep disturbances have been described in depression (e.g., the other choices, among others), early morning awakening has been most consistently linked with major depression.

14. **(B)** Increased cortisol in depression is one of the earliest observations in biological psychiatry, and is well borne out in subsequent studies. Catecholamines are decreased in depression as are sex hormones and immune function. Levels of MAOs are unknown.

15. **(C)** Bipolar I disorder clearly has a stronger genetic link than major depression and probably has the strongest genetic link of all the major psychiatric illnesses. Bipolar II disorder has a strong genetic link but not as strong as bipolar I disorder. Bipolar illness usually carries a poorer prognosis than unipolar depression. A higher percentage of patients with bipolar disease are eventually treated compared with patients with unipolar depression. Bipolar disorder has no gender predilection and has not been shown to be any more common in broad geographic areas.

16. **(C)** Antidepressants can precipitate or exacerbate mania in patients with bipolar disorder who are not infrequently first diagnosed as suffering from unipolar depression. SSRI levels have not been shown to correlate with efficacy. Because the paroxetine appears to have precipitated a mania, the drug should have been stopped. Insomnia would have likely resolved itself with the discontinuation of the SSRI and resolution of the manic episode. Starting two mood stabilizers at once is not supported by clinical trial evidence.

17. **(C)** Cyclothymia is cycling between hypomania and dysthymia. Treatment is the same as in bipolar disorder. Bipolar III disorder does not exist. Double depression occurs when a major depressive episode is superimposed on dysthymic disorder.

Bipolar II
(hypomania with ???)

Dr. Dunn said New literature says Bipolar III might be do to antidep.

18. **(B)** First-degree relatives of patients with bipolar disorder have a 25% risk of any mood disorder.

19. **(A)** Dangerous drug abuse should be ruled out first in this patient; cocaine is more acutely dangerous than LSD. She is on no medications, so she would have no reason to develop serotonin syndrome, a rare, severe adverse reaction to serotonergic drugs. Carcinoid tumor, another cause of serotonin syndrome, is equally unlikely. Hypochondriasis and specific phobia are seldom acutely life threatening.

20. **(C)** Porphyria is manifested not uncommonly by psychiatric (manic or psychotic appearing) symptoms. It rarely occurs without abdominal pain. Each of the other choices would have psychiatric symptoms less directly connected to the abdominal pain.

21. **(A)** Any type of hallucinations can be seen in delirium. In schizophrenia-spectrum illness, including brief psychotic disorder, one rarely sees hallucinations other than auditory. Nonauditory hallucinations, then, as a general rule, suggest delirium of some cause. Delusions are thoughts (fixed false beliefs) and do not include sensory phenomena like hallucinations. Conversion disorder does not usually show hallucinations of any sort.

22. **(B)** Klüver-Bucy syndrome presents with docility, lack of fear response, anterograde amnesia, hyperphagia, and hypersexuality. Pick disease is a form of dementia, often indistinguishable from Alzheimer disease, in which the frontal and temporal lobes are atrophied. *Arnold-Chiari syndrome* describes a condition with hydrocephalus and cerebellar anatomic and functional abnormalities. *Punchdrunk syndrome* describes an acquired movement disorder associated with traumatic damage to the substantia nigra. Möbius syndrome is congenital absence of the facial nerves and nuclei with resulting bilateral facial paralysis.

23. **(D)** Klüver-Bucy syndrome is most closely associated with severe damage to, or disconnectivity of, the amygdala bilaterally. The hippocampus, although important to short-term memory, is not directly involved with regulating aggression drives, sexual behaviors, and fear responses. The insula, found deep within the central sulcus, is medial to the temporal lobe and generally not considered a part of it. Superior temporal gyri are more generally involved with processing complex auditory information such as the understanding of language. The lateral ventricle is a CSF-containing space that has no direct neuropsychiatric functional role.

24. **(D)** This patient would meet the criteria for bulimia except that she missed three consecutive periods, which automatically places her in the category of anorexia. Her anorexia appears similar to bulimia, however, and she would likely be further qualified as having the binge eating-purging type of anorexia. Exercise can induce amenorrhea but other clues in this case indicate a more complex etiology of the loss of menses. OCD is often found comorbid with eating disorders in women, and indeed many of the food-associated behaviors in anorexia may seem similar to OCD-related rituals. In this case, all of the patient's symptoms are explained in the context of an eating disorder. Psychogenic gastritis is not a DSM-IV-TR diagnosis.

25. **(E)** As with many forms of starvation, the predominance of catabolic over anabolic processes tends to elevate BUN. Cortisol levels tend to be elevated in anorexia reflecting the stress state of the body. In anorexia, TSH responsiveness to TRH remains normal. Persons with anorexia also tend to be anemic. Serum growth hormone is often elevated in anorexia.

26. **(B)** Fluoxetine, an SSRI, is the treatment of choice for panic disorder with or without agoraphobia. Alprazolam, although commonly used for panic disorder, is a benzodiazepine that is effective in the short term but has considerable dependence liability. In addition, its short half-life may actually cause withdrawal states that mimic panic. Chlordiazepoxide is a long-acting benzodiazepine that is also effective in panic disorder but also carries some

dependence liability. SSRIs have been shown in trials to be as effective as benzodiazepines but without the abuse potential. Phenelzine, a monoamine oxide inhibitor (MAOI), has been shown to be effective in some studies in anxiety disorders but its side effect profile is regarded as problematic. Divalproex sodium has not been demonstrated to be effective for panic.

27. **(C)** This is one of the most important biological findings in affective disorder research. Studies show that in major depression, about half of all patients do not have blunted cortisol levels to an administration of dexamethasone the night before. This is thought to indicate abnormal feedback control in the hypothalamic-pituitary-adrenal axis in major depression. Patients with psychotic depression are even more likely to have poor dexamethasone suppression.

28. **(B)** About 30% of all patients with major depression do not show an increase of TSH with administration of TRH.

29. **(C)** Persons with schizoid personality are reclusive and do not mind the lack of social interaction. Agoraphobia is tied to the fear of panic symptoms in public. Such symptoms are not mentioned in this case. Persons with avoidant personality are shy and fearful of social rejection. However, their lack of socialization is distressing to them. Schizotypal persons can have schizoid features but they also have bizarre thinking. Patients with autism have pronounced deficits in language, communication, and socialization, which are not prominently reflected in this case of a woman who had uneventful but happy formative years.

30. **(D)** Studies show that most addicts do not experience a sufficient decrease of their cravings at less than 60 mg/day during initial treatment. The fear of bone decay and loss of libido are popular misconceptions about the effects of methadone. Although an opiate, methadone has a longer half-life than heroin (and thus a milder withdrawal syndrome) and is given in a treatment setting in which complete opiate detoxification is more likely to succeed if the

patient desires this route. There is no association of methadone treatment with Cushing syndrome.

31. **(A)** Cases of postpartum psychosis are considered to be a psychiatric emergency. Because of the immediate danger to the infant in this case, the patient requires admission to the hospital. While the other choices may certainly be appropriate in her management, protecting the baby is the first and most important matter. If a patient refuses admission, certification to a state hospital and/or involvement of Child Protective Services will likely be necessary.

32. **(B)** This patient's history is most consistent with a mood pattern defined by prolonged periods of hypomania (symptoms of mania not severe enough to cause occupational dysfunction or psychiatric treatment) and now a major depressive episode. Hypomania with major depression defines bipolar II disorder. In bipolar I disorder, the mania is more severe causing notable occupational dysfunction and usually contact with psychiatrists. This patient is in the midst of a major depressive episode but his history of mania indicates a bipolar diagnosis. This is an important distinction to make in diagnosis because improper treatment with antidepressants can precipitate a manic episode. Narcissistic personality disorder is an Axis II diagnosis. This patient does display impulsivity but impulse control disorder, not otherwise specified, can be diagnosed only after the exclusion of major mental illness such as bipolar disorder, which may have impulsive features.

33. **(B)** Dry mouth, dizziness (associated with hypotension), and urinary hesitancy are due to anticholinergic and adrenergic blocking effects of TCAs such as imipramine. Fluoxetine, an SSRI, is most often associated with gastrointestinal upset, sexual dysfunction, and agitation. Phenelzine, an MAOI, can be associated with hypotension but is less likely to have anticholinergic effects. Lithium is most often associated with polyuria, polydipsia, tremor, and mental confusion at higher doses. Divalproex sodium may cause gastrointestinal upset but is

otherwise commonly associated with sedation and tremor at higher doses.

34. **(B)** The classic triad of NPH is confusion, gait ataxia, and incontinence. Elevated opening pressure is not found in NPH (thus the "normal pressure" part of the diagnosis). Oculomotor difficulties are a part of the Wernicke-Korsakoff syndrome. Frontal release signs and perseveration are nonspecific findings common in demented patients.

35. **(A)** CT scan commonly reveals dilated ventricles thought to be the result of increased pressure waves impinging within the ventricular system. Normal ventricles would not be expected in NPH patients. Frontal sulcal widening is found in dementias that have underlying cerebral atrophy. Hypointensities found in subcortical areas are often indicative of lacunar strokes. Cerebellar atrophy is seen most often in congenital disorders and alcoholism.

36. **(A)** The patient's inability to quit drinking regardless of a desire to quit or knowledge of its negative aspects best differentiates dependence from abuse. Neither dependence nor abuse is determined based on quantity of alcohol consumed. The patient's history of drunk driving and gastric ulcer are both consequences of the abuse construct of DSM-IV-TR. The patient's statement that he cannot sleep when he tries to quit drinking does imply physiologic dependence but the alcohol dependence criteria can be met with a "without physiologic dependence" qualifier.

37. **(C)** Patients with alcoholism often are found to have elevated GGT on routine laboratory screening. They also may have an increased ALT and AST but with an increased AST/ALT ratio not increased ALT/AST. Patients with alcoholism also commonly have increased uric acid levels, macrocytic anemia, and increased serum triglycerides.

38. **(D)** This patient would meet the criteria for schizophrenia except the duration of his illness has been less than 6 months. Brief psychotic disorder may present with psychosis but the duration of the disturbance must be 1 month or less. This patient's delusions are too bizarre to meet the criteria for delusional disorder. Psychosis, not otherwise specified, is reserved for cases of psychosis in which the etiology may be related to substance abuse, a medical condition, or an endogenous psychotic illness of unknown duration.

39. **(A)** This patient has symptoms consistent with PTSD or acute stress disorder (i.e., traumatic event, intrusive memories of trauma, avoidance of reminders, hypervigilance), but the fact that the trauma was only 3 weeks prior means that she would be diagnosed with acute distress disorder. If her symptoms persist after 4 weeks, then she would be diagnosed with PTSD. Adjustment disorder most often represents a change in mood, anxiety, or conduct that happens after a nontraumatic event. In GAD, there is no associated trauma. The patient has no evidence of MDD.

40. **(C)** The lifetime incidence of suicide in patients with schizophrenia is about 10%, compared with less than 1% in the general population.

41. **(A)** Feelings and attitudes originating from the treater, evoked by the patient, are called *countertransference. Transference* denotes feelings and attitudes about the treater coming from the patient. *Empathy* is the ability of the treater to psychologically put himself in his patient's shoes and thereby understand his patient's thinking, feelings, or behavior. *Identification* is a rather unconscious incorporation of someone else's traits into one's own manner—for example, adolescents having hairstyles similar to admired rock stars. *Projection* occurs when one assigns emotions to another person in an attempt to psychologically cover up the presence of those emotions within himself. For example, the doctor in the case may tell his fellow resident that he believes that his female patient is attracted to him, when in actuality he is attracted to her.

42. **(E)** This patient displays symptoms of fear of loss and abandonment, intense interpersonal relationships, recurrent suicidal behavior or

threats, affective instability, and difficulty controlling intense anger. Patients with borderline personality disorder have depressive symptoms that may become full-blown as a result of their social isolation, but this scenario does not mention full criteria for major depression. Patients with histrionic personality disorder, like those with borderline personality disorder, may display excessive emotionality and attention seeking, but their core symptoms center around superficial seductiveness and theatricality. Patients with cyclothymia often present as a diagnostic question with regard to the possibility of a borderline personality diagnosis. This is because of their prominent mood instability and impulsivity, which happens in both disorders. In this case, the other criteria for a borderline diagnosis resolves this dilemma. Psychotic disorder, not otherwise specified, is reserved for more frank delusional symptoms of unclear etiology than are evident with this patient who is paranoid that "all the staff hates me."

43.   **(E)** Psychotherapy and steady social support represent the best long-term method for the management of borderline personality disorder. Dialectic behavioral therapy has gained recent popularity as a form of psychotherapeutic intervention for these patients. Neuroleptics, mood stabilizers, and antidepressants have all been shown to have some efficacy in treating target symptoms in some borderline patients. Benzodiazepines may treat anxiety in these patients but they have particular abuse liability in these impulsive patients.

44.   **(A)** Amnesia is a common side effect of ECT presenting in the form of short-term memory deficits. Anesthesia-induced respiratory dysfunction, fractures, and arrhythmias are rare side effects. Psychosis can be improved rather than worsened; indeed, ECT is regarded as most indicated in psychotic depressions.

45.   **(C)** For catatonic conditions, two or four ECT treatments may be effective. In major depression, 6–12 sessions are generally optimal for a good risk-benefit ratio of positive treatment effects versus memory impairment (which is more likely with 20 or 40 treatments). When ECT is given for psychosis or mania, 20 or more treatments may be necessary for a positive response.

46.   **(B)** This patient has recurrent thoughts that are distressing. They are conceived as a product of her mind and not as implanted messages, as may happen in schizophrenia. She attempts to ignore or suppress her symptoms by not explaining to her husband how she feels or by getting rid of all the knives in her kitchen. Impulse control disorder, not otherwise specified, is reserved for the inaction of impulses that are not as directly ego-dystonic (disturbing), as in this case, and that do not have an obsessional nonenacted (thinking) component. Obsessive-compulsive personality disorder is a pervasive character style marked by a pattern of preoccupation with orderliness, perfectionism, and mental and interpersonal control. These persons are often described as control freaks by laypersons and are noted to be particularly inflexible. Psychosis, not otherwise specified, is inappropriate because this patient has fair insight regarding her obsessional thinking. She does act on her thoughts and they are disturbing to her. She is thus not psychotic. This patient does not display a thinking style that is marked by magical thinking. There is no mention of a history of strangeness prior to the birth of her child. Therefore, schizotypal personality disorder is not appropriate.

47.   **(E)** Fluvoxamine and other SSRIs (paroxetine, fluoxetine, sertraline) are known for their antiobsessional effects as well as their antidepressant and antianxiety effects. Lorazepam, a benzodiazepine, may decrease anxiety but has no direct antiobsessional effects. Benztropine is an anticholinergic typically used to counter neuroleptic-induced extrapyramidal symptoms. Nortriptyline and other TCAs have not proven efficacious for OCD. Haloperidol is a typical high-potency neuroleptic that may be useful in forms of OCD in which there is a psychotic component. However, it does not ameliorate purely obsessional thinking.

48. **(C)** This patient's MSE is most consistent with delirium in that it is remarkable for relatively rapidly fluctuating memory, orientation, and attention. Also, her apparent dehydration and malnourishment provide evidence for an underlying medical cause of her mental status change. Amnestic disorder is not likely given this patient's shifts in attention and memory fluctuations. Cognitive disorder, not otherwise specified, is reserved for cases exclusive of dementia and delirium such as cases of traumatic brain injury. Although this patient would seem a likely person to have dementia because she came from a nursing home, her fluctuating mental status is indicative of a delirium. Dementias are diagnosed in the context of a relatively stable set of deficits on an MSE, and the underlying causes are rarely associated with acute medical insults. Importantly, however, the presence of dementia does predispose to delirium. Major depression can cause cognitive deficits on MSEs that are reversible with antidepressant treatment. These *pseudodementias*, like dementia, most often present as a more stable examination than is illustrated in this case.

49. **(C)** About one-third of all patients with depression respond to the surprisingly powerful placebo effect. However, this response is not as well sustained as in patients placed on antidepressant medications.

50. **(D)** Standard antidepressant therapies, including SSRIs and TCAs, have a positive response in 65–75% of patients.

51. **(A)** Schizophrenia, catatonic subtype, is defined by a predominance of symptoms that involve motor behaviors and nonverbal forms of communication such as facial expression. This category includes famous cases of waxy flexibility, *echolalia* (repeating another's words inappropriately), and *echopraxia* (repeating another's gestures inappropriately). Disorganized schizophrenia, traditionally known as *hebephrenia*, is notable for pronounced and severe thought disorder that can be relatively refractory to neuroleptic treatment. Such patients may present with a chief complaint as "I came to restore my tranquility so that I can get what's coming to me upside down." Patients with paranoid schizophrenia may be relatively high functioning between episodes of psychosis. They may have relatively little thought disorder and may not have other bizarre manners. The diagnosis of residual schizophrenia is reserved for patients who have not had prominent positive symptoms (primarily thought disorder and psychosis) for some time and present with primarily chronic negative symptoms (anergia, anhedonia, and flattened affect). A diagnosis of undifferentiated schizophrenia is reserved for cases in which the clinician cannot distinguish a subtype. Often, these cases present with mild components of all the types.

52. **(D)** Catatonic schizophrenia has always been the least prevalent subtype of schizophrenia according to most studies, but has also become increasingly rare in recent decades. It has been suggested that changes in diagnostic criteria may account for this finding. Additionally, some forms of mental illness that were diagnosed as catatonic schizophrenia may have been cases of neurosyphilis, which with antibiotics has become increasingly rare. It is possible also that the advent of neuroleptic and other modern medications may have extinguished catatonic symptoms in schizophrenic populations.

53. **(C)** There is no evidence of occupational or social dysfunction or marked distress caused by this patient's activities. Virtually all DSM-IV-TR diagnoses are qualified by these criteria. If the patient did describe such concerns, the diagnosis would most likely be sexual masochism, in which patients are aroused by psychologically or physically punishing acts by another person (or fantasies of punishment). In sexual sadism, the patient is aroused by giving such punishment (or fantasies of giving it) to others. Fetishism involves sexual arousal connected to nonliving objects. In frotteurism, the patient is sexually aroused by touching or rubbing up against a nonconsenting person.

54. **(C)** *Narcolepsy* is a disorder often affecting persons in their teens or twenties. It is a disorder

of REM sleep mechanisms that also affects dogs. Circadian rhythm sleep disorder is a sleep disorder caused most often by sleep scheduling changes such as jet lag or night-shift work. Dyssomnia, not otherwise specified, is reserved for sleep disturbances of unknown cause or causes associated with environmental disturbances such as those that produce prolonged sleep deprivation. Restless legs syndrome falls under this category. *Nightmare disorder* is diagnosed in the absence of other predisposing mental illness (e.g., PTSD) in which the patient has repeated nightmares causing significant distress. *Primary hypersomnia* is excessive daytime drowsiness or hours spent sleeping at night that is not better accounted for by an identifiable environmental or medical cause, substance abuse, or mental disorder (e.g., major depression). Additionally, it is not associated with specific stigmata of narcolepsy such as cataplexy or sleep paralysis.

55. **(D)** Methylphenidate has been shown to be useful in inhibiting onset of narcoleptic episodes, likely owing to the capacity for the drug to enhance CNS arousal mechanisms that inhibit REM-related mechanisms. Nighttime benzodiazepine regimens are not particularly effective for narcolepsy. Antidepressant treatment with TCAs has been found to be useful in combination with methylphenidate in some patients with narcolepsy. However, the efficacy of bupropion, MAOIs such as phenelzine, and SSRIs such as fluoxetine has not been well-studied.

56. **(E)** None of the listed medications have been proven completely safe in pregnancy, but studies of fluoxetine have led many psychiatrists to conclude that its benefits outweigh its risks. Haloperidol and chlorpromazine are Class C drugs by Food and Drug Administration (FDA) rating, signifying that adverse fetal effects have been seen in animals, but there are no human data available. Lithium is a Class D drug, meaning that there is known human fetal risk, but the drug may be used in a life-threatening situation or when clinical circumstances justify its use. Divalproex sodium is Category X, indicating that there is proven fetal risk in humans such that the risk outweighs the benefit.

57. **(C)** Positive prognostic factors include late onset of illness, obvious precipitating stressors, acute onset, good premorbid social and work function, marriage, family history of mood symptoms, and positive symptoms (hallucinations). Negative prognostic factors include early onset of illness, lack of precipitating stressors, insidious onset, poor premorbid social and work function, withdrawn/autistic behavior, positive family history of schizophrenia, poor social supports, negative symptoms (disorganized behavior, amotivation), neurologic symptoms, and history of perinatal trauma. Choice A is not true; although some patients may recover (often with the proper treatment), the majority do not spontaneously recover. Choices B and D may be possible scenarios but cannot be conclusively stated about the prognosis of this patient. There are, of course, no medications without risks.

58. **(C)** This patient's symptoms fit DSM-IV-TR criteria for PMDD. Her symptoms are not severe enough nor of sufficient duration (2 or more weeks) to diagnose MDD. The remittance of symptoms in the week after menses is typical of PMDD. In adults, dysthymic disorder is characterized by subthreshold depressive symptoms, for more days than not, over a 2-year period. The patient does not describe prominent anxiety symptoms making GAD unlikely. This is not just normal female behavior.

59. **(B)** This patient is displaying symptoms consistent with MDD. Asking about suicidal ideation and assessing suicide risk is extremely important in individuals with depressive disorders, as the risk of completed suicide is approximately 10–15%.

60. **(C)** Heroin overdose is most likely to have caused the clinical situation described. Cocaine use causes pupillary dilatation not constriction. PCP and alcohol intoxication may cause coma but both are associated with nystagmus rather than pupillary size changes. Inhalants are also known to cause coma but are not classically associated with pupillary constriction.

61. **(B)** Naloxone is used to reverse the acute effects of opiate overdose by blocking CNS opioid

receptors. Acetylcysteine is administered in acetaminophen overdose and deferoxamine is used in iron overdose. Methylene blue is used to treat methemoglobinemia. Methadone is used for the long-term maintenance of opiate addiction and would only worsen heroin overdose.

62. **(D)** This patient is suffering from symptoms of posttraumatic stress disorder (PTSD), an anxiety disorder consisting of reexperiencing symptoms (e.g., nightmares, flashbacks, intrusive thoughts), increased arousal (e.g., hyperstartle, hypervigilence, irritability), and avoidance/numbing. The best studied and most efficacious medications are considered to be the SSRIs. Antipsychotics, including the atypicals, should not be used as monotherapy, although may be used in conjunction, especially if there are associated psychotic symptoms. Benzodiazepines should be avoided in this patient population not only because of the significant comorbidity with substance addiction but also as they have not been found to be particularly effective. Mood stabilizers, such as lithium and valproic acid, occasionally are used in addition to SSRIs in order to target the mood lability or aggression sometimes seen in PTSD.

63. **(A)** This is an example of a case of panic disorder with agoraphobia inadequately treated with appropriate medication namely sertraline. Many mental illnesses including anxiety are best treated with a combination of pharmacology and psychotherapy. The best-studied psychotherapy for panic disorder is CBT. Eye movement desensitization and reprocessing (EMDR) is a specific therapy that has been developed for and studied in the treatment of PTSD. Insight-oriented therapy is a long-term dynamic therapy. Although it may be useful in some cases of panic disorder, it has not been as validated as CBT. Interpersonal therapy addresses relationships as a contributor of depression and is, therefore, used to treat individuals with MDD. The purpose of supportive psychotherapy is to strengthen the patient's defense mechanisms in order to return them to a previous level of functioning. It has not been adequately studied for panic disorder.

64. **(B)** This case best depicts a case of a patient who is feigning or producing symptoms of an illness to gain gratification from assuming the sick role. There is little reason to believe this act could help her achieve financial or other material gain as in malingering. In conversion disorder, patients are primarily preoccupied with the idea that they have an illness that presents with a constellation of neurologic symptoms that are usually not physiologic. In hypochondriasis, a patient believes that he or she has some particular medical diagnosis. It is the worry about this illness that causes much of the distress. Patients with somatoform disorder tend to have clusters of subjective symptoms over time affecting multiple possible organ symptoms or anatomic parts that do not usually correlate to any specific medical diagnosis.

65. **(B)** This patient meets criteria for a current manic episode with symptoms of psychomotor agitation, pressured speech, grandiose thinking, flight of ideas, and history of excessive spending as evidenced by his credit card debt. His history of good premorbid functioning and a remitted major depression are also consistent with a diagnosis of bipolar disorder rather than schizophrenia. Adjustment disorders present with an identifiable stressor creating a milder mood, anxiety, or behavioral disturbance than is present in this case. The patient's presentation of mania rules out major depression. In fact, although he may have future major depressive episodes, he should never be diagnosed with MDD due to the current episode of mania. This patient's history does not reveal an exposure to an acute severe psychological stressor and he does not present with symptoms of reliving past traumas, hypervigilance, and avoidance as in PTSD.

66. **(C)** Bipolar disorder usually presents in a range of ages from childhood to age 50, with a mean age of onset of 30.

67. **(C)** Classically, infarcts of the left frontal hemispheres (part of left middle cerebral artery distribution) present with depression whereas those of the right frontal hemisphere present

with euphoria, inappropriate indifference, or mania. Obsessive-compulsive behaviors present occasionally after diffuse bilateral frontal injury. Panic and anxiety symptoms have not been described as having any particular association with left middle cerebral artery strokes although such comorbid cases probably exist.

68. **(A)** *Hypnosis* is a state in which critical judgment is suspended and a person experiences alterations in perception, memory, or mood in response to suggestions. Hypnosis is not psychotherapy. It is better understood as a procedure that may be used as an adjunct to psychotherapy. Hypnosis should not be used if the therapist is not willing or able to treat the patient with psychotherapy, because it seems to help some patients talk about events that are otherwise too emotionally laden to be expressed. The judgment of whether these thoughts are repressed memories is controversial. Hypnosis cannot be tracked or mapped with an EEG.

69. **(E)** About 90% of cases of impotence in the age group 30–50 have a psychological etiology. After 50, the etiology becomes increasingly medically related to causes such as medications, diabetes, hypertension, and alcoholism.

70. **(E)** The serotonin metabolite designated 5-hydroxyindole acetic acid (5-HIAA) measured in the CSF has been shown to be lower than control groups in postmortem analysis of victims of suicide and patients with impulsivity and violence or aggression. No such associations have been established with the other neurotransmitters listed.

71. **(D)** Depression is the most common presenting psychiatric symptom in patients with multiple sclerosis. It may present during the course of mild progressive cognitive decline that is consistent with a subcortical dementia (slowing of mental processing, motor difficulties, blunted or inappropriate affect, relative preservation of language-dependent skills). Neuroimaging of these patients usually shows diffuse white matter plaques affecting the frontal lobes. Ventricular enlargement and cerebral atrophy

are associated with the most common form of cortical dementia, Alzheimer disease.

72. **(B)** The patient appears to be suffering from delirium. Although aggressiveness, memory deficits, psychotic symptoms, and uncooperativeness may be seen in either delirium or dementia, a fluctuation in the level of consciousness (i.e., from alertness to somnolence) is the hallmark for delirium.

73. **(E)** Generally speaking, patients with pronounced negative syndromes have greater social and occupational difficulty, refractoriness to medications, and more chronicity of illness compared to patients whose diseases are more episodic with acute psychotic exacerbations. Onset of symptoms late in life is a good prognostic indicator for patients with schizophrenia, as is good premorbid functioning. Patients who are married also do better than those who are single, possibly reflecting the advantages of social support in the marriage. Marriage is more likely be an option for those patients who are less socially impaired on account of having milder negative symptoms. Patients with a positive family history of affective disorders, rather than schizophrenia, have a better prognosis in schizophrenia. Generally speaking, the more schizophrenia-like the clinical picture and the family history, the worse the prognosis, and the more affective-like, the better the prognosis. The sudden-onset symptoms in schizophrenia, as opposed to insidious onset, is a good prognostic indicator, possibly because it reflects less chronicity of symptoms and a greater chance of medical or psychoactive agent-related psychosis.

74. **(C)** About 12% of children who have one parent with schizophrenia suffer from schizophrenia; the risk climbs to 40% if both parents have schizophrenia.

75. **(C)** Of all identical twin siblings with schizophrenia, about one-half of their twins also have schizophrenia. These data have served as important evidence that schizophrenia represents the result of a combination of environmental stressors and genetic vulnerability.

About 12% of dizygotic twins of schizophrenic patients also have schizophrenia. A nontwin sibling of a person with schizophrenia has about an 8% risk of having schizophrenia.

76. **(E)** There are a number of stigmata associated with schizophrenia that are not included in the diagnostic criteria. These include soft neurologic signs such as short-term memory deficits, unstable smooth-pursuit eye movements, and decreased ability to habituate to repeated sensory stimuli (sensory gating-abnormalities). In addition, patients with schizophrenia have difficulty in conceptualizing complex visual compositions. Patients with major depression, PTSD, OCD, and ADHD also have been shown to have short-term memory difficulties, but not the other stigmata mentioned.

77. **(C)** The most appropriate next step is to send the patient to the psychiatric emergency department. This patient is experiencing an acute episode of major depression and because of his suicidal ideation with thoughts of overdosing, he should be referred to the emergency department for further assessment while ensuring his safety. Telling the patient he will be fine, prescribing medication, or contacting his parents about transportation and a family meeting does not adequately address his immediate safety.

78. **(D)** The woman presents with a classic presentation for MDD. Having a depressive disorder significantly increases one's risk for suicide. Many other factors also increase the risk for completed suicide such as White race, male gender, older age, single/divorced, and being Protestant or Jewish religion.

79. **(A)** The most likely diagnosis is bipolar disorder classified in the DSM-IV-TR as a mood disorder in which the individual experiences symptoms of a depressive disorder and symptoms of mania independently during the course of the illness. The current episode exemplifies a manic episode with symptoms that include inflated self-esteem and grandiosity, pressured speech, a decreased need for sleep, and an impulsive shopping excursion without

considering possible consequences. A psychotic disorder like schizophrenia cannot be diagnosed because there is no indication of prominent psychotic symptoms (hallucinations, disorganized thought processes and speech) present for at least 6 months. Personality and anxiety disorder do not present with the classic signs of mania. There is no indication that she is making up her symptoms for some secondary gain.

80. **(C)** From the choices given, the patient was most likely taking either lithium or divalproex sodium, which are both mood stabilizers and both indicated for the treatment of bipolar disorder. Buspirone, an anxiolytic, and propranolol, a beta-blocker used occasionally for GAD and panic disorder, are not likely to have been prescribed for this patient's bipolar disorder. Ranitidine, although sometimes confused by patients for the benzodiazepine alprazolam, is an antacid. Changing the dose of zolpidem, a sleeping aid, would not account for her symptoms.

81. **(E)** The specific delusion referred to here is an idea of reference. The patient interprets an event as relating to him, even though it clearly does not. *Thought insertion* is a delusion in which the patient believes thoughts from some external entity are placed in his mind. *Somatic delusions* refer to a delusion about the patient's body, for example, a common belief is that one's body parts are diseased. *Thought broadcasting* is the belief that one's thoughts can be heard or somehow known by others without direct communication. *Paranoia* often colors many delusions and involves the belief that other people, agencies, or forces mean harm or danger to the patient. Any of the above delusions may include elements of paranoia.

82. **(C)** The choices in this question describe different patterns of amnesia. *Localized amnesia* refers to memory loss surrounding a discrete period of time, typically occurring after a traumatic event; in this case, the patient's amnesia results from learning of her husband's death. *Selective amnesia* involves the inability to recall certain aspects of an event, though other memories of the event

may be intact. Rarely, a patient may forget his or her entire preceding life (*generalized amnesia*) or forget all events following a trauma, except for the immediate past (*continuous amnesia*). *Retrograde amnesia* is any amnesia for events that come before a traumatic event.

83. **(B)** Having one parent with schizophrenia confers an increased risk of developing schizophrenia of approximately 12%. Having two parents with the illness further increases the risk to over 40%. Having a monozygotic twin with schizophrenia increases the risk to 40–50%.

84. **(B)** *Circumstantiality* involves a circuitous, over-inclusive answer that only eventually gets to the point as the patient demonstrates in this example. *Loosening of associations* is a response composed of a series of disconnected ideas. *Tangentiality* occurs when the patient strays off the point entirely never returning to the original intention of the answer. *Pressured speech* is a continuous, usually rapid, uninterruptible stream of ideas that may make sense but is often hard to follow. This patient's speech may be pressured but the question gives no clues to this. Pointless repetition of a word, a phrase, or an idea is *perseveration*. Generally, the speech of a schizophrenic patient may demonstrate any of these characteristics; his diagnosis provides no clue to the answer.

85. **(E)** A *pseudoseizure* is a psychogenically induced behavior that resembles epileptic activity. Although the syndrome may in some cases be motivated by secondary gain (as in malingering), it most often occurs in reaction to stress or in a setting of personality disorder, severe affective disorders, or conversion reactions. The other choices, which each represent true epileptic seizures, rarely, if ever, include purposeful, complex activity as is seen in this case. Often, patients with pseudoseizures have a concurrent seizure disorder, and it is quite difficult to sort out the true seizures from the pseudoseizures. Diagnosing pseudoseizure often requires demonstrating a normal EEG at the time of the pseudoseizure. The prognosis for pseudoseizures is quite poor.

86. **(D)** Abnormal sleep patterns are common in depression and may be the chief complaint of the depressed patient. Classically, increased *sleep latency* (difficulty falling asleep), early morning awakening, and increased wakefulness are seen. REM sleep tends to be redistributed so that most of it occurs in the first half of the night. REM latency (the period of time between falling asleep and starting REM sleep) decreases.

87. **(B)** *Narcolepsy* is a sleep disorder characterized by the tetrad of *hypersomnia* (excessive daytime somnolence), *cataplexy* (transient loss of motor tone associated with strong emotions), *sleep paralysis* (total or partial paralysis in sleep-wake transition), and *hypnagogic hallucinations* (vivid dream-like hallucinations occurring in the wake-sleep transition). *Hypnopompic hallucinations* occur in the sleep-wake transition. *Catalepsy* is a state of immobility sometimes seen in catatonic states.

88. **(D)** *Capgras syndrome* is the delusional idea that imposters have replaced once familiar persons. This belief is held despite the acknowledgment that the people appear exactly the same. *Doppelganger* is the belief in the existence of an identical counterpart. *Cacodemonomania* is the delusion of being poisoned by an evil spirit. *Folie à deux* is a delusion shared by more than one person, and *delusion of reference* is the ascribing of personal meaning or messages that are not intended.

89. **(A)** *Cotard syndrome* is a delusion that nothing exists (nihilism) or the person herself does not exist. The person may feel that her body has disintegrated or that she is dead. Occasionally, the belief may be so vivid that it can even be associated with the sensation of a rancid or rotting odor, which is quite unpleasant for the patient. It can be seen in schizophrenia or severe bipolar disorder. It can also be early evidence of Alzheimer disease. Capgras syndrome and Fregoli syndrome are both delusions but are opposite in content. Capgras syndrome is the belief that an imposter has replaced a familiar person, whereas *Fregoli syndrome* is the delusion that a person is taking the form of a number of

people or creatures. Cacodemonomania is the delusion that one is poisoned by an evil spirit. *Koro* is a traumatic fear that the penis is shrinking into the body cavity.

90. **(D)** *Formication* is a particular type of tactile hallucination in which one has the sensation of bugs crawling on or under the skin. It can be seen in cocaine intoxication and in major alcohol withdrawal. *Haptic hallucination* is another tactile hallucination in which one feels as if he is being touched, for example, by a phantom. *Hypnagogic* and *hypnopompic hallucinations* are not tactile hallucinations but are hallucinations experienced in the transition state from wakefulness to sleep and from sleep to wakefulness respectively. *Synesthesia* is a secondary sensation following an actual perception (e.g., the sensation of a color associated with taste). Synesthesia usually is secondary to neurologic disease or hallucinogen use, most notably LSD.

91. **(A)** All of the choices are possible side effects, either short term or long term, of neuroleptics. *Akathisia* is the subjective sensation of motor and mental restlessness. *Akinesia* is a dysfunction of slowed or absent movement that can be associated with pseudoparkinsonism in the setting of neuroleptics. A *dystonia*, like akathisia and akinesia, can occur acutely and involve muscle rigidity and spasticity. *Tardive dyskinesia* is a late-onset neurologic effect of neuroleptics and can include tongue and lip movements and choreic movement of the trunk or limbs. *Rabbit syndrome* is another late-onset side effect that involves fine, rhythmic movements of the lips.

92. **(B)** Both depersonalization and derealization can be seen in anxiety disorders. *Derealization* is the sense that one's surroundings are strange or unreal, and *depersonalization* is the feeling that one's identity is lost or the feeling of being unreal or strange. *Dereism* is simply mental activity not in accordance with reality. *Hypermnesia* is an abnormal recall of details. *Paresthesia* is an abnormal sensation such as tingling or prickling.

93. **(A)** This patient may be suffering from Wernicke-Korsakoff syndrome, a complication of long-term alcoholism. *Anterograde amnesia* is the loss of immediate or short-term memory. Patients are unable to form new memories. *Retrograde amnesia* is the loss of remote or previously formed memories. *Dissociative amnesia* is the loss of memory without the loss of ability to form new memories. It is usually associated with emotional trauma and is not due to drugs or a medical condition. *Prosopagnosia* is the inability to remember faces despite being able to recognize that they are faces. *Astereognosis* is the inability to recognize an object by touch despite the tactile sensations being intact.

94. **(E)** *Confabulation* is the fluent fabrication of fictitious responses in compensation of memory disturbance. *Clang associations* are the use of words based on sound and not with reference to the meaning. *Flight of ideas* is another form of speech in which one shifts rapidly from one idea to another but the relationship between the themes can sometimes be followed. *Hypermnesia* is the ability to recall detailed material that is not usually available to recall. *Logorrhea* is uncontrollable or excessive talking sometimes seen in manic episodes.

95. **(A)** All of these terms are used to describe speech. *Prosody* describes the melody, rhythm, or intonation of speech that carries its emotional quality. The lack of this type of emotional variation is called *aprosodic speech*. *Stuttering* is the disturbance of the fluidity of speech as in repeating sounds or syllables or using broken words. *Scanning speech* is irregular pauses between syllables, which also breaks the fluidity but does not cause the repeating of sounds or syllables. *Aphasia* is the inability to communicate by speech or language. *Dysphagia* is difficulty in swallowing.

96. **(C)** *Circumstantial speech* is the overuse of detailed information providing extraneous detail in a digressive manner to convey an idea. *Tangential speech* quickly moves off topic but can be followed and the patient never arrives at the point that is trying to be made. Flight of ideas is like tangential speech but the changes

in ideas or topics are more frequent and more abrupt; like tangential speech, the connections are still recognizable. In loosening of associations, the logical connections between ideas are completely lost; although proper grammar and words may be used, the speech is not logical or goal directed. *Derailment* refers to the abrupt interruption of an idea and then resuming after a period of time (a few seconds) to a new topic. This is usually without the patient's being aware of the switch in material.

97. **(A)** An *illusion* is a misperception of an actual stimulus, and a *hallucination* is the perception in the absence of a stimulus. *Micropsia* and *macropsia* are the misperceptions of objects being smaller or larger than they really are. *Palinopsia* is the persistence of the visual image after the stimulus has been removed.

98. **(B)** This patient suffers from OCD, an anxiety disorder characterized by recurrent obsessions (e.g., fear of contracting HIV) and/or compulsions (e.g., frequent hand washing), which cause significant distress or impairment in functioning. The neurophysiologic nature of this illness can be demonstrated through neuroimaging, which shows increased activity (metabolism) in the caudate nucleus, frontal lobes, and cingulum. These differences are actually reversed after adequate pharmacologic or behavioral therapy.

99. **(B)** *Circumlocution* is the substitution of a word or description for a word that cannot be recalled or spoken. *Confabulation* is the fluent fabrication of fictitious responses in compensation of memory disturbance. *Clang association* is the use of words based on sound and not with reference to the meaning. A *neologism* is a novel word that is used by a patient; *apraxia* is the inability to perform previously learned motor skills.

100. **(C)** *Anomia* is an inability to name objects outside of an aphasia. *Alexia* is the inability to read. *Apraxia* is the inability to perform previously learned motor skills. *Paralinguistic components of speech* refer to nonverbal communications such as facial expression and body movements.

Prosopagnosia refers to the inability to recognize faces despite perception of all the components.

101. **(A)** *Neurovegetative signs* are physiologic aspects of depression such as changes in sleep, bowel habits, and weight. *Conversion symptoms* are physical manifestations of underlying unconscious motivation or drives. *Catatonia* is a state of stupor, negativism, and rigidity. A neologism is a novel word that is used by a patient, and apraxia is the inability to perform previously learned motor skills. *Word salad* is an incoherent mix of words and phrases.

102. **(B)** *Sexual sadism* and *sexual masochism* are, respectively, the derivation of sexual pleasure from causing or receiving mental or physical abuse. *Exhibitionism* is exposure of the genitalia in public to an unwilling participant and usually occurs in men. *Transvestic fetishism* is arousal by cross-dressing. *Frotteurism*, the rubbing of genitals against another to achieve arousal and orgasm, is usually seen in men and is usually performed in crowded places.

103. **(E)** Paraphilias encompass a wide variety of maladaptive sexual behaviors and fantasies. *Frotteurism* is the syndrome of recurrent, intense sexual fantasies and behaviors involving touching or rubbing against a nonconsenting adult. Exhibitionism involves revealing one's genitals to unsuspecting strangers. *Pedophilia* is sexual fantasies and behaviors involving children. *Voyeurism* involves secretly watching someone involved in disrobing, nudity, or sexual behavior. *Fetishism* is a sexual attraction to an inanimate object.

104. **(A)** Koro, zar, and taijin kyofusho are all examples of culture-bound delusions. *Koro* is the worry that the penis is shrinking into the abdomen and is found in South and East Asia. *Zar* is the delusional possession by a spirit, and *taijin kyofusho* is the belief that one's body is offensive to others. *Kuru* is a slowly progressive neurologic disease leading to death, thought to be caused by an agent similar to Creutzfeldt-Jakob disease. *Capgras syndrome* is the delusional idea that imposters have replaced once familiar persons.

105. **(C)** *Voyeurism* is deriving sexual pleasure from watching another person or persons involved in the act of undressing or other sexually oriented activity. *Transvestic fetishism* involves being dressed in clothing of the opposite sex for sexual excitement. It is often present in heterosexual men and differs from transsexualism in that the person is usually comfortable and content with his gender identity. It is, however, possible to see these disorders concomitantly. Exhibitionism is another paraphilia and involves exposing one's genitalia to an unsuspecting audience. *Hermaphroditism* is not a paraphilia but is a rare disorder in which one possesses both male and female sexual characteristics.

106. **(A)** More than half a dozen well-controlled studies of schizophrenics have shown decreases in the size of the hippocampus, parahippocampal gyrus, and amygdala. The other regions mentioned in the question have not been conclusively shown to be altered in schizophrenia by MRI or CT scans.

107. **(C)** *Ideas of reference* is the delusion that others are focusing on you in some positive or negative way commonly seen in paranoid schizophrenia. For example, a patient might believe that the television is speaking directly to him. Formication is the sensation that bugs are crawling on one's skin. *Trichotillomania* is compulsive hair pulling accompanied by significant hair loss. *Reaction formation*, a defense mechanism, involves an unacceptable impulse being expressed as its opposite. Hallucinations are sensory phenomena that should not be confused with delusions.

108. **(E)** *Loss of ego boundaries* is commonly manifested as inappropriate conversational distance. Formication is the sensation that bugs are crawling on one's skin. Flight of ideas is the flow of nonconnected speech and thoughts; circumstantiality is speech and thoughts with identifiable connections between thoughts, but which drift off the point and ramble, eventually coming back to the point. Ideas of reference is the delusion that others are focusing on you in some positive or negative way.

109. **(B)** *Prodromal schizophrenia* is normally composed of increasing negative symptoms in the absence of positive symptoms. Negative symptoms do not include affective lability or become milder over time nor are they easy to tell apart from depressive symptoms. They include autistic features.

110. **(A)** This is a typical presentation for *mania*, an episode that seems to have been at least partially induced by treatment with an antidepressant (all antidepressants can induce or exacerbate mania). This patient's effect, like that of many patients with mania, is expansive and irritable. He is to a lesser extent guarded and suspicious but this does not capture the full picture of his mania. He is labile but hardly dysphoric, and he is euphoric but not bizarre. He is not euthymic.

111. **(B)** Although all of the other choices might explain part of his speech characterization, *pressured* is used to describe speech that is difficult to interrupt and at a fast rate.

112. **(A)** The locus ceruleus is the "alarm" center of the brain and is hyperactive in anxiety states. It is the center of most of the norepinephrine-containing neurons in the brain. The hippocampus, part of the limbic system, and the amygdala are involved in memory formation. The thalamus is the brain's relay center. The basal ganglia coordinate motor activity.

113. **(A)** The presence of the classic triad of confusion, gait ataxia, and incontinence suggests strongly that this patient is suffering from NPH. CT scan commonly reveals dilated ventricles thought to be the result of increased pressure waves impinging within the ventricular system. Normal ventricles would not be expected in NPH patients. *Frontal sulcal widening* is found in dementias that have underlying cerebral atrophy. *Hypointensities* found in subcortical areas are often indicative of lacunar strokes. *Cerebellar atrophy* is seen most often in congenital disorders and alcoholism.

114. **(D)** *Splitting* is the view that people around you are either all good or all bad. It is common

in patients with borderline personality disorder although there is no other evidence of that in this case. *Acting out* generally represents the enactment of a behavior coming from an impulse that had presented conflict to relieve the sense that the conflict exists at all. *Externalization*, a generalized form of projection, represents the tendency to believe in the existence of patterns of behavior in others that is really true about oneself. *Regression* is a return to patterns of relating, thinking, or feeling that had come before one's current developmental stage. For example, many medical students who return home act as if they are teenagers with regard to their parents or other hometown friends. *Sublimation* is the channeling of drives or conflicts into goals that eventually become gratifying. For example, some people remember being afraid of blood and hospitals and worked out these fears in medical school training.

plexy → puts Doctors in a "plex"

115. **(A)** *Cataplexy* is the sudden loss of muscle tone associated with stressful situations, a special stigmata of narcolepsy and points to the connection of this disorder with REM sleep mechanisms (which inhibit movement and muscle tone during REM sleep). Catalepsy and catatonia are used to describe bizarre movement and posture behaviors found in catatonic schizophrenia and some psychotic depressions. *Sleep jerks* and *primary atonia* are meaningless terms.

116. **(C)** This patient's reaction to paroxetine suggests that she had been on an MAOI. In patients already using an MAOI, blocking reuptake of catecholamines and indolamines with SSRIs can result in a potentially life-threatening drug interaction known as *serotonin syndrome*. Medications that block such reuptake include the SSRIs, TCAs, buspirone, and other antidepressants such as venlafaxine. Features of mild serotonin syndrome include tachycardia, flushing, fever, hypertension, ocular oscillations, and myoclonic jerks. Severe serotonin syndrome may result in severe hyperthermia, coma, autonomic instability, convulsions, and death; therefore, wait at least 14 days after discontinuing an MAOI before starting a serotonergic agent. Most serotonin

in the CNS is synthesized in the dorsal and medial raphe nucleus of the brain stem. The substantia nigra synthesizes dopamine and the locus ceruleus synthesizes norepinephrine.

117. **(C)** Conversion disorder is described as the often sudden onset of a singular neurologic deficit, often in the setting of stress. As in this case, there can be (often subconscious) guilt linkage to the development of the symptom.

118. **(A)** Characteristic features of borderline personality disorder, as demonstrated in this patient, include self-mutilative behavior (which can temporarily bring relief of emotional angst), emotional volatility, and instability of relationships with others, including tendencies to view others as either all good or all bad (also referred to as splitting). Borderline personality disorder often arises in patients who have histories of abandonment and/or abuse at a young age.

119. **(D)** Antisocial personality disorder describes individuals with long histories of disregard to the rights of others and dishonesty used in attempts to gain something for themselves. Often comorbid with substance abuse, this disorder is extremely common in prison inmates (30–50%). Schizotypal personality disorder is marked by a pattern of difficulty with close relationships as well as cognitive and perceptual disturbances. Schizoid personality disorder differs from schizotypal personal disorder by the absence of cognitive and perceptual disturbances.

120. **(B)** *Somatization disorder* describes the condition suffered by individuals who have a long history of multiple somatic complaints (gastrointestinal, sexual, and neurologic) that, despite exhaustive medical workups, have either no identifiable cause or are out of proportion to the medical findings. These patients often describe themselves as having been sickly all their lives and, presumably in their frustration with doctors' inability to find reasons for their problems, chronically doctor shop.

121. **(H)** The hallmark of hypochondriasis is the belief by a patient that he or she has a specific

medical illness. Patients with the disorder often interpret somatic complaints as signifying definite serious illness.

122. **(G)** *Factitious disorder*, Munchausen's type, describes the condition suffered by patients who intentionally produce signs and/or symptoms of medical illness. Commonly, patients are former health care workers or have such workers in their families.

123. **(I)** *Agoraphobia* describes the condition suffered by individuals who fear open, crowded spaces, particularly ones from which escape may be difficult. It is often comorbid with panic disorder as suggested by this patient's symptom of palpitations.

124. **(B)** This patient demonstrates a typical response to thiamine, namely, near complete resolution of his sixth nerve palsy, persistent nystagmus, and some improvement in his gait. However, as his acute delirium and apathy clear, an underlying inability to learn and retain new information emerges. This is known as *Korsakoff psychosis*; the amnestic state is best described as anterograde amnesia. Korsakoff psychosis is also caused by thiamine deficiency but is usually hidden by the acute delirium of Wernicke encephalopathy. Immediate memory and attention are normal; this is not true in delirium. Some degree of alcoholic dementia and Alzheimer disease may be present as well but the clinical setting most strongly points to Korsakoff syndrome.

125. **(C)** The encapsulated, fixed delusion seen here is typical of delusional disorder. The delusion in this illness is most often of the persecutory sort, as in this case, but may well be somatic, jealous, grandiose, and so on. Although this delusion is plausible, albeit unlikely, the delusions encountered in schizophrenia and brief psychotic disorder tend to be more bizarre and impossible, such as believing that others are controlling one's thoughts. Paranoid personality disorder does not present as a fixed, isolated delusion, rather, there is a more pervasive paranoia permeating many aspects of the patient's life. Patients with MDD with psychotic

features suffer from delusions or other psychotic symptoms that are mood congruent (e.g., "my organs are rotting").

126. **(A)** Somatization disorder is characterized by multiple physical complaints that cannot be explained by any objective physical findings. As in this case, patients' symptoms frequently date back many years and have prompted multiple doctor visits, even hospitalizations. Conversion disorder is a loss or deficit of motor or sensory function that is inconsistent with any known physiologic basis, for example, paralysis of both hands. Conversion disorders typically follow an identifiable stressor. Hypochondriasis is a fear of serious disease; it results from a hypervigilance and misinterpretation of normal bodily sensations. Malingering is the confabulation of symptoms with the conscious goal of personal gain, for example, using a doctor's diagnosis to get out of work. Factitious disorder is the purposeful production of signs or symptoms for the express purpose of becoming a patient (and assuming the sick role).

127. **(C)** The psychiatric disorder that carries the greatest risk for suicide in both men and women is a mood disorder. Although up to 15% of all alcohol-dependent persons commit suicide and up to 10% of schizophrenic patients commit suicide, the age-adjusted suicide rates for patients with mood disorders is estimated at 400 per 100,000 men and 180 per 100,000 women. Multiple sclerosis and cancer are distractors.

128. **(C)** Suicidal ideation is a serious manifestation of myriad disease processes. High-risk characteristics of suicidal persons have been studied extensively and predictive variables exist to assist the physician when called to assess suicidal ideation. Age 45 or greater is the most predictive factor. Alcohol dependence, rage or violence, prior suicidal behavior, and male gender follow in that order.

129. **(F)** Although this set of matching questions is not in United States Medical Licensing Examination (USMLE) Step 2 format, it tests concepts that are important both for ward

discussions and for understanding fundamental ideas. Schizophrenia is the most common illness in hospitalized psychiatric patients in the United States.

130. **(H)** Folie à deux is a shared delusion aroused in one person by the influence of another.

131. **(G)** Glucocorticoids (e.g., prednisone) are a common iatrogenic cause of reversible psychiatric symptoms such as depression and psychosis.

132. **(D)** Beta-amyloid plaque buildup is seen in Alzheimer dementia.

133. **(C)** Like alcohol, benzodiazepines have potentially extremely dangerous withdrawal syndromes, which have essentially identical clinical features (due to their near-identical actions on GABA modulation in the brain). The danger of withdrawal is even greater with the short-acting benzodiazepines (short-acting drugs in general cause more acute withdrawal) and alprazolam is one of the very shortest. Despite the profound discomfort of withdrawal from heroin and other opiates, opiate withdrawal is not life-threatening. Withdrawal from PCP is not well characterized.

134. **(E)** The Hamilton Depression Scale is a commonly used measure of depressive symptoms. The Rorschach Test is a projective test using inkblots, which measures perceptual accuracy, reality testing, and integration of affective and intellectual functioning.

135. **(F)** Dementia praecox was an early term for schizophrenia coined by Kraepelin.

136. **(J)** Korsakoff dementia (alcohol-induced persisting amnestic disorder) commonly evinces confabulation.

137–140. [137 (G), 138 (D), 139 (E), 140 (F)] *Lability* (A) refers to rapid fluctuations in affect, often between states of elation and sadness. *Irritability*

(B) refers to being easily brought to anger. *Dyscalculia* (C) is difficulty with simple arithmetic. *Verbigeration* (D) is repetitive and meaningless talking. *Dysarthria* (E) is difficulty with articulation. *Gustation* (F) is taste sensation. *Glossolalia* (G) is the ability to speak a new language suddenly. *Hypochondriasis* (H) is the misinterpretation of bodily symptoms leading one to erroneously believe he or she has a physical illness.

141–145. [141 (C), 142 (B), 143 (E), 144 (D), 145 (F)] Thought process disorders can be identified by the nature of the response. A *circumstantial thought* (A) finally reaches a point but after much unnecessary detail and digressions. It can be seen in disorders such as OCD, but can also be normal in some people. A *tangential thought* (B) differs from a circumstantial thought in that it never comes to a point, but like circumstantial thought it remains logically connected and can be followed. Flight of ideas (C) represents a change of direction every sentence or two, again with identifiable connections or associations tying them together. It is often a symptom of manic behavior and reflects underlying racing thoughts. Loosening of associations (D) is characterized by the lack of logical connections between ideas, but sentence structure remains intact. Another component of thought disorders, *clanging* or *clang associations* (E), is word choice based on sound and not meaning or semantics.
(F) Derailment Isoften associated with thought blocking then derail
In question 87, in the first sentence, the thoughts can be connected but do not reach a point. In question 88, the thoughts are more goal directed than in question 87 and this sentence is more consistent with tangentiality. In question 89, clanging is easily identified by word choice based on similar sounds rather than semantics. Associations between ideas are lost in question 90. Question 91 is a representation of thought blocking with derailment. The patient stops in one thought, pauses, and then resumes with an unrelated thought.

Somatic Treatment and Psychopharmacology
Questions

DIRECTIONS (Questions 1 through 74): Each of the numbered items in this section is followed by answers. Select the ONE lettered answer that is BEST in each case.

Questions 1 and 2

A 32-year-old man is admitted to a general hospital after ingesting an unknown quantity of phenelzine (Nardil) in a suicide attempt. After gastric lavage and administration of a charcoal slurry, he is transferred to the medical intensive care unit for monitoring. Twenty-four hours later, he begins to see horses running in the halls and pulls out his intravenous (IV) lines.

1. The most important treatment at this time should include which of the following?

    (A) chlorpromazine (Thorazine)
    (B) bretylium (Bretylol)
    (C) lorazepam (Ativan)
    (D) phenytoin (Dilantin)
    (E) meperidine (Demerol)

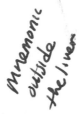
Mnemonic outside the liver

2. Twelve days after his suicide attempt, he receives venlafaxine (Effexor) to treat his depression. One hour after ingestion of the venlafaxine, he becomes tachycardic and diaphoretic and develops myoclonic jerks. This condition is known as which of the following?

    (A) neuroleptic malignant syndrome (NMS)
    (B) akathisia
    (C) serotonin syndrome

    (D) rapid-cycling bipolar disorder
    (E) opisthotonos

Questions 3 and 4

A 24-year-old woman presents to her primary care physician for a regular checkup. During the examination, her doctor notes a 15-pound weight gain. The patient complains that she always feels tired during the day despite sleeping from 8 PM to 9 AM daily. On further questioning, the physician learns that the patient feels sad and empty, often thinks about death, cannot concentrate at work, and lacks the energy to care for her two children. However, her mood picks up when her physician questions her about her children.

3. The most effective agent would be which of the following?

    (A) fluoxetine (Prozac)
    (B) nortriptyline (Pamelor)
    (C) phenelzine
    (D) sertraline (Zoloft)
    (E) trazodone (Desyrel)

4. Her physician initiates treatment with citalopram (Celexa). Which of the following is considered an adequate trial of this agent?

    (A) 2 weeks
    (B) 6 weeks
    (C) 3 months
    (D) 6 months
    (E) 8 months

Questions 5 and 6

While on call in a general hospital, you are called at 4:30 AM to evaluate a patient who wants to be discharged. Upon arriving on the floor, the nurse tells you he just pulled out his third IV of the day and started to swing the IV pole in the air while yelling profanities. He tells a nurse's aide he must capture the tiger that is loose in the parking lot. You quickly look at his chart and see that he is a 55-year-old man admitted 36 hours earlier for abdominal pain, nausea, and vomiting. His transaminases were elevated on admission, but his hepatitis profile is still pending. His orders are for acetaminophen (Tylenol) and Maalox as needed, normal saline at 125 cc/h, and nothing by mouth (NPO) for upper endoscopy in the morning.

5. The most appropriate initial medication at this time is which of the following?

   (A) oxazepam (Serax)
   (B) chlordiazepoxide (Librium)
   (C) haloperidol (Haldol)
   (D) chlorpromazine
   (E) disulfiram (Antabuse)

6. You speak briefly with this patient and are able to settle him down. His temperature is 102.1°F, pulse is 130 beats/min, and blood pressure is 220/120 mm Hg. The most appropriate medication and route should be which of the following?

   (A) labetalol (Normodyne) IV
   (B) haloperidol intramuscularly (IM)
   (C) haloperidol IV
   (D) lorazepam IM
   (E) lorazepam IV

Questions 7 and 8

A 32-year-old single woman presents to the emergency department escorted by her family after she revealed to them a plan to take a full bottle of acetaminophen and drink a bottle of wine in a suicide attempt. She claims that she cannot handle work any longer because her boss is trying to have her fired and her coworkers are helping him find fault in her work. She states they have even tapped her phone and are having her followed. Your detailed history reveals the following: She has never attempted suicide before and has never seen a psychiatrist. She was engaged to be married 2 years ago but her fiancé was killed in an auto accident. She has difficulty falling asleep at night and wakes up often during the night. She can no longer concentrate on her work. She does not enjoy painting as she once did. She has lost 10 pounds over the past 2 months without dieting. She denies hallucinations of any type. There is no significant family history of psychiatric illness.

7. You decide to prescribe a selective serotonin reuptake inhibitors (SSRI). After explaining the indications and side effects, she asks why it will take several weeks to see a significant improvement in her depression. What is the most likely mechanism for the delayed therapeutic response?

   (A) downregulation of postsynaptic 5-hydroxytryptamine-2 ($5-HT_2$) binding sites
   (B) upregulation of postsynaptic $5-HT_2$ binding sites
   (C) increased serotonin in the synaptic cleft
   (D) increased mitochondrial serotonin
   (E) downregulation of dopamine receptors

8. After 5 weeks of the treatment prescribed, the patient no longer has suicidal thoughts and is able to function well at work. She has begun to date again and is considering resuming a sexual relationship with an old boyfriend. The most common side effect of sexual function of the medications prescribed is which of the following?

   (A) anorgasmia
   (B) dyspareunia
   (C) decreased desire
   (D) vaginismus
   (E) female analog of premature ejaculation

Questions 9 and 10

A 25-year-old man presents to the emergency department accompanied by his family who report that the patient has not left his bedroom in 3 weeks. They report that he spends his day reading science fiction novels that they provide for him. He was once prescribed perphenazine (Trilafon), which they tell you seemed to help him, but he refuses to take it. On examination, you find him to be malodorous and disheveled. He is guarded when you speak with him. He does not make eye contact and he avoids looking at the television in the waiting room because, he says, he wants to prevent intruders from controlling his thoughts. After completing the examination, you admit him to the inpatient psychiatric unit.

9. Because the patient did not take the perphenazine, you decide to try fluphenazine (Prolixin). After 5 days, he is no longer afraid to look at the television but he spends much of the day pacing the floor. He claims he paces the floor because he does not like sitting in his room. His family informs you that he often walked the streets of his neighborhood when he was taking perphenazine. After reducing the fluphenazine to the lowest dose you feel he needs, he still paces the halls. Next, you do which of the following?

   (A) discontinue fluphenazine and try another agent
   (B) add propranolol
   (C) add lorazepam
   (D) add benztropine (Cogentin)
   (E) add diphenhydramine (Benadryl)

10. A 25-year-old White woman comes to your office complaining that whenever she takes the elevator in her boyfriend's building, she develops heart palpitations and breaks out into a cold sweat. The thought of being in the subway terrifies her. You tell her that you are planning to cure her by exposing her to those things that scare her most. Flooding is an example of what form of psychotherapy?

   (A) family therapy
   (B) couples therapy
   (C) psychodynamic psychotherapy

   (D) behavioral therapy
   (E) hypnosis

Questions 11 and 12

A 33-year-old mentally retarded male resident of a group home presents to the emergency department escorted by staff members who believe he has become confused and disoriented over the past few days. He has been a resident there for several years without incident, but last week his thioridazine was changed to haloperidol because of concerns about the long-term use of high doses of thioridazine. On examination, you find him to be disoriented to place and time; he is diaphoretic with a temperature of 105.8°F, a heart rate of 130 beats/min, and a respiratory rate of 20/min. His extremities are stiff. Routine laboratories reveal a white blood cell (WBC) count of 15,000/mL; blood urea nitrogen (BUN) 75 mg/dl, creatinine 1.2 mg/dl, and creatinine phosphokinase 2300 Iμ/L.

11. The most common serious complication this patient may experience is which of the following?

    (A) respiratory failure
    (B) pulmonary embolism
    (C) rhabdomyolysis
    (D) myocardial infarction (MI)
    (E) diffuse intravascular coagulation

12. The long-term consequence of high-dose thioridazine use that probably caused his physician to switch to haloperidol is which of the following?

    (A) tardive dyskinesia (TD)
    (B) priapism
    (C) retinal pigmentation
    (D) hyperprolactinemia
    (E) agranulocytosis

Questions 13 and 14

A 45-year-old unemployed investment banker presents to your office accompanied by his wife. He has been out of work for 1 month because he is afraid to take the train into work. He never had difficulty traveling until 2 months ago, when on a train during a family vacation, he suffered chest pain, shortness of breath, nausea, and a fear of dying. These symptoms lasted about 15 minutes. A workup by a cardiologist was negative. However, these symptoms, also accompanied by intense fear and a feeling of being detached from himself, have continued. He has had about two attacks a week and also has fear just thinking about returning to work because he fears he will die on the train. He tells you that he could not have come to see you without his wife's help.

13. A reasonable first choice of pharmacotherapy for this patient would be which of the following?

    (A) bupropion (Wellbutrin)
    (B) trazodone
    (C) propranolol
    (D) buspirone (BuSpar)
    (E) fluoxetine

14. The most potent antianxiety agent is which of the following?

    (A) alprazolam (Xanax)
    (B) buspirone
    (C) clonazepam (Klonopin)
    (D) chlordiazepoxide
    (E) diazepam (Valium)

Clonazepam → most potent antianxiety why its used for inpatients

Questions 15 and 16

A 22-year-old single male college music student reluctantly presents to your office on the request of his parents. His parents are worried because he has not been eating, talks constantly, and never seems to sleep. He says he has never felt better, he's writing several songs a day, and needs only a few hours of sleep. He believes he will be the next John Lennon and wants to get back to writing but he cannot stay focused long enough to answer any of your questions. He does not have any psychiatric history and denies using any substances.

15. The minimum initial laboratory data that should be obtained before starting treatment are which of the following?

    (A) serum creatinine, BUN and electrolytes, thyroid studies, urinalysis
    (B) liver function tests, serum creatinine, BUN and electrolytes
    (C) complete blood count (CBC) with differential
    (D) prothrombin and partial thromboplastin times
    (E) serum ammonia

16. You decide to start lithium. After starting the treatment, the patient sprains his ankle while exercising. His primary care doctor told him to take over-the-counter ibuprofen, which he started 2 days ago. His ankle still hurts, and he plans to continue taking the medication. You advise him to which of the following?

    (A) Increase the dose of ibuprofen.
    (B) Decrease the dose of ibuprofen.
    (C) Continue ibuprofen at the prescribed dose.
    (D) Switch to aspirin.
    (E) Stop the medication you prescribed.

Questions 17 and 18

A 9-year-old boy is brought to the physician because his parents have received a note from his second-grade teacher complaining that he is disruptive in class. His teacher believes he could achieve better grades if he could sit still and pay attention. His parents report he has always been an active child but does have difficulty getting along with other children in the neighborhood. In the examination room, he cannot sit still and has difficulty completing a task you have assigned. You decide to prescribe him methylphenidate (Ritalin).

17. The most common side effect of this treatment is which of the following?

    (A) difficulty falling asleep
    (B) daytime drowsiness

(C) slowed growth

✓ (D) increase in appetite

(E) decrease in systolic blood pressure

18. Treatment with this medication has been reported to exacerbate which of the following?

(A) bedwetting

(B) tics

✓ (C) poor impulse control

(D) reading difficulties

(E) myopia

Questions 19 and 20

A 9-year-old boy is brought to your office by his mother because of his "compulsions," which have worsened over the past year. She first noticed them last year when several times a day he would repeatedly blink his eyes and frown while clearing his throat. He continues to do this despite trying not to, and in addition, he often sticks out his tongue and smells his shirt while speaking with classmates. These "compulsions" have caused him to lose friends at school.

19. Pharmacologic blockade of which of the following receptors provides the greatest relief of these symptoms?

(A) norepinephrine

✓ (B) serotonin

(C) dopamine

(D) alpha2

(E) gamma-aminobutyric acid (GABA)

20. Which of the following agents is most effective to treat this disorder?

(A) amitriptyline (Elavil)

(B) haloperidol

✗ (C) clonidine (Catapres)

(D) alprazolam

(E) paroxetine (Paxil)

Tourette's you need strong dopamine

Questions 21 and 22

*blockade why
clonidine less effective than haloperidol*

You have been treating a 55-year-old man with schizophrenia for 20 years with haloperidol and benztropine.

Generally, he has done well and has not required major medication changes or hospitalizations. About 2 years ago, you noticed some lip smacking and tongue protrusions that did not bother him; however, now he also has odd, irregular movements of his arms that make it difficult for him to eat.

21. The syndrome that best describes these symptoms is which of the following?

(A) Meige syndrome

(B) anticholinergic toxicity

✓ (C) TD

(D) Huntington disease

(E) Sydenham chorea

TD ax mouth/lip and hands

22. The only medication that may improve these symptoms is which of the following?

✓ (A) benztropine

(B) trihexyphenidyl (Artane)

(C) olanzapine

(D) levodopa (Dopar)

(E) clozapine (Clozaril)

23. A 24-year-old married secretary has complained of dizziness, palpitations, and sweaty palms for the past 10 months. Sometimes, she also has extreme muscle tension in her neck that occurs both at work and at home. She has difficulty falling asleep and feels "edgy" most of the day. She also has difficulty concentrating at work. She has gone to a local emergency department three times because of the palpitations but nothing was found. Her family practitioner placed her on a hypoglycemic diet and referred her to a neurologist who found no abnormalities. She tells you she has many worries about her family but does not feel particularly depressed. Which of the following will provide the most immediate relief of her symptoms?

Super

(A) alprazolam

(B) fluoxetine

(C) bupropion

(D) buspirone

(E) imipramine (Tofranil)

24. A 22-year-old woman is admitted to a psychiatric unit after a serious suicide attempt. She has had many suicide attempts in the past with varying severity. Her arms are scarred by prior attempts at hurting herself. She had been a good student until high school, when she took up with a "fast" crowd, began abusing alcohol and marijuana, and ran away from home several times. She has had several intense, stormy relationships with men. Outpatient treatment has mostly consisted of her complaints to her therapist about her family. She usually calls her therapist daily about different crises; however, her therapist was on vacation during her most recent crisis. Which of the following classes of agents have been shown to be helpful for this patient?

    (A) tricyclic antidepressants (TCAs) and antipsychotics
    (B) SSRIs and antipsychotics
    (C) antipsychotics and benzodiazepines
    (D) anticonvulsants and stimulants
    (E) stimulants and SSRIs

25. A 36-year-old man is referred to you by his internist for evaluation of his eating disorder. He stands 6 feet 2 inches tall and had weighed 270 lb until he lost 90 lb last year because his wife thought he was "fat." Since losing weight, he is obsessed with becoming fat. He hates feeling full after a meal. Sometimes, he binges on junk food but always induces vomiting afterward. Now, he can no longer enjoy food and cannot stop dieting. Which of the following medications has shown success in treating such patients?

    (A) fluoxetine
    (B) mirtazapine (Remeron)
    (C) phenytoin
    (D) protriptyline (Vivactil)
    (E) quetiapine (Seroquel)

26. A 19-year-old woman is admitted to an inpatient psychiatric facility for her eating disorder. She weighs 82 lb and stands 5 feet 6 inches tall. She began dieting in high school to lose an unwanted 5 lb. Encouraged by compliments on her figure, she continued to lose another 10 lb. Her eating habits are ritualized: She cuts her food into small pieces and moves it around on her plate. She has an intense fear of being overweight. Which of the following statements most accurately reflects pharmacotherapy for this type of patient?

    (A) Successful pharmacotherapy should include appetite stimulants such as cyproheptadine (Periactin).
    (B) Pharmacotherapy generally has a limited role in the treatment of these patients.
    (C) High-dose chlorpromazine is useful in treating these patients.
    (D) Amitriptyline is useful in treating these patients.
    (E) Promotility agents such as cisapride (Propulsid) are useful in treating patients who purge.

27. A 36-year-old man whom you have treated for 8 months with paroxetine for his first episode of major depression has done very well. Because of the sexual function side effects, he decided to stop taking it 3 days ago without first informing you. Two days after he stopped it, he became irritable and even had a crying spell. He had the flu 2 weeks ago but the body aches, chills, and general lethargy have returned. Which of the following should you consider?

    (A) Start bupropion because it lacks sexual side effects.
    (B) Treat his flu symptomatically.
    (C) Consider a mood stabilizer for his irritability.
    (D) Restart the paroxetine and taper it off.
    (E) Prescribe phenytoin for seizure prophylaxis.

28. A 30-year-old man presents to a general hospital after ingesting 20 tablets of his prescribed carbamazepine (Tegretol) in a suicide attempt. He has no prior psychiatric history, but has a history of seizures. Your detailed history reveals several months of depressed mood, weight loss, anhedonia, sleeplessness, and difficulty

concentrating. Four days after admission, his carbamazepine level has returned to normal and has been restarted to treat his seizure disorder. Which of the following medications would be most appropriate for this patient?

(A) fluoxetine
(B) nefazodone (Serzone)
(C) paroxetine
(D) clomipramine (Anafranil)
(E) amitriptyline

Not "B" since long half life and can affect other drug metabolism.

Questions 29 and 30

A 65-year-old man presents to your psychiatric office on a referral from his primary care physician for evaluation of depression. He feels depressed and hopeless and has lost his appetite. He no longer enjoys seeing his grandchildren. It takes him several hours to fall asleep at night and he stays asleep only about 3 hours. He occasionally does not buy food because he is concerned about going broke; however, his family informs you that he is financially well off. He stands 6 feet tall and weighs 155 lb, much less than his usual 175 lb. Additionally, he feels guilty about becoming a burden on his family.

29. An antidepressant medication that might be useful to help him fall asleep at night is which of the following?

(A) diazepam
(B) diphenhydramine
(C) trazodone
(D) fluoxetine
(E) bupropion

30. A rare but troubling sexual side effect of this medication is which of the following?

(A) priapism
(B) premature ejaculation

(C) anorgasmia
(D) impotence
(E) gynecomastia

Questions 31 and 32

A 57-year-old man, whom you have treated for 20 years for bipolar disorder, is admitted to the general hospital with chest pain.

31. The hospital physician asks whether the lithium he is receiving can affect his electrocardiogram (ECG). You inform her that lithium has which of the following characteristics?

(A) has no effect on the ECG
(B) can prolong the PR interval
(C) can invert the T waves
(D) can prolong the QT interval
(E) can shorten the QT interval

32. The patient was found to have suffered from an MI and underwent angioplasty. He was discharged from the hospital on propranolol, losartan, topical nitroglycerin, hydrochlorothiazide, and one baby aspirin per day, in addition to his lithium. Prior to his MI, his lithium level was always 0.8 mmol/L on 900 mg/day of lithium carbonate. Now it is 1.3 mmol/L on the same dose. The most likely cause for this change is which of the following?

(A) decreased volume of distribution post-MI
(B) aspirin
(C) hydrochlorothiazide
(D) captopril
(E) propranolol

Questions 33 and 34

A 47-year-old male novelist feared contamination from anything he believed was dirty. In restaurants, he would use his own plastic utensils. Elsewhere, he would wear gloves or use paper towels to avoid touching "dirty objects." Upon returning home, he would wash his hands five times at night before going about his activities. If he accidentally touched anything prior to washing his hands, he would experience a vague uncomfortable feeling and would be unable to perform his usual nightly activities. As a result of these symptoms he was unable to have a meaningful social life.

33. The most effective agent for this syndrome is which of the following?

    (A) clomipramine
    (B) mirtazapine
    (C) clonazepam
    (D) phenelzine
    (E) olanzapine

34. You started treating this patient with fluoxetine at 60 mg/day 4 months ago. He no longer needs to wash his hands quite so often but still has an uncomfortable feeling when he touches "dirty things." Which of the following statements is most accurate regarding treatment at this point?

    (A) Buspirone is not effective as an augmenting agent.
    (B) Fenfluramine (Pendormin) has documented efficacy as an augmenting agent.
    (C) Lithium has documented efficacy as an augmenting agent.
    (D) Cingulotomy should be considered next.
    (E) Clozapine has been effective.

Handwritten margin note: OCD Buspirone is not effective; • Cingulotomy only severe cases of OCD this is not the case;

Questions 35 and 36

A 21-year-old college student has been hearing voices telling him to hurt himself for more than a year. Trials with the following agents have reduced the voices: chlorpromazine 1800 mg/day for 1 month, then haloperidol 60 mg/day for 6 weeks, then olanzapine

20 mg/day for 1 month. Despite a reduction in the voices, he remains isolated from family and friends. A trial of quetiapine also fails to decrease his isolation.

35. Which of the following agents should be tried next?

    (A) fluphenazine
    (B) risperidone
    (C) ziprasidone (Geodon)
    (D) clozapine
    (E) perphenazine

36. One of the leading theories for the efficacy of the above agent involves its action at which of the following receptors?

    (A) D_2
    (B) D_3
    (C) D_4
    (D) 5-hydroxytryptamine-1 (5-HT$_1$)
    (E) 5-hydroxytryptamine-3 (5-HT$_3$)

37. A 65-year-old man with major depression and hypertension presents to the emergency department because he fell to the ground after arising from a chair. He has no significant cardiac history and his ECG, electrolytes, and neurologic examination are unremarkable. His family reports that his physician recently started a new antidepressant but they do not know its name. Which of the following antidepressants is generally associated with this scenario?

    (A) bupropion
    (B) mirtazapine
    (C) nefazodone
    (D) imipramine
    (E) nortriptyline

38. A 35-year-old man with a history of seizures and hypertension has been treated for major depression with sertraline at 200 mg/day for 2 months with no improvement in symptoms. He is not acutely suicidal but he is frustrated by his lack of improvement. His primary care doctor has referred him to you for further evaluation. He has not had a seizure for years and

is not taking any anticonvulsant medications. At this time you should consider which of the following?

(A) adding lithium to his regimen
(B) adding thyroid hormone
(C) switching to imipramine
(D) switching to bupropion
(E) switching to venlafaxine

Questions 39 and 40

A 28-year-old woman whom you have treated for bipolar disorder informs you that she is 3 weeks pregnant and is anxious about the baby's health. You are treating her with lithium and she has not had a manic episode in 3 years.

39. Which of the following statements is correct regarding bipolar disorder and pregnancy?

(A) Lithium is safe after the first trimester and can be safely continued through birth.
(B) Divalproex sodium (Depakote) is a safe alternative to lithium.
(C) Carbamazepine is a safe alternative to lithium.
(D) Lithium substantially increases the risk of Ebstein anomaly of the tricuspid valves by 75%.
(E) Clonazepam does not carry an increased risk of major fetal malformations.

40. You are called to consult on an 85-year-old patient who has become combative, yelling, punching staff, and pulling out her IVs. She demands to leave but is too weak to get out of her hospital bed. Which of the following would be the most appropriate intervention at this time?

(A) diphenhydramine
(B) donepezil

(C) lorazepam
(D) orientation to her surroundings
(E) risperidone

Questions 41 and 42

A 67-year-old woman presents to your office for evaluation of a 20-lb weight loss over a 4-month period and insomnia for the past 4 weeks. Her daughter informs you that her mother no longer enjoys any of her hobbies and has been speaking lately about dying. They have already consulted an internist who performed an extensive medical workup, including chemistries, blood count, thyroid studies, gastrointestinal imaging, and endoscopy all of which were normal.

41. You would like to start an antidepressant medication but would like to minimize adverse side effects while exploiting other side effects. Which of the following agents has a side effect profile that may be beneficial?

(A) nefazodone
(B) fluoxetine
(C) nortriptyline
(D) mirtazapine
(E) bupropion

42. Upon further history, you learn that antidepressants have failed in several previous trials. You would like to start a TCA. Which of the following would preclude using such an agent?

(A) lacunar infarcts
(B) treatment with the antihypertensive amlodipine
(C) left bundle branch block on ECG
(D) urinary retention
(E) estrogen replacement therapy

Questions 43 and 44

A 72-year-old man is admitted to a general hospital's intensive care unit because of altered mental status. His medical workup has revealed pneumonia and congestive heart failure (CHF). On the second hospital day, he is agitated and pulls out his IV access. He also has been noted to speak out loud with no one in the room. His level of consciousness seems to wax and wane. He does not have a psychiatric history and is not allergic to any medications. Besides his CHF and pneumonia, he does not have other comorbid conditions.

43. Which of the following agents would be the most appropriate to administer for his agitation?

    (A) thioridazine
    (B) chlorpromazine
    (C) lorazepam
    (D) olanzapine
    (E) haloperidol

44. Which of the following agents would be least likely to cause orthostatic hypotension?

    (A) haloperidol
    (B) perphenazine
    (C) thioridazine
    (D) risperidone
    (E) quetiapine

haloperidol is more specific for only
Dopamine receptors
and why its least likely
to cause orthostatic hypotension;

Questions 45 and 46

A 32-year-old man presents to your clinic after losing his job because he was intoxicated while working. He has been drinking daily since he was 16 years old. He was able to complete college and went to work full-time right after graduation, but has lost several jobs since. After the loss of his last job, his wife threatened to leave him if he does not get help.

45. Which of the following agents can be used to sensitize him to the effects of alcohol?

    (A) metronidazole (Flagyl)
    (B) fluoxetine
    (C) flumazenil (Romazicon)
    (D) disulfiram
    (E) naloxone (Narcan)

46. Further history reveals that he does not have a mood disorder. He tells you that often he simply cannot control his craving to have another drink. Which of the following agents has shown some success in decreasing cravings for alcohol?

    (A) fluoxetine
    (B) disulfiram
    (C) naltrexone (ReVia)
    (D) bupropion
    (E) diazepam

Questions 47 and 48

A 36-year-old woman is referred to you by her primary care physician for management of anxiety and fear that has persisted for several months. She reports that she was raped and held hostage on a boat for several days by two armed men. During this, she experienced intense fear for her life. Since then, she has had intense stress whenever she is near the water and has frequent nightmares. She cannot recall details of the ordeal but tries to avoid driving her car within sight of the ocean, which has been difficult because of the location of her home. She feels detached from her husband and family and has abandoned plans to pursue her career as a painter. She has difficulty falling asleep and is easily startled by phone calls. She no longer goes to public places alone.

47. Which of the following agents is believed to help relieve the numbing symptoms she is experiencing?

    (A) alprazolam
    (B) fluoxetine
    (C) carbamazepine
    (D) thioridazine
    (E) naltrexone

48. Whenever she drives near the water, which is unavoidable, she experiences intense anxiety, fear, and palpitations, and feels that she is reexperiencing her abduction. Which of the following agents may help reduce these symptoms?

    (A) olanzapine
    (B) naltrexone

(C) perphenazine ✓

(D) divalproex sodium

(E) clonidine

49. You have been asked to evaluate an 80-year-old male nursing home resident because of a change in mental status. The nursing staff reports that he has been a patient there for about a year without any problems until about 1 month ago when he was having difficulty sleeping. The staff physician prescribed lorazepam 2 mg at bedtime; however, he was still unable to sleep. He started wandering during the day and has been restricted to his room. Because he remains agitated during the day, they have been giving him lorazepam 2 mg every 6 hours for agitation. His other medications include hydrochlorothiazide 25 mg/day, digoxin 0.125 mg every other day, diltiazem (Cardizem) 240 mg sustained release daily, and transdermal nitroglycerin 0.4 mg/h. His electrolytes are normal except for a potassium of 3.4 mmol/L. A recent digoxin level is not available. The first intervention you should consider is which of the following?

(A) stopping the room seclusion ✓

(B) replacing the potassium

(C) tapering the lorazepam

(D) checking the hydrochlorothiazide level

(E) monitoring orthostatic vitals

Elderly person on BZ First thing you do is start tapering since that can lead to delerium

Questions 50 and 51

A 64-year-old man presents to your office, accompanied by his wife, complaining of memory loss. He is a retired stockbroker who can no longer recall stock quotes like he did several years ago. His wife has become both concerned and annoyed because he seems to immediately forget whatever she has told him. These memory problems have slowly progressed over several years and recently he has had difficulty getting dressed. <u>More than once, he has put his underwear on over his pants.</u> His wife has

also noted that he speaks much less than he once did over dinner. He does not have any medical illnesses.

50. Which of the following agents may play a role in improving his memory?

(A) fluoxetine

(B) trazodone

(C) aspirin ✓

(D) donepezil (Aricept)

(E) pemoline (Cylert)

51. On further questioning, his wife reports that he does not sleep well at night and wanders around the house. He then sleeps for a large part of the day. Which of the following would be useful to control this behavior?

(A) trazodone ✓

(B) haloperidol

(C) lorazepam

(D) triazolam (Halcion)

(E) chlorpromazine

Questions 52 and 53

A 25-year-old man is brought into the emergency department lethargic and stuporous. He responds only to painful stimuli, wakes up briefly and yells, then goes back to sleep. Ambulance personnel report that they found him near a house known for drug trafficking. There is no evidence of physical injury.

52. Which of the following medications should he receive first?

(A) dextrose and flumazenil

(B) dextrose, flumazenil, and naloxone

(C) dextrose, flumazenil, naloxone, and thiamine

(D) dextrose and naloxone ✓

(E) dextrose, naloxone, and thiamine

No evidence of BZ overdose since the pt would Not be able to yell briefly.

53. The patient is treated and a urine toxicology screen is positive for the presence of opioids. When he is more alert, he informs you that he has been using IV heroin daily for several weeks. His last use was about 8 hours ago. His heroin use escalated several weeks ago from snorting to IV use when he no longer felt a good "high" from snorting. He has never detoxified before. He has no other comorbid medical conditions and he does not abuse alcohol. To detoxify him, many clinicians might use which of the following?

(A) clonidine
(B) propranolol
(C) methadone
(D) naloxone
(E) chlordiazepoxide

54. A 45-year-old woman presents to your practice with depression. Her mother recently passed away from lung cancer and her father died 4 years ago from lung cancer. She has seen therapists to help with her grief but she continues to have symptoms of major depression 6 months after her mother's death. Despite several attempts to quit smoking, she still smokes two packs of cigarettes a day. Which of the following should be considered as pharmacotherapy for her depression and smoking?

(A) imipramine
(B) bupropion
(C) buspirone
(D) trazodone
(E) phenelzine

55. A 52-year-old man who has poorly controlled diabetes is referred to you for evaluation of medication noncompliance. You learn that he cannot fall asleep at night and has no energy during the day. His appetite is gone and he does not enjoy activities as he once did. Overall he feels depressed. Additionally, he has been experiencing chronic pain in his feet, which is not relieved by analgesics. Which of the following may help his mood and his pain?

(A) alprazolam
(B) citalopram

(C) amitriptyline
(D) bupropion
(E) nefazodone

56. A 47-year-old woman presents to your office for psychiatric care because she has just relocated to your town. She has a history of bipolar disorder, but her prior psychiatrist recently stopped her lithium because she developed thyroid autoantibodies. She complains of being irritable and not able to sleep for several weeks. She tells you that her thoughts are racing and you have a difficult time redirecting her answers. However, she believes her biggest problem is her facial pain, which was diagnosed as trigeminal neuralgia and has not improved with analgesics. A medication that may potentially help both conditions is which of the following?

(A) lithium
(B) amitriptyline
(C) fluoxetine
(D) gabapentin (Neurontin)
(E) thyroxine

57. A 33-year-old woman with a history of schizophrenia has recently started treatment with olanzapine. She has tolerated the medication well and is living in a group home, anticipating moving into her own apartment. She no longer hears voices and no longer has a desire to hurt herself. Which of the following side effects of olanzapine is most likely to interfere with her continued use of the drug?

(A) increased prolactin
(B) increased excitability
(C) weight gain
(D) agranulocytosis
(E) development of cataracts

58. A 42-year-old male with schizophrenia is being treated for an acute exacerbation of his auditory hallucinations. As is his pattern, he responds very favorably to medications while hospitalized, but when he is discharged forgets to take them regularly. This results in a cycle of subsequent worsening of his psychosis and rehospitalization. He is currently taking

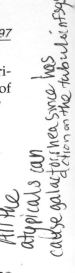

oral risperidone and tolerating it well with good efficacy. Which of the following would be the most appropriate step in his treatment?

(A) begin oral haloperidol
(B) begin Risperdal Consta
(C) continue the current regimen
(D) cross-taper with clozaril
(E) cross-taper with olanzapine

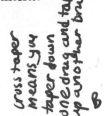

cross-taper means you taper down one drug and taper up another drug

Questions 59 and 60

A 76-year-old man who has felt depressed for several months presents to your office for evaluation. He has had weight loss, decreased appetite, and no interest in his hobbies, and cannot concentrate on your cognitive examination. He has passing thoughts of dying. He admits that he frequently hears voices telling him that he is going to die soon. You have decided to start an antidepressant and risperidone at 0.5 mg bid.

59. Which of the following side effects of risperidone should be monitored for?

(A) agranulocytosis
(B) leukocytosis
(C) anticholinergic side effects
(D) orthostatic hypotension
(E) weight loss

D

risperidone is the "dom" well of water so leads to orthostatic hypotension

60. As his dose of risperidone increases, the likelihood of which of the following can also be expected to increase?

(A) extrapyramidal side effects
(B) leukocytosis
(C) anticholinergic effects
(D) agranulocytosis
(E) weight loss

A

61. A 26-year-old woman who gave birth to her first child 2 months ago presents to your office on a referral for evaluation of depression. She is not breast-feeding. She has a history of depression from before her pregnancy and her depression is usually accompanied by voices that tell her to harm herself. In the past, she has

responded well to nortriptyline and risperidone. Which of the following is a side effect of risperidone that could possibly limit its use?

(A) weight gain
(B) galactorrhea
(C) sedation
(D) akathisia
(E) parkinsonism

B

All the atypicals can cause galactorrhea since has action on the tubuloinfundibular

Questions 62 and 63

A 58-year-old man arrives in your office complaining of impotence. He suffers from hypertension but does not have cardiac disease, renal disease, glaucoma, or a history of peptic or duodenal ulcers.

62. Which of the following drugs is best for the treatment of impotence?

(A) paroxetine
(B) citalopram
(C) molindone (Moban)
(D) diphenhydramine
(E) yohimbine *(yo-him-bine)*

63. If the patient is taking clonidine for hypertension, which of the following drugs would directly inhibit clonidine's mechanism of action?

(A) paroxetine
(B) citalopram
(C) molindone
(D) diphenhydramine
(E) yohimbine *(yo-him-bine)*

64. A 45-year-old woman who travels often to Europe from the United States presents to your office complaining of not being able to fall asleep at night after she arrives in Germany. Which of the following is the first line of treatment for insomnia?

(A) diphenhydramine
(B) trazodone
(C) clozapine
(D) benzodiazepines
(E) amitriptyline

Questions 65 and 66

A 60-year-old man presents to your office complaining of the sudden onset of palpitations, sweating, shaking, shortness of breath, choking, and feeling that he is "going crazy." He has been seen by his cardiologist who has ruled out a cardiac etiology. The patient fears future attacks.

65. Which of the following is the safest drug with which to treat panic disorder?

    (A) fluvoxamine (Luvox)
    (B) imipramine
    (C) phenelzine
    (D) bupropion
    (E) selegiline (Eldepryl)

66. If the patient's symptoms were due to a cardiac etiology and he subsequently became depressed, which antidepressant would be the most dangerous?

    (A) amitriptyline
    (B) sertraline
    (C) amphetamines
    (D) bupropion
    (E) venlafaxine

67. A 33-year-old woman with a diagnosis of chronic paranoid schizophrenia has been maintained on haloperidol since she was diagnosed at age 24. In your office, she says she has not had her period in several months, has diminished sex drive, has been unable to conceive, has been discharging milk from her breasts, and has suffered pain on sexual intercourse. Assuming that these complaints are caused by her antipsychotic medication, which of the following is most likely to explain her symptoms?

    (A) increased adrenocorticotropic hormone (ACTH) levels
    (B) decreased prolactin levels
    (C) increased prolactin levels
    (D) increased serotonin levels
    (E) increased dopamine levels

68. A 24-year-old man is hospitalized because he has been hearing voices for 6 months telling him to kill himself and fears he may act on them. He appears unkempt and lost his job 2 months ago. You decide to prescribe haloperidol for this patient's psychotic symptoms, which resolve enough for him to be discharged. On a follow-up visit to your office, he reports that his hallucinations have improved but that he "can't sit still" and feels like he needs to be constantly in motion. The patient intermittently stands up and walks around your office as you interview him. This patient most likely has which of the following?

    (A) acute dystonic reaction
    (B) akathisia
    (C) NMS
    (D) mania
    (E) obsessive-compulsive disorder (OCD)

69. You are seeing a 19-year-old male college student whose roommates say has been "creeping them out." He was always withdrawn, but has built himself a wall around his bed and frequently yells at his roommates for trying to poison him. After taking a complete history, you diagnose schizophrenia. What is the most important consideration in choosing antipsychotic medications?

    (A) renal function
    (B) the presence of negative symptoms
    (C) gender
    (D) onset of action
    (E) side effect profile

70. You have been treating a 33-year-old woman with bipolar disorder for 3 years. In preparation for a planned pregnancy, and because she has never demonstrated behavior that would put her or others in danger, you have tapered off her medications but see her frequently in case of a manic episode. Two months into her pregnancy, she presents to your office with pressured speech and the belief that her baby is

Jesus Christ. Her husband says he is concerned because she has stopped taking her prenatal vitamins and is acting bizarrely. Which of the following is the safest intervention to consider to treat her symptoms?

(A) lithium carbonate
(B) divalproex sodium
(C) chlorpromazine
(D) electroconvulsive therapy (ECT)
(E) diazepam

71. You are the consult-liaison psychiatrist on call for the trauma surgery team. You are asked for to see a man who was hit by a car and severely injured. He is unable to give a history but an acquaintance who accompanied him to the hospital reports that he is a drug user. He has track marks on his arms. Which of the following classes of drugs do you tell the surgeons is the most dangerous when abruptly withdrawn?

(A) opiates
(B) sedative-hypnotics
(C) stimulants
(D) psychedelics
(E) cannabinoids

Questions 72 and 73

A 44-year-old man with a history of alcoholism is brought to the emergency room. You get a report from a family member of the patient that he "has been living off booze and drugs and nothing else for weeks." The emergency department nurse is about to go in to draw blood from the patient and offer him food.

72. What is the most important thing to do next for this patient?

(A) Be sure liver function tests are included in the blood draw.
(B) Listen for a murmur.
(C) Administer lorazepam prophylactically for probable agitation.
(D) Administer thiamine.
(E) Get a vitamin B$_{12}$ level.

Sidenote liver func test not needed now since elevated in acute setting

73. How will this man's underlying condition be best treated in the acute medical setting?

(A) benzodiazepines
(B) barbiturates
(C) clonidine
(D) phenytoin
(E) disulfiram

74. You are seeing a 56-year-old man with a history of hepatitis C and alcoholism. He tells you that would like to quit drinking and wants to detox first. In a patient with alcoholism in whom you suspect impaired liver function, which of the following is the most appropriate drug to treat withdrawal symptoms?

(A) phenobarbital (Luminal)
(B) chlordiazepoxide
(C) lorazepam
(D) alprazolam
(E) clonidine

Benzo safe to use for liver as since metabolised

Clonidine is for heroine withdrawal

DIRECTIONS (Questions 75 through 84): Each group of items in this section consists of lettered headings followed by a set of numbered words or phrases. For each numbered word or phrase, select the ONE lettered heading that is most closely associated with it. Each lettered heading may be selected once, more than once, or not at all.

Questions 75 through 79

For each vignette, pick the medication most likely to be associated with the side effect.

(A) lithium
(B) divalproex sodium
(C) paroxetine
(D) haloperidol
(E) gabapentin
(F) pimozide (Orap)
(G) ziprasidone (Geodon)
(H) perphenazine
(I) clozapine
(J) carbamazepine

Clozapine can cause DM and fat's why last resort in Schizophrenia;

75. A 14-year-old boy being treated for Tourette disorder is started on citalopram and is seen to have an increase of 11 msec in his QTc values on ECG.

76. A 51-year-old woman being treated for schizophrenia develops diabetes.

77. An 11-year-old girl being treated for major depressive disorder reports frequent suicidal ideation.

78. A 34-year-old woman being treated for bipolar I disorder develops acute pain in her abdomen and is diagnosed with pancreatitis

79. The WBC count of a 27-year-old man being treated for schizophrenia drops to 3000/mL.

Questions 80 through 84

(A) fluoxetine
(B) alprazolam
(C) trazodone
(D) paroxetine
(E) risperidone
(F) haloperidol
(G) olanzapine
(H) lithium
(I) citalopram
(J) divalproex sodium
(K) sertraline

80. A 42-year-old man stops his antidepressant. Two days later, he experiences a feeling of hopelessness, has difficulty sleeping, and feels quite anxious.

81. A 34-year-old man has been noncompliant with medications in the past. You want to be able to give him a depot injection of an antipsychotic.

82. A 36-year-old woman being treated for bipolar disorder finds herself urinating very frequently.

83. You are treating a 45-year-old veteran with a history of alcoholism for posttraumatic stress disorder (PTSD) and he asked you for something to help him sleep.

84. Several months after starting on a new antipsychotic, a 32-year-old patient's total cholesterol increases from 210 to 230 mg/dL.

DIRECTIONS (Questions 85 through 89): Each of the numbered items in this section is followed by answer choices. Select the ONE lettered answer that is BEST in each case.

Questions 85 and 86

You are treating a 28-year-old single woman for a first episode of major depression with sertraline. Two months after starting treatment with you, the patient reports that she feels "back to normal" and asks when she can stop the medication you initially prescribed.

85. You tell her that she can safely stop the medication

(A) now
(B) in 2 months
(C) in 4 months
(D) after 10 months
(E) after 5 years

86. She returns 3 months after starting treatment and reports a poor sexual relationship with her boyfriend. Which of the following antidepressants could be considered in place of your original therapy if the sexual dysfunction becomes intolerable?

(A) bupropion
(B) fluvoxamine
(C) fluoxetine
(D) clomipramine
(E) citalopram

Questions 87 and 88

You are treating a 28-year-old man with a 6-year history of schizophrenia who lives with his parents. The patient has had a number of debilitating side effects, such as severe extrapyramidal symptoms, from traditional antipsychotics including haloperidol. His family is worried about weight gain, which the patient has experienced on olanzapine. You discuss clozapine with the patient and his family and they agree to try the medication. You have initiated treatment slowly and he has shown some improvement; however, he has been producing a large amount of saliva and drool soaking his shirts.

only main SE of
atypicals is ↑sugar ↓↑cholesterol;

87. You should

    (A) stop treatment with clozapine
    (B) initiate propranolol
    (C) initiate propylthiouracil
    (D) increase the dose of clozapine
    (E) initiate amantadine (Symmetrel)

88. In addition to the above side effect, the patient develops an increase in his resting heart rate. An ECG revealed a sinus tachycardia without other changes from his baseline. This has been repeated several times over the past month and the heart rate remains elevated. You should consider which of the following?

    (A) stopping treatment with clozapine
    (B) initiating benztropine
    (C) checking creatinine phosphokinase levels
    (D) initiating treatment with propranolol
    (E) initiating treatment with labetalol

89. A 21-year-old single female college student is brought to the university health service by her roommates. She makes it clear to you that she does not think there's anything wrong with her, but her roommates tell you that they "can't deal with her anymore" because she never sleeps and "never shuts up." The woman tells you that's just because she has discovered an important mathematical proof that she just must finish writing. She's sure that the university will grant her tenure as soon as they see the proof, although she has trouble staying on the topic when you start to ask questions about it. She has not seen a psychiatrist before, and a urine toxicology screen, which she consents to "to prove I'm not crazy," is negative. The most appropriate agent for initial and maintenance treatment of this patient is which of the following?

    (A) clonazepam
    (B) lithium
    (C) topiramate (Topamax)
    (D) haloperidol
    (E) gabapentin

90. A 34-year-old electrical engineer complains to his doctor that he has been feeling suicidal. He feels guilty over the breakup of his marriage, cannot concentrate, feels hopeless and helpless, and has a subjective feeling of sadness and depression. He has lost 25 lb in the last 3 months because his "appetite isn't the same." A diagnosis of depression is made and he is started on an antidepressant. Which symptom can be expected to improve most quickly?

    (A) guilt
    (B) hopelessness and helplessness
    (C) decreased concentration
    (D) suicidality
    (E) decreased appetite

91. The patient is a 59-year-old female with chronic schizophrenia, undifferentiated type, as well as poorly controlled diabetes mellitus and hypertension. She has been treated for over 35 years with various typical antipsychotics, and although she is on an adequate dose, she still has residual psychotic symptoms and has now begun to develop involuntary blinking and tongue rolling movements. She is agreeable to switching to an atypical antipsychotic. Which of the following medications would be the most appropriate for this patient?

    (A) aripiprazole
    (B) clozapine
    (C) olanzapine
    (D) quetiapine
    (E) risperidone

92. Jane is a 20-year-old prostitute who has been using cocaine regularly for greater than 3 years. Over the past 12 months, she finds that she has had to use increasing amounts of cocaine in order to obtain the same level of "high." Which of the following terms best describes this effect?

    (A) tolerance
    (B) dependence
    (C) addiction
    (D) withdrawal
    (E) abuse

[handwritten left margin: If Both parents are manic-depressive the pt must also be manic depressive ... 2 of the misanswer.]

93. A 25-year-old woman is sent to a psychiatrist for evaluation. She has felt "tired" for the past 2 1/2 months, with associated crying spells, difficulty falling asleep, diminished appetite with a 10 lb weight loss, and feelings of guilt over many aspects of her life. She hasn't been able to enjoy pursuits that had given her pleasure, and she has been distracted at work, making many "silly" mistakes. Although she feels like she has "no hope," she denies any suicidal ideation. She denies past psychiatric or medical history, and she drinks 2 glasses of wine per week. She admits both parents were diagnosed with "manic-depression" and are on unknown medications for it. Which of the following would be the most appropriate treatment for this patient?

   (A) aripiprazole
   (B) carbamazepine
   (C) ECT
   (D) lamotrigine
   (E) venlafaxine

94. A 40-year-old woman with a history of psychotic depression resistant to many trials of antidepressant medication is being considered for ECT. Which of the following conditions is an relative contraindication to ECT?

   (A) pregnancy
   (B) degenerative joint disease
   (C) hypertension
   (D) recent MI
   (E) psychotic depression

Questions 95 and 96

95. The patient is a 23-year-old obese male newly diagnosed with schizophrenia. He was first admitted to the inpatient unit 2 months ago where he was stabilized on haloperidol 10 mg bid and he is following up for his outpatient appointment. Upon evaluation, he is cooperative but does not expand on his answers. He denies feeling depressed but also denies enjoyment of activities. He sleeps approximately 5 hours per night. He admits to lingering auditory hallucinations telling him derogatory things, but he denies any commands. While he

no longer believes he is the Messiah, he still wonders if cars are following him near his group home. His Mental Status Examination is notable for psychomotor retardation and a flat affect. He admits to suicidal ideation without plan or intent and denies homicidal ideation. Consideration is given to switching to quetiapine. Which of the following symptoms would be the most appropriate to target for switching medication in this patient?

   (A) anhedonia
   (B) hallucinations
   (C) obesity
   (D) paranoia
   (E) suicidality

96. After discussion with the patient, it is decided to change medications to quetiapine, with a target dose of at least 400 mg daily. Which of the following switching methods would be the most appropriate?

   (A) Initiate quetiapine at 50 mg bid and increase while tapering haloperidol.
   (B) Initiate quetiapine at 200 mg bid while tapering haloperidol.
   (C) Initiate quetiapine at 200 mg bid and taper haloperidol after 4 weeks.
   (D) Simultaneously discontinue haloperidol while initiating quetiapine at 50 mg bid.
   (E) Taper haloperidol and then initiate quetiapine at 50 mg bid.

[handwritten: Antipsychotics you taper one down and start other at minimum dose and titrate up.]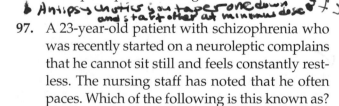

97. A 23-year-old patient with schizophrenia who was recently started on a neuroleptic complains that he cannot sit still and feels constantly restless. The nursing staff has noted that he often paces. Which of the following is this known as?

   (A) parkinsonism
   (B) dystonia
   (C) tremor
   (D) TD
   (E) akathisia

98. A 35-year-old woman with a history of seizures is diagnosed with bipolar disorder and started on lamotrigene. Which of the following side

effects would be the most important to educate the patient about?

(A) aplastic anemia

✓ (B) hypertension

(C) memory loss

(D) rash

(E) TD

99. A 19-year-old man is diagnosed with schizophreniform disorder and is given an intramuscular injection of haloperidol. Later, the patient is found arching forward. On physical examination, stiffness of the neck and back muscles are noted. How is this dystonia best described?

(A) opisthotonos

✓ (B) torticollis

(C) laryngospasm

(D) oculogyric crisis

(E) pleurothotonos

Ans→ torso muscles —abd + thorax

100. The patient is a 59-year-old woman, with a past medical history of hypercholesterolemia, diabetes, and diabetic neuropathy, who presents to her primary care doctor with the chief complaint of "headaches." Upon further interview, she states her symptoms began after the death of her husband 5 months ago. Since that time, she has felt "empty," with poor sleep, fatigue, decreased concentration, and wishes she "would die so I can join him." Her review of systems is remarkable for the above complaints plus ongoing "sharp pins and needles" in her extremities. Her physical examination is unchanged and her blood sugars have been relatively well-controlled. Which of the following would be the most appropriate treatment for her symptoms?

(A) bupropion

(B) duloxetine

Only Duloxetine is approved
For DM and depression
double "D's."

(C) fluoxetine

(D) mirtazapine

(E) reassurance

101. A 44-year-old married patient with a history of recurrent major depressive disorder presents to a psychiatrist after stopping his sertraline 1 month ago. Although it has been effective in the treatment of his depression, he has had increasing difficulty maintaining an erection, and this has caused friction and conflicts with his wife. He is concerned, however, that he will have a relapse of his depressive symptoms if not medicated. Which of the following would be the most appropriate treatment for this individual?

(A) begin mirtazapine

(B) begin paroxetine

(C) begin venlafaxine

(D) no treatment

(E) restart sertraline

Note
venlafaxine
can lead to
HTN and
HTN induced
erethie Dys.

Questions 102 and 103

102. A 36-year-old man is started on bupropion (Zyban/Wellbutrin) for depression. He returns 2 weeks later and states that he feels that his mood has improved slightly and that he has more energy. He has also noticed that his sexual desires have become insatiable. He notes a dramatic increase in his sexual energy and is masturbating frequently despite having intercourse up to two times per day with his wife. Which of the following is the best term to describe this patient's insatiable sexual desire?

(A) hypervigilance

(B) hypermnesia

(C) satyriasis

(D) sexual sadism

(E) sexual masochism

103. The patient is switched to fluoxetine (Prozac) after the bupropion was stopped. One week later, he calls complaining of an inability to sleep. He is able to fall asleep but awakens within 2 hours and is unable to return to sleep. The patient is started on trazodone (Desyrel) for this problem. Three days later, he calls complaining of a painful erection that he cannot get rid of even after several hours. Which of the following best describes the condition of the patient following the initiation of trazodone?

    (A) parapraxis
    (B) priapism
    (C) nymphomania
    (D) satyriasis
    (E) libido

104. A 35-year-old married female is being followed by a psychiatrist for her first episode of major depression. She is prescribed citalopram 40 mg daily and has been in remission for 3 months. She now complains of the new onset of decreased libido and this is causing her a moderate amount of distress. Which of the following would be the most appropriate to add to her current regimen?

    (A) bupropion
    (B) desipramine
    (C) lithium
    (D) tranylcypromine
    (E) venlafaxine

105. A 27-year-old married female, 13 weeks pregnant, is referred to a psychiatrist for evaluation. She has no past psychiatric or medical history, but she believes that her mother also suffered from depression. Over the past 5 weeks, she has become increasingly "sad," with almost daily crying spells, middle insomnia, anergia, and anhedonia. More concerning, however, is that she has had "no interest" in eating, and she has lost 10 lb. Although she denies a specific plan for suicide, she feels no hope for the future and doesn't care "if I live or die." Which of the following would be the most appropriate treatment?

    (A) amitriptyline
    (B) cognitive-behavioral therapy
    (C) duloxetine
    (D) ECT
    (E) fluoxetine

Questions 106 through 109

Use the list below to identify the proper term for each question.

    (A) inhalants
    (B) withdrawal
    (C) tolerance
    (D) abuse
    (E) dependence
    (F) formication
    (G) intoxication
    (H) cannabis
    (I) post-hallucinogen perception disorder
    (J) amotivational syndrome
    (K) cannabis

106. A 45-year-old man presents to the emergency department in delirium tremens. He complains of bugs crawling on his skin.

107. A 14-year-old boy is brought to you by his mother. She states that he has no motivation and is failing in school. The boy admitted to his mother that he has been smoking marijuana. To what class of substances does marijuana belong?

108. A 21-year-old man presents to the emergency department after "huffing gas." The patient claims that he feels disconnected from reality and is frightened. After about 20 minutes, these effects diminish. Petroleum fumes are in what group of substances?

109. A 54-year-old man states that he continues to use alcohol despite having lost his family and job. He often drives his car while intoxicated and recently was arrested in a barroom brawl. The fact that this patient continues to drink alcohol despite adverse effects indicates that he has which substance problem?

Questions 110 through 121

Use the following terms to match the correct response to the questions below.

- (A) galactorrhea
- (B) agranulocytosis
- (C) blepharospasm
- (D) opisthotonos
- (E) torticollis
- (F) rabbit syndrome
- (G) NMS
- (H) obstructive jaundice
- (I) gynecomastia
- (J) pigmented retinopathy
- (K) orthostatic hypotension
- (L) pseudoparkinsonism
- (M) akathisia
- (N) TD
- (O) constipation
- (P) retrograde ejaculation
- (Q) double depression
- (R) kindling

110. A 27-year-old man with paranoid schizophrenia notices the development of breasts, a decreased libido, and not ejaculating with orgasm. He is being treated with thioridazine (Mellaril). The development of breasts is due to the blockade of dopamine receptors in the tuberoinfundibular tract.

111. A 35-year-old man taking thioridazine finds himself unable to ejaculate.

112. A 35-year-old woman you are treating for an active dysthymic disorder develops major depression.

113. A 22-year-old African American man on clozapine (Clozaril) for 3 months reports a sore throat and fever. A CBC is obtained with a WBC count of 1000/mm³ with 1% granulocytes.

114. A 43-year-old man with schizophrenia is on haloperidol. He is noted to have a flexed posture, festinating gait, resting tremor, and bradykinesia.

115. The same 43-year-old man was continued on haloperidol despite his side effects and after several years developed choreic movements of the trunk and limbs along with lip smacking and tongue movements.

116. A 21-year-old man with psychosis was started on haloperidol at high doses. Eight days into his treatment, he developed fever, generalized rigidity, diaphoresis, and altered mental status.

117. A 32-year-old woman with bipolar disorder suffers a severe depressive decompensation 1 month after a minor decompensation.

118. A 26-year-old man being treated with high-dose thioridazine is found on ophthalmologic examination to have peppery pigmentation of the retina. Despite discontinuation of the medication, the pigmentation continues and the patient eventually suffers total blindness.

119. A 22-year-old man complains of severe restlessness and agitation after starting on a neuroleptic. He complains that he cannot sit still and paces constantly.

120. A 26-year-old patient with schizophrenia is started on chlorpromazine (Thorazine). After 1 week, he complains of flu-like symptoms. A CBC is obtained and is normal. After another week, the patient develops a yellowish color to his skin and sclera.

121. A 45-year-old patient with schizophrenia is started on a high dose of chlorpromazine. The next day, he complains of being light-headed every time he stands. On examination, he is noted to have a significant decrease in blood pressure and an increase in heart rate. You speculate that this is secondary to the alpha1-adrenergic blockade.

α 1 blockade — orthostatic hypo
the two low potency
neuroleptics "C T"

Questions 122 and 123

122. You are called in the middle of the night by the surgical service to see a 52-year-old man who was admitted to the hospital 36 hours earlier for an emergency appendectomy. The man is very agitated and is talking nonsense to the nursing staff who is unable to calm him down. You suspect alcohol withdrawal. Which of the following is the receptor most closely associated with these symptoms?

    (A) dopamine-2 (D_2)
    (B) dopamine-4 (D_4)
    (C) GABA-A
    (D) GABA-B
    (E) 5-HT$_2$

123. This syndrome usually occurs at which of the following times?

    (A) within the first 12 hours after admission
    (B) within the first 2 days after admission
    (C) within the first 5 days after admission
    (D) within the first 10 days after admission
    (E) anytime during this admission

Answers and Explanations

1. **(C)** Phenelzine and tranylcypromine are the only nonselective monoamine oxidase inhibitors (MAOIs) currently approved for use in the United States. They are extremely dangerous in overdose and, after a brief asymptomatic period of 12–24 hours, may produce hyperpyrexia and autonomic excitability sufficient enough to cause rhabdomyolysis. Supportive care should be instituted. If delirium develops, small doses of IV benzodiazepines should be used. Lorazepam is preferred because of its short elimination half-life. Neuroleptics, especially short-acting agents such as chlorpromazine, should be avoided because of their tendency to contribute to hypotension. If ventricular arrhythmias develop, they can be treated with lidocaine. Bretylium may contribute to the adrenergic crisis and should be avoided. Phenytoin may be used if seizures develop. Meperidine should be avoided because it may contribute to the adrenergic crisis. Other medications that are contraindicated with MAOIs include stimulants, decongestants, amine precursors such as L-dopa and L-tryptophan, and the antihypertensives methyldopa, guanethidine, and reserpine.

2. **(C)** Blocking reuptake of catecholamines and indolamines in patients already using an MAOI can result in a potentially life-threatening drug interaction known as serotonin syndrome. Medications that block such reuptake include the SSRIs, TCAs, buspirone, and other antidepressants such as venlafaxine. Features of mild serotonin syndrome include tachycardia, flushing, fever, hypertension, ocular oscillations, and myoclonic jerks. Severe serotonin syndrome may result in severe hyperthermia, coma, autonomic instability, convulsions, and death; therefore, wait at least 14 days after discontinuing an MAOI before starting a serotonergic agent. Rapid-cycling bipolar disorder is an affective disorder and NMS is an idiosyncratic reaction to neuroleptic drugs. Akathisia and opisthotonos are both extrapyramidal side effects of neuroleptics.

3. **(C)** This patient is likely suffering from a major depressive episode. Because of her weight gain, hypersomnia, and mood reactivity, her depression has atypical features. Although atypical features respond best to MAOIs such as phenelzine, these medications are rarely used because of the potential risk of a fatal hypertensive crisis when eating certain tyramine-containing foods. SSRIs such as fluoxetine and sertraline are also beneficial even though response rates to SSRIs may not match those of the MAOIs. Because of their favorable safety profile, SSRIs have become a first-line treatment in major depression. TCAs such as nortriptyline are less effective than MAOIs for atypical depression. Trazodone inhibits serotonin reuptake and may also be serotonomimetic.

4. **(B)** Approximately 50% of patients who meet criteria for major depression recover after treatment for 6 weeks with an adequately dosed antidepressant. Initially, sleep may improve within the first 2 weeks; however, this response may not be predictive of efficacy. Substantial effects may not be seen for 4 weeks, and maximal effects may require up to 8 weeks of treatment.

5. **(A)** Alcohol withdrawal should be strongly considered in this patient. Benzodiazepines are the drug of choice for control of alcohol

withdrawal symptoms and for prophylaxis against withdrawal seizures and the potentially life-threatening delirium tremens. Long-acting benzodiazepines such as chlordiazepoxide and diazepam are appropriate; however, both are extensively metabolized by the liver. Because this patient has elevated transaminases, oxazepam or lorazepam, which only undergoes glucuronidation prior to elimination, is preferable. A high-potency antipsychotic agent such as haloperidol may be necessary to help control this patient. However, low-potency antipsychotics, such as chlorpromazine, should be avoided because they may lower the seizure threshold. Disulfiram is used to treat alcohol dependence not acute alcohol withdrawal.

6. **(E)** This patient has delirium tremens, which is a medical emergency. He should be transferred to an intensive care setting where IV benzodiazepines can be administered with greater safety. The IV route is preferred in this situation to ensure adequate absorption. Haloperidol can be used for its sedative effect but it should not take the place of a benzodiazepine. Similarly, IV labetalol may be useful in the intensive care unit but it should not replace a benzodiazepine.

7. **(A)** The precise mechanism of action of SSRIs in depression is not fully understood. Acutely, they enhance serotonergic neurotransmission by permitting serotonin more time to bind at the postsynaptic terminal. However, because therapeutic effect of SSRIs may take several weeks, this acute effect is likely not responsible for the improvement seen in depression. One leading theory is that they cause downregulation of postsynaptic 5-HT$_2$ receptors. However, not all SSRIs have been shown to do this, so the answer is likely much more complicated. SSRIs can inhibit the dopamine system accounting for the anecdotal reports of SSRIs causing extrapyramidal side effects. However, this is probably unrelated to their effectiveness in depression.

8. **(A)** Anorgasmia is the most common reported sexual dysfunction side effect in women taking SSRIs such as sertraline.

9. **(B)** Akathisia, an extrapyramidal side effect of neuroleptics, can be difficult to distinguish from anxiety in a psychotic individual; however, based on observation and history from his parents, akathisia should be strongly considered and empiric treatment attempted. Onset usually begins between 5 and 60 days after initiation of treatment but can occur after just one dose. First, the neuroleptic dose should be reduced as much as possible. In general, anticholinergic agents such as benztropine are used to treat extrapyramidal symptoms. In the absence of other extrapyramidal side effects, however, many clinicians would start treatment with a beta-blocker such as propranolol. Antianxiety agents such as lorazepam are generally not helpful. Diphenhydramine is helpful in acute dystonias but not in akathisia.

10. **(D)** Flooding is an exposure technique that is commonly used in behavior therapy. The premise is confrontation with the feared symptom. *Couples* and *family therapy* are designed to modify relationships between the patient and others in his or her social constellation. *Psychodynamic psychotherapy* is a form of therapy informed by psychodynamic processes. *Hypnosis* is a sleep-like state induced by a therapist that has been of some use in uncovering psychodynamic processes and in behavioral modification such as stopping smoking.

11. **(C)** Rhabdomyolysis is the most common serious complication of NMS, occurring in up to 25% of patients in one series. Dialysis may be required to protect patients from renal failure. Creatinine phosphokinase is usually elevated in NMS but there are no specific laboratory findings. All of the other listed complications have been reported but with less frequency.

12. **(C)** Retinal pigmentation is known to occur when thioridazine is used in high doses (>1000 mg/day). It may not remit when thioridazine is discontinued and it can lead to blindness. The other choices can occur with all neuroleptics.

13. **(E)** This patient is suffering from panic disorder with agoraphobia. There are many medications that have proven benefit for this condition

including TCAs, SSRIs, MAOIs, and high-potency benzodiazepines. Of the agents listed, only fluoxetine, an SSRI, is one of them. Bupropion, an antidepressant with dopamine activity, is not effective. Trazodone, an antidepressant with mixed serotonergic effects, has shown conflicting results. Buspirone, a partial 5-HT$_{1a}$ antagonist with antianxiety activity, is not effective. Propranolol, a beta-adrenergic blocker, may help to alleviate the physical symptoms such as tachycardia but does not prevent the attack.

14. **(C)** Clonazepam is the most potent benzodiazepine listed. Using 1 mg of lorazepam for the equivalent dose in milligrams, the potency relationship of some common benzodiazepines is as follows: clonazepam 0.25 mg, triazolam 0.25 mg, alprazolam 0.5 mg, diazepam 5 mg, clorazepate (Tranxene) 7.5 mg, chlordiazepoxide 10 mg, and flurazepam (Dalmane) 30 mg. Flumazenil is a benzodiazepine antagonist. Buspirone is a nonbenzodiazepine anxiolytic that is generally considered to be less potent.

15. **(A)** These are the minimum initial laboratory studies required before initiating lithium treatment. Because lithium is a Group IA monovalent ion, the kidney handles it much as it does sodium. Ninety-five percent of lithium is excreted unchanged through the kidneys. Therefore electrolytes, creatinine, BUN, and urinalysis are required to check kidney function. Thyroid studies are required because lithium inhibits the synthesis of thyroid hormone and its release from the thyroid. A CBC is optional. Lithium may cause a benign elevation in the WBC. Liver function tests should be performed prior to initiating treatment with divalproex sodium. Rare cases of fatal hepatotoxicity have been reported with divalproex sodium. Divalproex sodium may also elevate serum ammonia levels, but this is rare.

16. **(D)** The recommendation should be to switch to aspirin. In some individuals, nonsteroidal anti-inflammatory agents (NSAIDs) cause an increase in lithium levels. Therefore, these agents should be used with caution in patients taking lithium and avoided if possible. Aspirin and sulindac, however, do not affect lithium levels and are therefore safe for use with lithium.

17. **(A)** Difficulty falling asleep and decreased appetite are the two most common side effects of methylphenidate. Stimulants have been reported to slow growth; however, it is believed to be less common with methylphenidate and dose related. When drug holidays are given, a growth rebound is seen. Methylphenidate may cause an increase in systolic blood pressure.

18. **(B)** Stimulants have been frequently reported to exacerbate the tics associated with Tourette disorder and some studies have warned that they should not be given to children with tics or a family history of Tourette disorder. However, some recent studies have identified frequent comorbidity of attention deficit hyperactivity disorder (ADHD) and Tourette disorder.

19. **(C)** Dopamine D$_2$ receptor antagonism provides the greatest relief of symptoms in children suffering from Tourette disorder. Pharmacologic treatment is strictly symptomatic and is not curative. An alpha2-agonist, not antagonist, would provide some relief but it is not as effective as D$_2$ receptor antagonism.

20. **(B)** Haloperidol is the only medication listed that is a strong antagonist at the D$_2$ receptor. Another agent that is nearly as effective as haloperidol is pimozide. Clonidine, which is an alpha2-agonist, is also used in Tourette disorder but it is clearly less effective than haloperidol. However, because clonidine is not a neuroleptic, it lacks extrapyramidal side effects and the associated long-term sequelae. Additionally, it may be useful in patients with ADHD and Tourette disorder.

21. **(C)** The most likely syndrome is TD, a movement disorder that may occur after long-term treatment with neuroleptic medication such as haloperidol. It consists of a number of abnormal and involuntary movements such as lip smacking, facial grimacing, and choreoathetoid-like movements of the limbs and trunk. In Huntington disease, a dominant genetic disorder, the involuntary movements

are accompanied by a progressive dementia. Sydenham chorea, associated with rheumatic fever, occurs in children. *Meige syndrome* is an oral facial dystonia involving blinking and chin thrusting, sometimes lip pursing or tongue movements, and occasionally shoulder movement. Anticholinergic toxicity, which usually presents as delirium, is not present.

22. **(E)** It was once believed that if patients developed signs of TD, they would progress to severe dyskinesias. Recent evidence, however, indicates that most patients stabilize and may spontaneously improve even if they continue taking the antipsychotic. However, the only medication that may improve these symptoms is clozapine.

23. **(A)** This patient likely has generalized anxiety disorder (GAD). Benzodiazepines are the most effective medications for quickly reducing symptoms of GAD. All benzodiazepines are effective and the choice should be based on potency, half-life, and side effects. Alprazolam has an intermediate onset, a half-life of 6–20 hours, and does not have active metabolites. Buspirone is effective for reducing symptoms but does not work as quickly as benzodiazepines. The tricyclic agent imipramine and SSRIs such as fluoxetine also have anxiolytic properties but also do not work as quickly as benzodiazepines. Bupropion does not have anxiolytic properties.

24. **(B)** This patient likely has the Axis II diagnosis of borderline personality disorder. This disorder can be extremely difficult to treat. SSRIs, particularly fluoxetine, have been shown to reduce the impulsiveness and affective instability in these patients, and antipsychotics such as haloperidol have been shown to decrease the impulsiveness and psychotic thinking. One recent study used low-dose clozapine in a small sample of patients with severe borderline personality disorder and found it to be beneficial. Anticonvulsants such as divalproex sodium may help to modulate intense fluctuations in affect but stimulants have not been shown to be effective in borderline personality disorder.

TCAs carry a heightened risk in these patients because of their potential lethality in overdose.

25. **(A)** This patient is suffering from bulimia nervosa, purging type, and several studies have shown that fluoxetine can help these patients. Many believe it is related to the high incidence of comorbid depression in this population. TCAs, such as protriptyline, have not been as effective. Because electroencephalographic abnormalities have been found in patients with bulimia, phenytoin has been tried but it does not appear to be effective.

26. **(B)** Unless there is a comorbid psychiatric disorder such as OCD or depression, pharmacotherapy generally has a limited role in the treatment of anorexia nervosa. Reports on the usefulness of cyproheptadine to stimulate appetite have been mixed. Generally, these patients already have a good appetite. One study suggested that high-dose chlorpromazine is useful, but the results have not been duplicated. The TCA amitriptyline and the promotility agent cisapride are not useful in anorexia nervosa. In particular, cisapride should be avoided because patients with anorexia nervosa are already at high risk for arrhythmias, which can be worsened by cisapride.

27. **(D)** This patient likely has SSRI discontinuation syndrome, which may occur within 1–3 days of abruptly stopping an SSRI. The most common physical symptoms are dizziness, nausea and vomiting, fatigue, lethargy, and flu-like symptoms. Psychological symptoms are anxiety, irritability, and crying spells. Paroxetine may cause this because of its short half-life and lack of an active metabolite. Fluoxetine has an active metabolite with a half-life ranging from 4 to 16 days, and, therefore, does not require tapering. The discontinuation syndrome is not known to be lethal; however, restarting the paroxetine and tapering it is a reasonable choice.

28. **(C)** This patient has major depression requiring antidepressant treatment. SSRIs are a good first choice; however, fluoxetine has been reported to increase carbamazepine levels. Paroxetine

has not been reported to increase carbamazepine levels. Nefazodone does increase carbamazepine levels, perhaps through interaction with the cytochrome P-450 3A3/4 isoenzyme. Clomipramine and amitriptyline are both TCAs that have substantial anticholinergic side effects. TCAs are more dangerous in overdose than are SSRIs as well.

29. **(C)** Trazodone is an antidepressant medication, unrelated to other antidepressant drugs (except nefazodone), which affects the serotonin system by weak reuptake inhibition and antagonist activity at 5-HT$_{1a}$, 5-HT$_{1c}$, and 5-HT$_2$ receptors. Some clinicians have questioned its efficacy in severe illness but its use as an adjunct to help with sleep in depressed patients is growing. Some SSRIs can be activating, such as fluoxetine, and trazodone can help with sleep in these patients. Bupropion does not cause significant drowsiness. Diazepam is a benzodiazepine and diphenhydramine is an antihistamine although both have been used to help with sleep. Both should be avoided in the elderly if possible.

30. **(A)** Priapism, though rare, has been reported with trazodone use. The manufacturer has reported the incidence of any abnormal erectile function to be about 1 in 6000 men. This side effect usually occurs within the first month of treatment but can occur at any time. Any abnormal erectile function should prompt discontinuation of the medication.

31. **(C)** Lithium often causes T-wave flattening or inversion on ECG, but the changes are usually not clinically significant. Sinus node dysfunction and first-degree atrioventricular (AV) block are rare but are the most commonly reported cardiac side effects of lithium. Lithium toxicity can cause sinoatrial block, AV block, AV dissociation, bradyarrhythmias, ventricular tachycardia, and ventricular fibrillation.

32. **(C)** Thiazide diuretics can increase lithium levels owing to decreased lithium clearance. Other agents that can increase lithium levels are the diuretics ethacrynic acid, spironolactone, and triamterene; NSAIDs except aspirin and sulindac; the antibiotics metronidazole and tetracycline; and angiotensin-converting enzyme inhibitors.

33. **(A)** Clomipramine, a TCA with potent serotonin reuptake inhibition, is the most widely studied agent with efficacy in OCD. Several SSRIs, including fluoxetine, fluvoxamine, sertraline, and paroxetine, have demonstrated efficacy in OCD. Other tricyclic agents are not as effective as clomipramine probably because they lack the potent serotonin reuptake inhibition of clomipramine. Clonazepam may be used for anxiety associated with OCD but it is not effective in treating the underlying disorder. Mirtazapine is an antidepressant that is a central alpha2-antagonist, leading to increased norepinephrine and serotonin release, and an antagonist of both 5-HT$_2$ and 5-HT$_3$. However, it has not been used in OCD. Phenelzine is an MAOI that is not used in OCD. Olanzapine is an atypical neuroleptic. Neuroleptics generally are not effective in OCD.

34. **(A)** Just like treatment of refractory depression, treatment of refractory OCD is largely based on case reports and clinical preferences. There are very few controlled blinded trials in refractory OCD. Several open label studies reported buspirone was effective as an augmentation to SSRIs or clomipramine; however, a double-blind controlled study found no benefit to the addition of buspirone. There are case reports of fenfluramine and lithium as effective augmenting agents but these findings require validation and fenfluramine has been withdrawn from the U.S. market. Some studies found that clozapine in patients with schizophrenia worsened OCD symptoms. Cingulotomy, a surgical procedure, should be reserved for severe refractory cases.

35. **(D)** This patient is suffering from command auditory hallucinations, which have not sufficiently responded to adequate trials of two typical neuroleptic agents, chlorpromazine and haloperidol, and one atypical neuroleptic agent, olanzapine. Therefore, a trial of clozapine is warranted. Clozapine was the first atypical neuroleptic and has been found to be superior to typical neuroleptics in reducing

both positive and negative symptoms. It may also improve cognitive deficits in patients with schizophrenia. Fluphenazine and perphenazine are both typical neuroleptics like haloperidol and chlorpromazine. Risperidone is considered an atypical neuroleptic but the rate of response in refractory patients is less than that with clozapine. Ziprasidone, approved by the U.S. Food and Drug Administration in August 2004, is like olanzapine in that it has 5-HT$_{2a}$ and D$_2$ receptor antagonist properties.

36. **(C)** Clozapine acts at many receptors, including D$_1$, D$_2$, and D$_4$; histamine-1; muscarinic; alpha1-adrenergic; and serotonin types 5-HT$_2$, 5-HT$_{2c}$, and 5-HT$_3$. Efforts to identify the exact mechanism of antipsychotic action of clozapine have revealed at least two possibilities. Unlike typical neuroleptics, it has much more potent antagonism at the D$_4$ receptor compared to the D$_2$ receptor, especially in the limbic system. This has led to speculation that the D$_4$ receptor may mediate psychotic symptoms. It also has activity at the 5-HT$_2$ receptor, activity that typical neuroleptics lack.

37. **(D)** TCAs, including imipramine and nortriptyline, block various receptors, including muscarinic, alpha1- and alpha2-adrenergic, dopaminergic, and histaminergic, to varying degrees. As a class, their blockade of alpha1-receptors is generally believed to be responsible for any orthostatic hypotension that may occur especially in the elderly. Nortriptyline has relatively less alpha1-blocking potency and some clinicians prefer it over other tricyclics in the elderly. Bupropion and mirtazapine are not associated with orthostatic hypotension. Trazodone can cause orthostatic hypotension from alpha1-blockade; however, nefazodone has a lower affinity and is expected to have a lower incidence of orthostatic hypotension.

38. **(E)** Treatment of refractory depression remains controversial. Unlike evidence for initial selection of antidepressant therapy, there is little well-controlled evidence regarding treatment of refractory depression. Selection is based largely on clinical practice and side effect profile. This patient has had an adequate trial of an

SSRI without response. Lithium and thyroid augmentation of antidepressants have been well worked out; however, this patient has not even had a partial response to augment. Additionally, these options are generally reserved for patients who have failed multiple trials of other medications. Imipramine, a TCA, has the accompanying anticholinergic side effects typical of this class, which make it a less desirable choice. Bupropion is an effective agent; however, the risk of seizures in patients without a seizure history is 0.6–0.9% at doses greater than 200 mg/day. At low doses, venlafaxine inhibits only serotonin reuptake, but at doses greater than 225 mg/day, it also inhibits norepinephrine reuptake distinguishing it from the SSRIs. In 3–13% of patients, venlafaxine has caused a sustained increase in supine diastolic blood pressure.

39. **(E)** All of the commonly used mood-stabilizing medications, except clonazepam (a benzodiazepine), appear to carry an increased risk of fetal malformations or a potential deleterious effect on later cognitive development. Use of lithium during the first trimester increases the risk of cardiac malformations, including Ebstein anomaly, to 7.7%. A fetal echocardiogram should be done between weeks 16 and 18 of pregnancy. Lithium may be used in the second and third trimesters but it should be stopped peripartum because of the rapid fluid shifts and changes in glomerular filtration. Carbamazepine increases the risk of neural tube defects and divalproex sodium increases the risk of intrauterine growth retardation and neural tube defects.

40. **(E)** It is not unusual for delirious patients to become hostile or combative posing a risk to themselves or other hospital staff. Low-dose atypical antipsychotics, such as risperidone, are very effective in reducing agitation in delirious patients. Diphenhydramine should be avoided as the anticholinergic effects may actually worsen the delirium and confusion. Donepezil is an anticholinesterase inhibitor used for dementias. Although benzodiazepines can be used for agitation in delirium, they may overly sedate or conversely disinhibit the

patient further. Orientation to surroundings is often additionally helpful in delirium but it will not immediately calm the patient.

41. **(D)** Mirtazapine is an antidepressant whose pharmacologic profile is different from other available agents. It is a central alpha2-adrenergic antagonist and an antagonist of 5-HT$_2$ and 5-HT$_3$ receptors as well as H$_1$ receptors. Because it blocks alpha2-receptors, it leads to enhanced serotonin release but blockade of 5-HT$_2$ and 5-HT$_3$ leads to relative enhancement of 5-HT$_1$ activity giving it a different side effect profile than SSRIs. For example, it tends to increase appetite and cause weight gain compared to placebo. Also, its H$_1$ antagonism causes sedation. However, at higher doses, alpha2-adrenergic blockade also leads to increased norepinephrine release, which may counteract the H$_1$-mediated sedation. In this patient, use of mirtazapine to exploit its potential increased appetite and sedation side effects should be considered.

42. **(C)** TCAs produce several cardiovascular side effects, the most significant being a quinidine-like effect slowing cardiac conduction. Some clinicians avoid TCAs if there are any ECG changes. Certainly, if there are changes in conduction, such as a prolonged QT interval, widening of the QRS complex, or AV conduction abnormalities, TCAs should be avoided. In overdose, they can produce heart block, widen the QRS complex, cause a bundle branch block, and cause tachyarrhythmias; however, even at therapeutic concentrations, they may have adverse effects on cardiac conduction. TCAs may be used in patients with prior cerebral infarctions. Amlodipine and estrogen replacement are not contraindications. TCAs may exacerbate urinary retention from anticholinergic effects but this is not a contraindication.

43. **(E)** This patient is likely delirious and prompt identification and treatment of the underlying cause is indicated. To help control the agitation that may accompany delirium, low-dose haloperidol is frequently used. Haloperidol does not treat the delirium, however. It is used most frequently because it is the most potent of the typical antipsychotics, therefore, requiring

lower doses with fewer anticholinergic or orthostatic side effects. Additionally, low-potency agents such as chlorpromazine or thioridazine are not only associated with orthostatic hypotension and anticholinergic side effects but also with prolongation of the QT interval. Olanzapine is not used in the intensive care setting partly because it is not available in a parenteral form. Lorazepam may help sedate the patient but it will not help his psychosis.

44. **(A)** Of the typical neuroleptics listed (haloperidol, perphenazine, and thioridazine), haloperidol is the most potent and has the least activity at alpha1-receptors. Therefore, it is the least likely to cause orthostatic hypotension. The atypical agents listed (risperidone and quetiapine) have activity at alpha1-receptors and are both associated with orthostatic hypotension.

45. **(D)** The metabolism of ethyl alcohol involves a two-step enzymatic process. The first enzyme, alcohol dehydrogenase, metabolizes ethanol to acetaldehyde, which is quickly metabolized by aldehyde dehydrogenase. Disulfiram inhibits aldehyde dehydrogenase resulting in an accumulation of acetaldehyde. Acetaldehyde causes facial flushing, tachycardia, hypotension, nausea and vomiting, and physical discomfort. Therefore, a patient on disulfiram has an incentive to remain abstinent. Obviously, disulfiram works only if patients continue to take it. Metronidazole is an antibiotic that has a disulfiram-like reaction but is not used for this purpose. Flumazenil is a benzodiazepine antagonist. Fluoxetine does not sensitize against alcohol use. Naloxone is an opioid antagonist.

46. **(C)** Multiple neurotransmitter systems have been investigated in attempts to control alcohol cravings. One system that may play a role is the opioid system. Naltrexone is an opioid antagonist that has been shown to decrease the number of days a person with alcohol dependence drinks and to increase the time before relapse of heavy drinking. Treatment of depression with an agent such as fluoxetine or bupropion may help control drinking if a comorbid depression exists but use of antidepressants in the absence of a mood disorder has not been

effective. Disulfiram is an alcohol-sensitizing agent. Diazepam is a benzodiazepine that may treat withdrawal symptoms but has not been shown to decrease cravings.

47. **(B)** This patient is likely suffering from PTSD. Several studies have found that SSRIs were useful in reducing the numbing symptoms of PTSD. In one trial with rape victims, fluoxetine reduced symptoms of reexperiencing, avoidance or numbing, and hyperarousal. Further double-blind controlled trials are needed to confirm these findings. Benzodiazepines have not been useful for these symptoms. Antipsychotics such as thioridazine have generally not been useful, although some clinicians are beginning to try the atypical neuroleptics. Anticonvulsants are not routinely used but some studies found that carbamazepine reduced the reexperiencing and arousal symptoms. Naltrexone, an opioid antagonist, has not been extensively studied in PTSD.

48. **(E)** Open-label trials of the antiadrenergic agent clonidine (an alpha2-adrenergic agonist) have demonstrated decreases in symptoms of reexperiencing and hyperarousal. Double-blind controlled trials are needed to confirm these findings.

49. **(C)** Elderly patients can be sensitive to the adverse effects of benzodiazepines. This patient is taking 8 mg/day of lorazepam, which is a large dose. Slowly tapering the lorazepam while investigating other causes of delirium is a reasonable first step. A digoxin level might be useful because high levels of digoxin can affect mental status. Hydrochlorothiazide levels are not measured.

50. **(D)** This patient may be suffering from Alzheimer dementia. He has clear cognitive decline and, although reversible causes of cognitive impairment should be investigated, there is no indication that any reversible cause is present. Two cholinesterase inhibitors have been approved for use in Alzheimer dementia: donepezil and tacrine (Cognex). There does not appear to be an indication for fluoxetine in this patient. Aspirin or trazodone will not improve cognitive

ability. Pemoline is a stimulant that does not appear to be indicated in this case.

51. **(A)** Trazodone is a serotonergic agent frequently used in the elderly to help with sleep and in turn may help this patient's occasional wandering behavior. It can cause orthostatic hypotension and should therefore be used with caution in those with risk factors for bleeding. Benzodiazepines should generally be used with caution in the elderly. They may actually make behavior worse and may contribute to delirium. If necessary, starting doses should be much lower than recommended. Chlorpromazine and haloperidol are neuroleptics that should also be used carefully in the elderly. Chlorpromazine, a low-potency neuroleptic, has substantial side effects including extrapyramidal symptoms and anticholinergic properties that may exacerbate other problems such as urinary retention and confusion. Haloperidol is a high-potency neuroleptic that may cause substantial extrapyramidal symptoms. Additionally, elderly patients may develop TD much more rapidly than younger patients might.

52. **(E)** Patients who present with altered levels of consciousness need to be medically managed, evaluated, and treated for several reversible causes. These include hypoglycemia, opioid overdose, and alcohol intoxication. Airway protection and monitoring of air exchange and cardiovascular status are required. Several treatments that should be immediately considered include IV dextrose, usually D_{50}, to treat hypoglycemia; thiamine to guard against the development of Wernicke-Korsakoff syndrome when giving the dextrose to an alcoholic patient with thiamine deficiency; and naloxone, an opioid antagonist, to reverse the effects of opioid intoxication. Flumazenil is a benzodiazepine antagonist that should not be used before obtaining further history because it may theoretically lower the seizure threshold.

53. **(A)** Detoxification from heroin can usually be managed with clonidine. Clonidine, a central alpha2-agonist, suppresses the sympathetic response to the heroin withdrawal and helps to

control agitation and autonomic instability, such as elevated blood pressure and heart rate, seen in opioid withdrawal. It does not take away heroin craving. Some centers use methadone for heroin withdrawal but some authors advise against methadone for detoxification in patients who have never detoxified before because of the success of clonidine detoxification. Propranolol is not used for heroin detoxification. Naloxone would not be appropriate beyond the initial resuscitation efforts. Benzodiazepines may be helpful as adjuncts to control anxiety, but they are not sufficient.

54. **(B)** Bupropion (Wellbutrin, Zyban) is an antidepressant that has been shown to be effective as part of a smoking cessation program. The mechanism of action is unclear, but it is believed to have an affect on dopaminergic transmission. Giving up cigarettes may be extremely difficult for a patient who is also suffering from major depression; however, starting bupropion during the depression may help her to quit smoking after she has recovered from her depression.

55. **(B)** Several TCAs have been used to treat chronic pain, including amitriptyline and nortriptyline. Using such an antidepressant in this patient may have the added benefit of reducing the chronic pain. However, TCAs, as compared with SSRIs, are more lethal in overdose and generally have more side effects, particularly anticholinergic and cardiovascular. SSRIs may play a role in chronic pain management so as a first-line therapy they are a better choice.

56. **(D)** Gabapentin is an anticonvulsant that has been reported to be modestly effective in bipolar disorder as well as in neuropathic pain disorders, although it is important to note that it has not been approved for bipolar disorder. Gabapentin has not been studied as extensively as lithium, valproic acid, or even carbamazepine; however, it has been shown to be more efficacious than placebo in a few studies. Additionally, it has been used to treat neuropathic pain, such as trigeminal neuralgia. In this patient, who is demonstrating hypomanic

symptoms, it could potentially treat both disorders.

57. **(C)** Weight gain is a side effect of most neuroleptic medications, traditional and atypical; however, it has been particularly troubling for olanzapine. For most patients, the weight gain can be modest (5–15 lb), but for some it can be particularly troubling, necessitating discontinuation of the medication. Elevated prolactin is a side effect of typical antipsychotics and less common with olanzapine. Agranulocytosis is a rare side effect of clozapine. Olanzapine is likely to cause sedation and is usually administered in the evening. As an antipsychotic with mood-stabilizing properties, it is useful for both psychotic disorders and bipolar disorder. Olanzapine is not associated with increased excitability or cataracts.

58. **(B)** The patient is a good candidate for Risperdal Consta. He responds favorably to and tolerates oral risperidone; however, he suffers exacerbations due to poor compliance. Depot haloperidol is not as good a choice given his positive response to risperidone and greater likelihood of TD. Continuing his current regimen or switching to another oral atypical such as olanzapine will likely only lead to a continuation of the vicious cycle of relapse. As he is not treatment refractory, clozaril is not appropriate in this case.

59. **(D)** Risperidone is an atypical antipsychotic agent that has potent 5-HT_{2a} antagonist properties as well as D_2 antagonism and alpha1-adrenergic blocking activity. Because of the alpha1-blocking activity, it may cause orthostatic hypotension. It may cause weight gain not weight loss. Unlike clozapine, hematologic effects do not require routine monitoring. It does not cause significant anticholinergic effects.

60. **(A)** Atypical antipsychotic agents, like clozapine and risperidone, are considered atypical because of their decreased propensity for causing extrapyramidal side effects and presumably a reduced risk of TD. Unfortunately, only clozapine appears to truly obey this rule. The other atypical antipsychotic agents all appear to have some degree of extrapyramidal side

effects. Risperidone seems to have the greatest propensity for extrapyramidal side effects and at doses greater than 6 mg/day may cause extrapyramidal side effects comparable to haloperidol.

61. **(B)** Antipsychotic agents, in addition to blocking dopamine receptors in the nigrostriatal system (causing extrapyramidal symptoms) and the mesolimbic system (decreasing hallucinations), may also block dopamine in the tuberoinfundibular system, thereby, increasing prolactin levels and causing galactorrhea especially in women. Risperidone may raise prolactin levels 100-fold. Olanzapine has not been demonstrated to raise prolactin levels significantly.

62. **(E)** Yohimbine, used to treat impotence, can cause elevated blood pressure and heart rate and should not be used by patients with cardiac or renal disease, glaucoma, or a history of ulcers. In fact, paroxetine and citalopram are antidepressants that can cause impotence. Molindone is an antipsychotic. Diphenhydramine is an antihistamine.

63. **(E)** Clonidine is a centrally acting alpha2-agonist. In contrast, yohimbine is an alpha2-antagonist. Clonidine decreases norepinephrine by stimulating the alpha2-autoreceptor. Yohimbine increases norepinephrine by blocking the alpha2-autoreceptor.

64. **(D)** Benzodiazepines are considered the first-line agents for the treatment of primary insomnia. Short-acting agents such as temazepam are useful in helping patients fall asleep and not remaining drowsy the next day. Diphenhydramine and trazodone are often used for insomnia and are effective medications. However, these can leave patients feeling drowsy the next day. Clozapine and amitriptyline are sedating but have serious side effects and should not be used for primary insomnia.

65. **(A)** Fluvoxamine is an SSRI. As a group, the SSRIs have fewer side effects and are safer than the tricyclics and the monoamine oxidase (MAO) "a" inhibitors. Fluvoxamine, imipramine, and

phenelzine have all been shown to be effective in the treatment of panic disorder. The first-line agents are the SSRIs because of their better side effect profile. Bupropion, an antidepressant with a dopaminergic mechanism, and deprenyl, an MAO "b" inhibitor, have both been shown to be ineffective in the treatment of panic disorder.

66. **(A)** The TCAs have been shown to increase mortality in cardiac patients because of their quinidine-like effects and tendency to increase heart rate and decrease blood pressure. Sertraline is safe for patients with cardiac disease and affords the fewest drug-drug interactions of the SSRIs. As a class, the amphetamines have been found to be safe in patients with cardiac illness. There may be minor changes in blood pressure and pulse; patients should be monitored closely. Bupropion is safe in cardiac patients. Venlafaxine can increase the blood pressure an average of 8–10 mm Hg but this effect is dose related. At doses less than 150 mg qd, clinically significant changes are relatively rare. Doses above 300 mg/day are the highest risk but most patients tolerate this dose without increases in blood pressure.

67. **(C)** Haloperidol's mechanism of action is dopamine receptor blockade (D_2). Dopamine inhibits prolactin secretion. Because haloperidol prevents dopamine from binding to the dopamine receptor, prolactin secretion is unopposed. The symptoms the patient is experiencing are common effects of elevated prolactin levels. Haloperidol does not increase ACTH, serotonin, or dopamine levels to clinically significant levels and the symptoms described are not associated with ACTH, serotonin, or dopamine.

68. **(B)** This patient most likely has akathisia, which is a neuroleptic-induced side effect. Patients generally experience subjective feelings of restlessness and can be seen swinging their legs, rocking back and forth while sitting, pacing, and rapidly alternating between sitting and standing. Acute dystonias are characterized by contraction of muscles resulting in abnormal movements or postures, such as spasms of the jaw, abnormal positioning of the

head, or difficulty swallowing. The onset of acute dystonia usually develops within the first week of initiating a neuroleptic medication. NMS is a life-threatening complication involving muscle rigidity and dystonia as well as autonomic symptoms such as elevated temperature, increased heart rate, and increased blood pressure. Akathisia can sometimes be mistaken for anxiety or mania, but in this case there are no other signs (such as delusions of grandeur, decreased need for sleep, increased energy, or hypersexuality) to indicate a manic episode. There is no evidence of OCD, feeling as though one must always be in motion is not a compulsion.

69. **(E)** When starting a patient on antipsychotic medication (neuroleptics), the most important consideration is the side effects the patient will experience. Compliance with medication is usually a major issue and there is a general tendency to want to "get off on the right foot." Renal function is less important with neuroleptics because they are cleared principally by the liver. The presence of negative symptoms may steer a clinician toward the atypical antipsychotics but today these are often chosen because of their superior side effect profile. Gender and onset of action do not typically guide the choice of neuroleptic.

70. **(D)** Lithium and valproic acid are indicated as first-line agents for the treatment of bipolar manic episodes. Antipsychotic agents like chlorpromazine are important for the treatment of psychosis, sometimes associated with mania, but are not considered effective as single agents. Fluoxetine is an antidepressant that may actually activate patients with bipolar disorder and precipitate a manic episode. Ideally, all medications should be discontinued during pregnancy, but in many instances they are necessary. Considering the risk-benefit ratio is important. Low-potency antipsychotics (chlorpromazine), lithium, and valproic acid are all associated with an increased risk of congenital abnormalities, especially when taken during the first trimester. The benzodiazepines are associated with an increased risk for oral clefts after first-trimester exposure. However, this

remains controversial. ECT has been used in pregnancy for more than 50 years and its safety and efficacy is well documented.

71. **(B)** Cessation or a reduction in sedative, hypnotic, or anxiolytic medications that have been used heavily or for a prolonged period of time may result in a withdrawal syndrome characterized by symptoms that develop within hours to a few days after cessation or reduction. Autonomic hyperactivity, orthostatic hypotension, muscle weakness, tremor, insomnia, nausea, vomiting, auditory/visual/ tactile hallucinations, agitation, or anxiety may occur. By far, the most serious sequelae are grand mal seizures or delirium. As many as 75% of patients may experience grand mal seizures on the second or third day of withdrawal and two-thirds of these patients have more than one seizure. Delirium may develop between the third and eight day of withdrawal. Minor symptoms may persist for up to 2 weeks.

72. **(D)** Serious chronic alcoholics often take in calories from little else besides alcohol and are thus at risk for thiamine deficiency. If a thiamine-deficient patient is given food, he or she can develop Wernicke encephalopathy from the body's attempts to metabolize glucose in the absence of thiamine pyrophosphate. Although the other choices are important concerns, none are of the acute significance of thiamine deficiency.

73. **(A)** This man is probably suffering from alcohol withdrawal. Benzodiazepines and alcohol have near identical modes of action in their modulation of GABA receptors in the brain. This similarity makes benzodiazepines a sensible and popular choice for treatment of alcohol withdrawal. Much less commonly (although more common in the distant past), barbiturates (which also act on GABA) and clonidine (which modulates autonomic instability) are used. Phenytoin is not used and disulfiram is used to encourage alcohol abstinence by its inhibition of aldehyde dehydrogenase.

74. **(C)** In cases of suspected liver impairment, it is advisable to use a benzodiazepine minimally

metabolized by the liver of which there are two: lorazepam and oxazepam. Other benzodiazepines, such as those listed, are mostly metabolized by the liver and could thus quickly build to toxic levels. Phenobarbital and clonidine are no longer used to treat alcohol withdrawal.

75–79. [75 (F), 76 (I), 77 (C), 78 (B), 79 (I)] Psychiatric drugs can have serious side effects, some of which are the subjects of "black box" warnings on prescribing information packets. Pimozide is known to interact with a number of medications including citalopram. Although haloperidol, perphenazine, ziprasidone, and clozapine are all antipsychotics used to treat schizophrenia, only clozapine is a member of the class of newer atypical antipsychotics known to cause hyperglycemia and lead to the development of diabetes. After a controversial set of hearings on the subject of children and antidepressants in the United Kingdom and United States in 2003 and 2004, regulators decided there was enough evidence to show that some of the SSRIs, including paroxetine, may increase the risk of suicidal thoughts in children. Although lithium, carbamazepine, divalproex sodium, and gabapentin are all used to treat bipolar disorder, only valproic acid carries a warning of an increased risk of pancreatitis. Finally, although carbamazepine and clozapine can both cause agranulocytosis, the only one of these drugs that would be used primarily for schizophrenia is clozapine.

80–84. [80 (D), 81 (E), 82 (H), 83 (C), 84 (G)] Although fluoxetine, trazodone, paroxetine, citalopram, and sertraline are all antidepressants, paroxetine is the only such medication with a short enough half-life that it produces a significant withdrawal syndrome after just 2 days. Haloperidol, clozapine, risperidone, and olanzapine are all useful in the treatment of schizophrenia, but only haloperidol and risperidone, of these choices, are available in a depot injection. Risperidone is preferable because it is an atypical with a better side effect profile. Lithium and divalproex sodium are both used to treat bipolar disorder, but it is lithium that causes nephrogenic diabetes insipidus, which is suggested by

question 82. Finally, alprazolam is an effective sleeping aid but it is wise to avoid using it and other benzodiazepines in a patient with a history of alcoholism because of the affinity of such drugs to the GABA receptors implicated in alcohol dependence. Trazodone, an antidepressant, is an effective sleeping aid that is not habit forming. Olanzapine has been shown to increase cholesterol levels in about 10% of patients after 14 weeks of treatment.

85. **(D)** The recommended length of treatment of a first episode of unipolar depression is at least 6 months and usually on the scale of 8–12 months, and possibly longer, depending on patient factors such as family history of mood disorder, severity and duration of the depressive episode, and comorbid psychiatric symptoms such as anxiety and substance abuse. Discontinuation within the first 16 weeks of treatment is associated with a high risk of relapse.

86. **(A)** Bupropion is the one antidepressant listed that does not cause sexual dysfunction. Fluvoxamine, fluoxetine, and citalopram are all SSRIs that have been reported to cause varying degrees of sexual dysfunction. Clomipramine is a TCA that has a greater incidence of sexual dysfunction than other TCAs, possibly due to its potent serotonin reuptake inhibiting properties.

87. **(C)** Sialorrhea is a common side effect of treatment with clozapine. It can be extremely bothersome to the patient and others but does not usually require discontinuation of treatment. Often, behavioral measures are sufficient, such as the use of lozenges or placing a towel on the patient's pillow at night. Anticholinergic agents such as propylthiouracil often help to reduce the volume of saliva. Propranolol is useful in the treatment of akathisia and amantadine may be helpful in the treatment of parkinsonian symptoms.

88. **(D)** Patients on clozapine often develop a persistent sinus tachycardia that does not require cessation of treatment. Often, the tachycardia resolves without necessitating further intervention; however, should it persist, it may be treated with the beta-antagonist propranolol.

Clozapine has significant alpha-receptor blockage, which often causes orthostatic hypotension, requiring a gradual titration of the dose. Because of this, labetalol would not be appropriate as it may exacerbate this side effect. Benztropine is an anticholinergic agent that will not help the tachycardia. There is no reason to check creatinine phosphokinase levels, which might be expected to be high in NMS.

89. **(B)** This patient presents with signs and symptoms suggestive of a first manic episode. Lithium and divalproex sodium remain the mainstay of initial and maintenance treatment of bipolar I disorder. The use of anticonvulsants such as gabapentin and topiramate are being utilized for bipolar disorder but they are not drugs of first choice. Neuroleptics, such as haloperidol, and benzodiazepines, such as clonazepam, may be used with lithium or divalproex sodium initially; however, they are not routinely used as maintenance treatment.

90. **(E)** The neurovegetative symptoms can be remembered by a mnemonic, **SIGECAPS**, developed by Dr Carey Gross: **S**leep disorder, **I**nterest deficit (anhedonia), **G**uilt, **E**nergy deficit, **C**oncentration deficit, **A**ppetite disorder, **P**sychomotor retardation, and **S**uicidality. Such symptoms tend to respond first with antidepressant treatment. This is why it is a common wisdom in psychiatry that the person who begins to recover from depression may be at greater risk for suicide than when he is at the height of his depression. As he starts to function better physiologically, he may be more capable of carrying out a suicidal impulse.

91. **(A)** All of the second-generation antipsychotics have a lower incidence of TD when compared to the typical antipsychotics. Although they all have warnings regarding the increased risk of diabetes and hyperlipidemia (metabolic syndrome), they are believed to cause it at different rates, so this is often a factor in choosing a particular antipsychotic medications. The least likely are aripiprazole and ziprasidone followed by risperidone and quetiapine. The most likely are olanzapine and clozapine.

92. **(A)** The need for increasing amounts of a drug to achieve the same effect or a diminishing effect achieved through the use of the same amount of a drug describes *tolerance*. *Withdrawal* is a syndrome of behavioral, emotional, and physiologic signs and symptoms that occur in a setting of the discontinuation of a drug. Dependence and abuse both require more history and clinical information than is offered in this question. *Dependence* on a drug requires that its use causes significant impairment, anguish, or devastation to the individual and, despite this, the patient continues using. The presence of withdrawal on discontinuation and tolerance frequently help make a diagnosis of substance dependence. *Abuse* is similar in that use causes significant problems for the patient, but use of the drug is generally more infrequent than is found in dependence and consequently does not involve tolerance and withdrawal symptoms.

92. **(D)** The patient is currently suffering from a major depressive episode but her significant family history of bipolar is likely to increase her risk for mania as well. Antidepressants such as venlafaxine or even ECT may provoke a manic episode in vulnerable patients. Lamotrigine, an antiseizure medication, has been approved and recommended for the treatment of bipolar depression. Although atypical antipsychotics (e.g., aripiprazole) and mood stabilizers (e.g., carbamazepine) may also be used, they are not likely to be as effective as lamotrigine in monotherapy for depression.

93. **(A)** All of the second-generation antipsychotics have a lower incidence of TD when compared to the typical antipsychotics. Although they all have warnings regarding the increased risk of diabetes and hyperlipidemia (metabolic syndrome), they are believed to cause it at different rates so this is often a factor in choosing a particular antipsychotic medications. The least likely are aripiprazole and ziprasidone followed by risperidone and quetiapine. The most likely are olanzapine and clozapine.

94. **(D)** ECT has relatively few contraindications and in some cases is preferred for its rapid

onset of action. However, because of the cardiovascular effects of ECT, a history of a recent MI (within the past 6 months) is a relative contraindication. Another relative contraindication is the presence of a clinically significant intracranial space-occupying lesion because of the risk of brain stem herniation. ECT may be performed during pregnancy. The most common complaints patients have following ECT are impairments in both anterograde and retrograde memory. Although most memory problems resolve, some may persist indefinitely.

95. **(A)** Atypical, or second-generation, antipsychotics are being used first line in the treatment of schizophrenia. While they are likely at least as effective as typical neuroleptics for the positive symptoms of schizophrenia (hallucinations, delusions, paranoia, disorganization), they are believed to be more effective for the negative symptoms (such as anhedonia, amotivation, flat affect, etc). The newer antipsychotics can also cause significant weight gain in some patients. Only clozapine has been demonstrated to reduce suicidality in individuals with schizophrenia.

96. **(A)** Beginning quetiapine at a low dose and gradually increasing while simultaneously tapering haloperidol (a cross-taper) is the most appropriate switching strategy. Starting at the target dose may cause significant side effects such as sedation and orthostasis, which may lead to poor compliance. Discontinuing the haloperidol completely or tapering it before the quetiapine is at a therapeutic level may lead to a relapse or worsening of psychotic symptoms.

97. **(E)** A subjective feeling of restlessness and a need to constantly move about and pace is known as *akathisia*, a common side effect of neuroleptic medication that can occur soon after such medications are started. The other choices listed are also neuroleptic side effects. *Parkinsonism* refers to symptoms evoked by neuroleptics that are commonly seen in Parkinson disease. Parkinsonian symptoms include tremor (a 3–6-cycle/second motion), akinesia (or bradykinesia), and rigidity.

Dystonias are uncontrolled muscle contractions. *TD* is a rhythmic, involuntary movement of the tongue, jaw, trunk, or extremities appearing months to years after the initiation of neuroleptic therapy.

98. **(D)** Although there are various side effects of lamotrigine, the most dangerous is that of a severe rash, which can develop into Stevens-Johnson syndrome. Beginning at a low dose and slowly tapering reduces the risk significantly. Aplastic anemia is a rare side effect of carbamazepine. Hypertension can occur in higher doses of venlafaxine. Short-term memory loss is not uncommon after receiving ECT. TD is a long-term side effect of antipsychotics although much less likely with newer medications such as aripiprazole.

99. **(A)** All of these are types of dystonic reactions that are induced by the use of neuroleptics. *Opisthotonos*, also known as *arc de cercle*, is a spasm of the neck and back that causes the patient to arch forward. *Torticollis* is a spasm of the neck muscles that usually brings the neck to one side or another but can also pull forward or backward. *Pleurothotonos*, also known as *Pisa syndrome*, is a leaning posture induced by the spasm of the torso muscles. *Oculogyric crisis* is simply the spasm of the extraocular muscles. The most alarming of these dystonias is *laryngospasm*, which is the spasm of the muscles controlling the tongue and the throat. This can lead to respiratory distress.

100. **(B)** Although any of the listed antidepressants will treat her depression adequately, only duloxetine, a combined serotonin-norepinephrine reuptake inhibitor, which has demonstrated efficacy in and been approved in the treatment of both depression *and* diabetic neuropathy. Given her major depressive disorder, reassurance would not be appropriate or efficacious.

101. **(A)** With the exception of mirtazapine, bupropion, and nefazodone, the antidepressants all can cause significant sexual dysfunction, including decreased libido, erectile dysfunction, and anorgasmia. Given the recurrent nature of his illness, no treatment would likely lead to a

relapse of his major depression, and restarting sertraline would be likely to cause the same problems and lead to noncompliance.

102. **(C)** *Satyriasis* is a man's insatiable need for sexual gratification. *Hypervigilance* is often used in anxiety disorders and is simply an increased awareness of internal or external stimuli. *Hypermnesia* is the ability to recall detailed material that is not usually available to recall. *Sexual sadism* and *sexual masochism* are deriving sexual pleasure from causing or receiving mental or physical abuse respectively.

103. **(B)** *Priapism* is a painful, prolonged erection that can be seen as an uncommon side effect of trazodone in men. *Parapraxis*, a slip of the tongue, is also known as a *Freudian slip*. *Nymphomania* is insatiable sexual desire in a woman and *satyriasis* is its counterpart in men. *Libido* refers to sexual energy.

104. **(A)** Sexual dysfunction (e.g., decreased libido, erectile dysfunction, anorgasmia) is not uncommonly seen with SSRIs and other antidepressants in the treatment of depression. Many other psychotropic medications such as antipsychotics or lithium may also cause sexual dysfunction. Bupropion is one of the few antidepressants, which causes little to no sexual dysfunction, and, in fact, it has been found to reverse the side effect when added to treatment.

105. **(D)** Given the time it takes for antidepressant medications to become effective, ECT is considered the treatment of choice when rapid antidepressant action is desired (e.g., refusal to eat/drink, severe suicidality, catatonia). There are no absolute contraindications and it is very safe during pregnancy as well. The other antidepressants have not been proven safe in pregnancy and cognitive-behavior therapy alone would not be appropriate for treating a severe depression disorder.

106–109. [106 **(F)**, 107 **(J)**, 108 **(A)**, 109 **(D)**] *Inhalants* **(A)** are volatile substances that have rapid-onset intoxicating effects. *Withdrawal* **(B)** is a set of signs and symptoms, physical and psychiatric, that are associated with drug cessation.

Tolerance **(C)** is the need for higher doses of a drug needed for intoxication. *Abuse* **(D)** is drug use in spite of adverse consequences related to the substance. *Dependence* **(E)** is a physical or psychological need to continue taking a drug. *Formication* **(F)** is the feeling of bugs crawling on the skin. *Intoxication* **(G)** is represented by behavioral, cognitive, or perceptual changes taken in relationship to drug ingestion. *Hallucinogens* **(H)** are a group of drugs administered by various routes that cause perceptual changes. *Posthallucinogen perception disorder* **(I)** is also known as a flashback. It is characterized by a distressing return of perceptual changes without the ingestion of hallucinogens. *Amotivational syndrome* **(J)** is a lack of drive or motivation usually associated with drug use, especially marijuana. Marijuana has its own classification in the *Diagnostic and Statistical Manual of Mental Disorders, Fourth Edition, Text Revision* (DSM-IV-TR), cannabis **(K)**, and is not considered among the hallucinogens.

110–121. [110 **(I)**, 111 **(P)**, 112 **(Q)**, 113 **(B)**, 114 **(L)**, 115 **(N)**, 116 **(G)**, 117 **(R)**, 118 **(J)**, 119 **(M)**, 120 **(H)**, 121 **(K)**] Antipsychotics, also known as neuroleptics, can cause a wide variety of side effects. These side effects can be broken down into some of the following categories for an easier approach. The dopaminergic side effects include those that are due to the blockade of the natural dopamine inhibition of prolactin release from the anterior pituitary causing *galactorrhea* (lactation; **A**) and *gynecomastia* (breast development; **I**). The dopaminergic side effects also include those that arise from the dopamine blockade in the basal ganglia causing extrapyramidal and other side effects such as *blepharospasm* (spasm of the eyelids; **C**), *opisthotonos* (spasm of the neck and back causing an arched posture; **D**), and *torticollis* (spasm of the sternocleidomastoid; **E**). The blockade of D_2 receptors in the basal ganglia can also cause *pseudoparkinsonism disorder* **(L)** resembling Parkinson disease, characterized by muscle rigidity and a short festinating gait, and *TD* **(N)**, a disorder of abnormal involuntary movements caused by prolonged use of neuroleptics. *Akathisia* (subjective or observable restlessness; **M**) and *rabbit syndrome* (rapid movement of the lips; **F**) are also highly distressing side effects related to the dopaminergic system.

Another side effect that can be caused, especially by high-potency neuroleptics such as haloperidol, is *NMS* (**G**). This is characterized by hyperthermia, change in mental status, and increased muscle tone. It can lead to renal failure following dehydration and a rise in muscle breakdown products (creatine kinase levels are typically elevated), pulmonary complications, and death.

Clozapine and chlorpromazine can both cause *agranulocytosis* (**B**), a dangerous side effect that sometimes produces symptoms of sore throat and fever. The drug must be stopped immediately. *Constipation* (**O**) is a complicating side effect of some antipsychotics with anticholinergic effects. This troublesome side effect can often be relieved with use of a laxative. *Orthostatic hypotension* (**K**), a drop in blood pressure while standing, is a side effect from alpha1-adrenergic blockade. This is especially troublesome with chlorpromazine and clozapine and is best handled by raising doses slowly. *Obstructive jaundice* (**H**) is rare and occurs mainly with chlorpromazine. Symptoms are fever, nausea, malaise, and pruritus. *Pigmented retinopathy* (**J**) is observed with uses of high doses of thioridazine and is best detected with a good ophthalmologic examination. Another side effect that can decrease compliance with antipsychotics is *retrograde ejaculation* (**P**). Orgasm may be achieved but ejaculation is abnormal with retrograde propulsion of the semen.

Double depression (**Q**) occurs when a major depressive episode is superimposed on dysthymic disorder. It is thought to affect as many as 40% of patients with MDD and to carry a poorer prognosis. *Kindling* (**R**), based on a model of neural activity in which repeated subthreshold stimulation of a given neuron results in discharge of an action potential, is a theory that suggests that one decompensation can lead to a second episode.

122. (**C**) In the CNS, GABA is an inhibitory neurotransmitter. At the postsynaptic GABA-A receptor, GABA facilitates chloride ion influx into a cell via a chloride channel resulting in inhibition of that neuron. Alcohol and benzodiazepines both allosterically modulate the GABA-A receptor to facilitate GABAergic inhibition. Abrupt removal of alcohol or benzodiazepines after prolonged use results in a relative deficit of GABAergic inhibition, which can lead to anxiety, insomnia, delirium, and seizures. GABA-B is the site of action of the muscle relaxant baclofen. Alcohol does not act at the dopamine or serotonin receptors.

GABA -B → Baclofen   GABA A balcohol

123. (**C**) Alcohol withdrawal can take the form of minor withdrawal symptoms such as tremulousness, withdrawal seizures, or withdrawal delirium, formerly known as delirium tremens. Minor withdrawal symptoms can last for several days. Withdrawal seizures are rarely focal and usually occur within 48 hours after alcohol consumption ceases. Delirium tremens most often occurs within 96 hours of cessation of drinking; therefore, 5 days is the most correct response.

CHAPTER 5

Psychological Treatment and Management
Questions

DIRECTIONS (Questions 1 through 42): Each of the numbered items in this section is followed by answer choices. Select the ONE lettered answer or completion that is BEST in each case.

Questions 1 and 2

A 34-year-old married man comes into your office complaining of being "overcome" with discrete episodes of palpitations, sweating, shortness of breath, "choking," abdominal discomfort, and feelings of impending doom. He goes on to say that he was a football player in high school and was never scared of anything. Now, he says, he is starting to avoid driving for fear of being locked in the car when he has one of these "attacks" and not being able to get out. All of his friends say that he is "losing it," and he wants to know if you think he is.

1. What would be the most appropriate response?

   (A) "Yes, you are."
   (B) "No, you are not."
   (C) "Why do you want to know?"
   (D) "What do you think?"
   (E) Ask him what he means by "losing it."

2. He goes on to say that he will not take medication for these episodes. What therapy is generally most effective in treating panic disorder?

   (A) psychodynamic psychotherapy
   (B) cognitive-behavioral therapy
   (C) couples therapy
   (D) family therapy
   (E) paradoxical therapy

3. A 43-year-old man is chastised at work. When he comes home, his friend asks him how his day went. He responds angrily saying that a "real friend wouldn't be so nosy." What is the name of this defense mechanism?

   (A) denial
   (B) displacement
   (C) isolation of affect
   (D) intellectualization
   (E) humor

4. A 20-year-old woman diagnosed with borderline personality disorder thinks of her therapist as "the best person in the world." The next week, the therapist announces that he will be going on vacation. The patient then says that he is "the worst person in the world." What is the defense mechanism that allows people to see others as either all good or all bad?

   (A) splitting
   (B) intellectualization
   (C) repression
   (D) devaluation
   (E) idealization

5. A 16-year-old boy has just lost his mother and father in a car accident. In your office, he talks philosophically about death and its implications. When asked how he feels about his parents' death, he responds by saying that "it is the nature of things to pass away." This patient's inability to talk directly of his emotional experience concerning personal losses is an example of which defense mechanism?

(A) lying
(B) projection
(C) intellectualization
(D) denial
(E) suppression

Questions 6 and 7

A 44-year-old woman with schizophrenia is struggling with paranoia, auditory hallucinations, and delusions. She lives with her mother but has a poor relationship with her. She tells you that everyone wants her to spend a lot of money and buy drugs.

6. Which of the following would be the best response?

(A) "Well, deciding for yourself is best."
(B) "If you buy drugs, I'll call the police."
(C) "Perhaps we should look at what your mother would think about that."
(D) "Why do you think everyone wants you to do that?"
(E) "No, they don't."

7. You decide that supportive therapy would be helpful to this patient. Which of the following is a goal of supportive therapy?

(A) personality change
(B) correcting faulty ideas
(C) the reestablishment of psychic homeostasis through the strengthening of defenses
(D) exploring the feeling of meaninglessness in life
(E) investigating the freedom of individuals

8. A 32-year-old psychiatry resident is in psychoanalysis. He is lying on the couch and saying whatever comes to mind. This is an example of what analytic technique?

(A) repression
(B) speakeasy
(C) countertransference
(D) transference
(E) free association

9. A psychotherapist finds herself getting angry at a patient after the patient reports beating up his little brother. The psychotherapist is exhibiting what phenomenon?

(A) countertransference
(B) transference
(C) resistance
(D) interpretation
(E) extinction

10. In an acute inpatient psychiatric ward, the resident psychiatrist is in charge of leading a group consisting of patients admitted to the ward. In the morning, she asks each patient in turn to comment on his or her goals for treatment. What is the name of this technique of group psychotherapy?

(A) go-around
(B) free association
(C) feedback
(D) interpretation
(E) resistance

Questions 11 and 12

A 29-year-old health professional entered group therapy wanting to know why he was unable to stay in a long-term relationship with a woman. A handsome man, he said that women found him attractive and he did not understand why he should restrict himself to one person. However, he was bored with the attention and felt empty inside. At work, he was very competitive with his male colleagues. In the group, members pointed out to him that whenever he was criticized by other men in the group, he made advances toward women in the group. These advances sometimes continued outside the group, but he lost interest when he felt better.

11. What is the name of this defense mechanism?

   (A) idealization
   (B) acting out
   (C) abreaction
   (D) ventilation
   (E) catharsis

12. Compared with inpatient groups, which of the following is a treatment objective most characteristic of outpatient groups?

   (A) crisis intervention
   (B) return to previous level of functioning
   (C) personality change and reconstruction
   (D) stabilization of psychotic symptoms
   (E) discussing current feelings regarding alcohol detoxification and heart disease

Questions 13 and 14

You have been assigned to lead various groups that help patients who suffer from personality disorders. To accomplish this task, you need to know which personality disorders are appropriate for group psychotherapy. In addition, you need to know which personality disorders benefit from combined individual and group psychotherapy.

13. Which of the following personality disorders is best treated with combined individual and group psychotherapy because of intense transferences and countertransference that develop in a single mode of treatment?

   (A) borderline personality disorder
   (B) avoidant personality disorder
   (C) schizotypal personality disorder
   (D) antisocial personality disorder
   (E) schizoid personality disorder

14. Patients with narcissistic personality disorder are best treated with combined individual and

group psychotherapy. Which of the following reasons is most consistent with why this is true?

   (A) Wounds to self-image while in the group can be examined supportively in individual therapy.
   (B) These patients need as much attention as they can get.
   (C) These patients deplore the attention of others and need exposure to overcome this.
   (D) These patients constantly believe others are conspiring against them.
   (E) These patients need much structure to occupy their time.

Questions 15 and 16

A 29-year-old woman has been depressed for 2 months prior to seeking medical attention. She believes that nobody likes her even though she is always cordial and there is nothing that she can do to change the way other people perceive her. She adamantly refuses to take antidepressants. You believe that cognitive therapy is indicated for this patient.

15. Which of the following cognitive profiles most reflects the profile seen in depression?

   (A) negative view of self, experience, and future
   (B) fear of being fat and unattractive
   (C) concern about serious, insidious medical disorders
   (D) view of others as biased, manipulative, and devious
   (E) fear of physical or psychological danger

16. According to cognitive psychology, what are automatic thoughts?

   (A) thoughts that impede free association
   (B) thoughts that cannot be changed
   (C) thoughts at the edge of conscious awareness that regularly precede unpleasant feelings
   (D) genetically determined thoughts
   (E) thoughts that every human ought to have

Questions 17 and 18

A 45-year-old man presents to the outpatient clinic handicapped by a fear of parking lots and fields. This fear started 4 months prior to this visit. At the beginning of cognitive therapy, he says that his behavior is constantly being scrutinized and criticized by other people. He says that he cannot change his behavior because if he does others will think that he is a fool.

17. What would be the most appropriate response from the therapist?

   (A) "That's silly. People will not think you are a fool."
   (B) "Yes, I can see that."
   (C) "What makes you think that others are constantly scrutinizing your behavior?"
   (D) "How can you possibly think other people care enough about you to constantly scrutinize your behavior?"
   (E) "Well, maybe you are a fool. Have you ever thought of that?"

18. Which of the following statements best describes the view of cognitive therapy regarding the role of cognition in psychiatric disorders?

   (A) Cognitive distortions are always the cause of various psychiatric syndromes.
   (B) Cognitive distortions are never the cause of various psychiatric syndromes.
   (C) Correcting cognitive distortions is always sufficient to correct symptomatology.
   (D) Although cognitive distortions are not necessarily the ultimate cause of psychiatric syndromes, correcting distortions can be an effective intervention in psychiatric syndromes.
   (E) Correcting cognitive distortions never completely alleviates symptoms.

Questions 19 and 20

An 18-year-old man presents to your office complaining that he cannot pass a movie theater without stopping, going inside, and buying candy. This behavior is troublesome to him and interferes with

his daily activities causing him to be constantly late to other appointments. You decide to help the patient with behavior therapy.

19. Which of the following does behavior therapy attempt to change?

   (A) maladaptive thoughts underlying a maladaptive behavior
   (B) neurobiology
   (C) how a patient perceives the environment
   (D) maladaptive behaviors seen in a particular syndrome
   (E) underlying conflicts in an attempt to change behavior

20. Which of the following best describes behavior therapy?

   (A) a long-term assessment of relational issues
   (B) a set of procedures designed to change maladaptive thoughts
   (C) a set of procedures designed to enhance the learning of adaptive behaviors and the unlearning of maladaptive behaviors
   (D) hypnosis
   (E) a technique used to resolve unconscious conflicts

21. A 39-year-old man presents to your office complaining of headaches, which you diagnose as tension headaches. As part of this patient's treatment, you decide to use behavior therapy. Which of the following behavior techniques is used in the reduction of tension headaches?

   (A) stress reduction
   (B) stimulus control
   (C) systematic desensitization
   (D) aversive stimuli
   (E) negative reinforcement

Questions 22 and 23

A 23-year-old woman broke up with her boyfriend of 8 months 1 month before presenting to your office complaining of depression. Currently, she is just starting to date someone else. Given that her episode meets criteria for a major depressive episode, you decide to use both medication and interpersonal psychotherapy.

22. Which of the following is the major focus of interpersonal psychotherapy?

    (A) character change
    (B) clarifying communication patterns
    (C) interpreting transference
    (D) hypnosis
    (E) pointing out resistance

23. Which of the following best represents the hypothesis on which interpersonal psycho-therapy rests?

    (A) In addition to any biological diathesis, certain interpersonal problems predispose one to depressive disorders, complicate their course, or interfere with recovery.
    (B) Unconscious conflicting psychic processes need to be resolved.
    (C) Maladaptive behaviors may be changed by examining cognitive errors.
    (D) Maladaptive behaviors may be changed by positive reinforcement.
    (E) Maladaptive behaviors may be changed through the power of suggestion.

Questions 24 and 25

A 22-year-old college student presents complaining of having no goals in life, not doing as well as he could in school, and desiring but having no serious long-term romantic relationship. He has not chosen a major and says that his indecision is paralyzing him from moving on with the rest of his life. After discussing various forms of psychotherapy with the patient, you recommend psychoanalysis and he agrees.

24. Why does it take four or five treatment sessions per week to have a successful analysis?

    (A) It is difficult for patients to sustain a transference and keep their defenses lowered with fewer sessions.
    (B) Analytic patients are more seriously mentally ill and therefore need more time.
    (C) Analytic patients are typically more seriously mentally ill and therefore need less time.
    (D) Analysis is based on a supportive model of therapy.
    (E) Analysis is a quick therapy.

25. What is the major tool of treatment in psycho-analysis?

    (A) interpretation of transference
    (B) altering maladaptive behaviors
    (C) altering cognitive errors
    (D) interpreting dreams
    (E) solving interpersonal problems

Questions 26 and 27

A 50-year-old man is in psychoanalysis because he feels ineffective in his professional and personal relationships.

26. Which of the following best defines the analytic term *dynamic*?

    (A) the notion that all mental phenomena are the result of a continual interaction of forces that oppose one another
    (B) the notion that mental phenomena reveal themselves at various levels in the psyche
    (C) the notion that personality and its subsequent development has a historical aspect
    (D) the notion that the psyche is organized into functional units called the id, ego, and superego
    (E) fun, interactive, and pleasant

27. How are dreams useful in psychoanalysis?

(A) Dreams are interpreted by the analyst to subliminally influence the minds of patients.

(B) Dreams are used to alter cognitive errors.

(C) Dreams provide information about psychic conflicts.

(D) Dreams are used to change behavior.

(E) Dreams represent the conscious framework for behavior.

Questions 28 and 29

You are seeing a 50-year-old man who suffers from generalized anxiety disorder for cognitive-behavioral therapy. He is having a hard time with the restructuring of maladaptive thoughts. You decide that hypnosis may be helpful as an adjunctive therapy for this patient.

28. Which of the following is most needed for a successful hypnosis?

(A) a skillful hypnotist

(B) a patient who is highly responsive to suggestion

(C) a quiet room

(D) a skilled induction technique

(E) creative ability

29. Hypnosis is best used as an adjunctive therapy within a psychotherapeutic relationship. In which of the following is hypnosis a relative contraindication?

(A) intractable hiccups

(B) anxiety disorders

(C) pain disorder

(D) treatment of warts (specifically verrucae planae juvenalis)

(E) psychotic disorders

Questions 30 and 31

A 14-year-old girl is brought by her mother to see you. The mother says that the patient has been depressed for the last year. You learn that 1 year ago, the patient's mother and father began divorce proceedings and are currently still living together. Also, 1 year ago, the patient's younger brother was born. You suspect that there are significant environmental stressors that are contributing to this patient's depression and decide that a trial of family therapy is warranted.

30. Family therapy is based on which of the following theories?

(A) Individual therapy is inappropriate for someone in a family.

(B) When families are dysfunctional, look for the individual who is causing the trouble.

(C) Families that live together fight together.

(D) The familial dynamic can help to explain individual psychopathology.

(E) Role playing can explore a patient's interpersonal relationships, personality makeup, and conflicts.

31. After further questioning, it becomes clear that the patient's mother is also depressed. Which of the following is the greatest risk factor for depression for women with chronic depression?

(A) marital status and satisfaction

(B) being single

(C) age over 30 years

(D) low income

(E) high-fat diet

Questions 32 and 33

A 9-year-old boy with attention deficit hyperactivity disorder (ADHD), predominantly hyperactive type, presents to your office accompanied by his mother. He is currently on methylphenidate (Ritalin) and they both wonder if there is something else that can be done to help the patient. You recommend behavior therapy.

32. Which of the following best illustrates how behavioral therapy would help this patient?

(A) reinforcing attention to various tasks necessary for learning and ignoring disruptive behaviors

(B) interpreting a transference

(C) positively reframing a negative experience

(D) focusing on the patient's interpersonal relationships

(E) focusing on maladaptive communication techniques in the family

33. Which of the following represents a behavioral tool that is helpful for patients with ADHD?

    (A) a well-timed interpretation of maladaptive behaviors

    (B) a report card of various behaviors that can be rewarded at home by parents

    (C) clozapine (Clozaril)

    (D) methylphenidate

    (E) positively reframing a negative experience

Questions 34 and 35

A 25-year-old man in his fourth year of medical school presents to your office complaining of not being able to remain in a relationship with a girlfriend for longer than 3 months. He says that he would like an insight-oriented therapy, and you agree that this form of therapy would help him. You decide to treat this patient with brief psychodynamic psychotherapy.

34. Which of the following factors best predicts a positive outcome with brief psychodynamic psychotherapy?

    (A) gender

    (B) age

    (C) motivation for change

    (D) marital status

    (E) socioeconomic status

35. Which of the following most distinguishes brief psychodynamic therapy from other forms of therapy?

(A) correcting cognitive errors

(B) interpreting many different conflicts

(C) modifying maladaptive behaviors

(D) interpreting resistance

(E) identification of a focal conflict

Questions 36 and 37

A 20-year-old man is currently in college and has completed his first semester of the sophomore year. Halfway into his second semester, his grades drop from As to Fs over a 3-month period. He becomes increasingly isolated and paranoid, believing that the government is after him because he has solved all theological problems through direct communication with God. He is started on olanzapine (Zyprexa) 10 mg by mouth (PO) daily and is tentatively diagnosed with schizophreniform disorder. He recovers after 4 months but has another relapse 6 months later in the absence of elevated, irritable, or depressed mood. He is given a diagnosis of schizophrenia.

36. Which of the following is most indicated for the treatment of this patient's schizophrenia?

    (A) psychoeducation alone

    (B) medication alone

    (C) family therapy

    (D) psychoanalysis

    (E) a combination of psychoeducation, medication, and family therapy

37. Which of the following therapies is usually not indicated for the treatment of psychotic disorders?

    (A) behavioral therapy

    (B) psychoanalysis

    (C) supportive psychotherapy

    (D) family therapy

    (E) group psychotherapy

Questions 38 and 39

A 33-year-old woman presents to the emergency department saying that she wants to kill herself. She is hopeless and feels helpless. She has a plan to overdose on pills that she has stockpiled at home.

38. Other than severe hopelessness, which of the following cognitive difficulties do suicidal patients characteristically exhibit?

    (A) personalization
    (B) begging the question
    (C) rigid, black-or-white, either-or thinking that limits problem-solving options
    (D) selective abstraction
    (E) circular reasoning

39. Which of the following forms of psychotherapy would be most appropriate to help this patient think of alternatives to suicide?

    (A) behavioral therapy
    (B) cognitive therapy
    (C) interpersonal psychotherapy
    (D) hypnosis
    (E) paradoxical therapy

40. A psychiatry consult is called on a patient who, in a variety of ways, is making the nursing staff angry at him. He became enraged during this hospitalization when he was told that he has a terminal illness. What defense mechanism is being demonstrated?

    (A) denial
    (B) sublimation
    (C) intellectualization
    (D) projective identification
    (E) reaction formation

41. Which of the following statements best characterizes a 34-year-old man being treated with systematic desensitization?

    (A) Reciprocal inhibition is key to his treatment.
    (B) Allowing this patient to use his imagination is far more effective than exposing him to the actual situation that engenders anxiety.

    (C) Psychoanalytic theory is the most important underpinning of this treatment.
    (D) It is likely that he is in treatment for depression.
    (E) He is being confronted directly with the feared situation and will eventually grow immune to the anxiety it produces.

42. During his session, a patient receives mainly empathetic reassurances from his psychiatrist. This best exemplifies which type of psychotherapy?

    (A) existential
    (B) dynamic
    (C) biological
    (D) supportive
    (E) cognitive-behavioral

DIRECTIONS (Questions 43 through 49): Each set of items in this section consists of a list of lettered headings followed by several numbered words or phrases. For each numbered word or phrase, select the ONE lettered option that is most closely associated with it. Each lettered option may be selected once, more than once, or not at all.

Questions 43 and 44

    (A) conditioning
    (B) insight
    (C) therapeutic alliance
    (D) schema
    (E) real relationship
    (F) anxiety
    (G) posttraumatic stress disorder
    (H) projection
    (I) transference neurosis or transference
    (J) countertransference
    (K) projective identification
    (L) biofeedback
    (M) undoing
    (N) negative reinforcement
    (O) punishment
    (P) operant conditioning
    (Q) splitting

43. You are seeing a 26-year-old woman who complains of migraines. She is otherwise healthy. You explain to her that you would like to try a technique in which you give her information on muscle tension and temperature.

44. You are seeing a 45-year-old man in analysis four times per week. After about 6 months, the man tells you that you are the center of his universe.

Questions 45 through 47

    (A) negative reinforcement
    (B) positive reinforcement
    (C) desensitization
    (D) avoidance
    (E) extinction
    (F) conditioned avoidance
    (G) flooding
    (H) reciprocal inhibition
    (I) hypnosis
    (J) modeling

45. You prescribe disulfiram (Antabuse) to a 56-year-old patient.

46. To train a 4-year-old boy to say "thank you," his mother gives him a sweet whenever he does.

47. To train a 4-year-old boy not to bite his classmates, his mother puts soap in his mouth whenever he does.

Questions 48 and 49

    (A) Sigmund Freud
    (B) Franz Anton Mesmer
    (C) Josef Breuer
    (D) Jean-Martin Charcot
    (E) Friedrich Nietzsche

48. Who is considered the father of psychoanalysis?

49. Who is considered the father of modern hypnosis?

Answers and Explanations

1. **(E)** Although it would be tempting to reassure this patient that he is not "going crazy," it is better to find out what he specifically means by "losing it." He could mention a specific fear that would be important for you to help him clarify or address. Asking the patient why he wants to know or asking "what do you think" is easily interpreted as an insulting and patronizing statement that does nothing to enhance doctor-patient trust.

2. **(B)** Cognitive-behavioral therapy is actually the combination of two therapies: cognitive therapy and behavioral therapy. Cognitive therapy would help the patient to think about his symptoms as misinterpretations. For example, his feelings of impending doom, although frightening, do not actually predict the end of his life. An example of behavioral therapy is exposure. The premise is to expose patients to feared situations while maintaining a safe atmosphere. For example, a therapist could accompany the patient to the car to precipitate symptoms. In the controlled atmosphere, the patient can separate the connection of feared symptoms with the specific environment. In paradoxical therapy, developed by Bateson, the therapist suggests that the patient engage in the behavior with negative connotations (e.g., a phobia or compulsion). The efficacy of cognitive-behavioral therapy is more established than that of paradoxical therapy. Couples therapy is not indicated here because we have no evidence that the root of the patient's disorder is a conflict with a significant other; similarly, family therapy is not indicated. Psychodynamic psychotherapy is a form of therapy informed by psychodynamic processes.

3. **(B)** *Displacement* is a defense that transfers a feeling about, or a response to, one object onto another object. *Denial* is a defense that keeps out of conscious awareness an aspect of external reality or subjective distress that is too uncomfortable for the person to accept. *Isolation of affect* involves detachment of feelings from a particular idea or experience. *Intellectualization* is a defense in which the individual favors abstract thinking over dealing with the disturbing feelings of an idea or experience. *Humor* is considered a defense mechanism that emphasizes the amusing or ironic aspects of the stressor.

4. **(A)** *Splitting* occurs when an individual is unable to see others moderately; that is, people's actions are either all good or all bad. Intellectualization is a defense that utilizes excessive abstract thinking or generalizations to control threatening emotions. *Repression* is a defense that expels disturbing wishes, thoughts, or experiences from conscious awareness. The feeling component may remain but be divorced from the idea. *Devaluation* is a defense that attributes excessive negative qualities to another. *Idealization* is a defense that attributes excessive positive qualities to another.

5. **(C)** This is an example of intellectualization, a defense that utilizes excessive abstract thinking or generalizations to control threatening emotions. *Lying* is not considered a defense mechanism. Denial is a defense that keeps out of conscious awareness an aspect of external reality or subjective distress that is too uncomfortable for the person to accept. *Projection* is a defense whereby a thought, feeling, or idea

that is unacceptable to the person is falsely attributed to another person. *Suppression* is a defense in which one intentionally avoids thinking of distressing thoughts, feelings, ideas, or experiences.

6. **(D)** The best strategy in any communication is to try to gain clarity. Asking this patient why she believes what she does may lead nowhere or it may very much help understand this thought. Choice A may be helpful in some situations and certainly has a positive ring to it. However, this patient's comment is an implicit question. She is asking for help and genuinely does not know what to do. Hiding behind pithy maxims is not helpful. Choices B and C are coercive and block communication. Giving supportive guidance is appropriate in this situation, but coercion is never appropriate in a therapeutic relationship. Choice E is not coercive but blocks communication. This may be the content that needs to be heard but it abruptly terminates communication and could sacrifice a more insightful, empowering response.

7. **(C)** The goal of supportive therapy is not to break down the defenses to achieve a more optimal level of functioning. This would be a long-term goal of psychodynamic psychotherapy. Supportive therapy's goal is the strengthening of current defense mechanisms. Through supportive care, the patient can learn to cope with difficult problems using already established abilities. Personality change is a goal of psychodynamic psychotherapy, and correcting faulty ideas is the expressed goal of cognitive therapy. Exploring the feeling of meaninglessness in life and investigating the freedom of individuals are goals of existential psychotherapy.

8. **(E)** This is an example of free association. Freud believed that all mental activity is causally related, meaning that free associations are not truly random. They follow logically, but the missing connection is being held down or repressed unconsciously by defenses. *Repression* is a defense mechanism that expels disturbing wishes, thoughts, or experiences from conscious awareness. *Transference*, in strict terms, is the reexperiencing of past experiences with the analyst in the setting of psychoanalytic psychotherapy. Countertransference is the analyst's response to this. However, these terms have come to mean the transferring of emotions and feelings that one has from one's past to the physician or care provider in the case of transference and the physician toward the patient in countertransference. A speakeasy was an underground bar during Prohibition.

9. **(A)** *Countertransference* is the conscious or unconscious emotional reaction of the therapist to the patient. Transference is the conscious or unconscious emotional reaction of the patient to the therapist based on a past relationship the patient had with a significant other person. *Resistance* is unconscious opposition to full disclosure of feelings or ideas. *Interpretation* is insight offered by the therapist regarding patterns of thought or behavior. *Extinction* is the reduction in frequency of a learned response as a result of the cessation of reinforcement, and is a term frequently used in learning theory.

10. **(A)** The *go-around* is a technique frequently used in inpatient groups. By having each patient comment on a plan, theme, mood, behavior, or idea, active participation by all members is ensured, and other members of the group can benefit from various ideas presented. The go-around also helps patients to feel that they are not the only ones with difficulties. *Free association* is used in psychoanalytically oriented groups. These groups are largely outpatient groups whose members can tolerate and effectively use this technique. Members are encouraged to be spontaneous with their thoughts and feelings, and the therapist assists in pointing out common themes and possible connections. *Feedback,* a cardinal feature of group psychotherapy, comes from peers as well as from the leader. Feedback from peers in the group can be a powerful stimulus for insight and change. Interpretation is the offering of insight that allows patients to gain an understanding of conflicts and motivations that contribute to their behavior. Resistance is the unconscious opposition to full disclosure of thoughts or feelings.

11. **(B)** *Acting out* is characterized by behaviors that distract a patient who needs to relieve tension or gratify needs through activity rather than verbalization of uncomfortable feelings in the group. Idealization is a defense that attributes excessive positive qualities to another. *Abreaction* is a process by which repressed material, particularly a painful experience of conflict, is brought back to consciousness. In the process, the person not only recalls the experience but relives the experience, which is accompanied by the appropriate emotional response. *Ventilation* (also known as *self-disclosure*) is the expression of suppressed feelings, ideas, or events to other group members; this relieves a sense of sin or guilt. *Catharsis* is expression of ideas, thoughts, and suppressed material that is accompanied by an emotional response that produces a state of relief in the patient.

12. **(C)** Personality change and reconstruction are goals of psychoanalytically oriented outpatient groups. This type of significant change is virtually impossible in an inpatient group. Crisis intervention, return to previous level of functioning, and preparation for outpatient therapy are all objectives for inpatient group psychotherapy. Certain outpatient groups can also help with these objectives so that inpatient hospitalization may be averted. If a patient has heart disease and needs alcohol detoxification, inpatient detoxification is indicated.

13. **(A)** Patients with borderline personality disorder develop intense transferences in individual treatment. This can impede the work of psychotherapy. Transference is usually diluted in group psychotherapy because of the number of people. The group can offer stability and moderation to the extreme ways of seeing others that distort borderline perceptions. The combined modes of treatment, individual and group, offer the patient with borderline personality disorder a higher probability for personality change. Patients with borderline personality disorder are known for their intense personal relationships, self-destructive behaviors, anger management issues, and poor senses of self-image. Schizotypal patients are known for their quirkiness and seemingly

magical thinking styles. Unlike the patient with schizotypal personality disorder, the patient with avoidant personality disorder longs for relationships yet is morbidly shy and fears them. Schizoid personality disorder is marked by bizarre behavior and withdrawal.

14. **(A)** This is one of the strongest reasons for combining the two forms of therapy. In individual therapy, patients can reflect on what their feelings are in the group and the responses of others to them from the group. Choice B is true of this personality disorder but is not a reason to combine therapies. Choices C, D, and E are not characteristic of narcissistic personality disorder.

15. **(A)** The cognitive triad of depression is a belief that oneself is ineffective, the world is a hostile place, and nothing one can do will ever change anything. The other choices are cognitive profiles typical of various psychiatric syndromes. Fear of being fat and unattractive is typical of anorexia nervosa and bulimia nervosa. Concern about serious, insidious medical disorders is typical of hypochondriasis. Seeing others as biased, manipulative, and devious is typical of paranoid states. Fear of physical or psychological danger is typical of anxiety disorders.

16. **(C)** *Automatic thoughts* are constant ways of perceiving situations and oneself in relation to the environment. They can be thought of as a given way of evaluating events. Cognitive therapy aims to identify negative automatic thoughts and then change them so that individuals do not constantly view themselves or their environment in a negative light. Automatic thoughts are not genetically determined. They have not always been present and can be changed. There is no moral imperative from automatic thoughts and they do not impede free association.

17. **(C)** One of the reasons that this is the best of the possible responses is that it is a question. Patients with cognitive distortions often take their view of the world as a given. They do not question their perspectives. Asking a question invites patients to examine their perspectives and thereby become open to the possibility that their thoughts may be inaccurate. Choices D

and E are also questions but are authoritarian and punitive not to mention insulting. To have the best outcome in any form of therapy, there must be a good relationship or alliance between the patient and therapist. Choices A and B have not been supported by any evidence. Choice B is ambiguous—to which part of the question are you responding? The patient may not think you are awkwardly trying to be supportive but may believe that you are insulting him. Choice A is dangerous—a patient should not be called "silly."

18. **(D)** This question is meant to emphasize that although correcting cognitive distortions may have symptomatic benefit, it should not be inferred that cognitive distortions are the ultimate cause of the psychiatric syndromes. The other choices are wrong because of the "always" or "never" used in the question. The other choices can be true at times but are not always true or false.

19. **(D)** Behavior therapy is focused on behaviors, not on possible underlying factors that cause behaviors. Behavior therapy is a here-and-now approach to maladaptive behaviors. It may utilize information surrounding the emergence of a particular maladaptive behavior to construct a behavior modification plan. Although behavior therapy can and does change neurobiology, this is not its expressed goal. Changing maladaptive thoughts underlying a maladaptive behavior and changing how the patient perceives the environment involve perspectives more appropriate for cognitive therapy. Changing underlying conflicts in an attempt to change behavior is a description of the goals of psychodynamic therapy.

20. **(C)** *Behavior therapy* is a set of procedures designed to enhance the learning of adaptive behaviors and the unlearning of maladaptive behaviors. In a strict sense, it is not designed to uncover or alter unconscious conflicts using hypnosis or other methods. It is also a short-term therapy.

21. **(A)** Stress reduction and biofeedback are used to reduce the frequency and the severity of each headache. They are equally effective in accomplishing this goal. Stimulus control is used in the treatment of insomnia. Stimulus control procedures are used to narrow the stimuli associated with sleep onset. Systematic desensitization is a technique used in asthma, in which the patient becomes relaxed and visualizes typical situations that precipitate asthma attacks. Substance withdrawal syndromes are examples of the aversive stimuli and consequently negative reinforcement that lead to decrease in substance use.

22. **(B)** The major focus of interpersonal psychotherapy is communication analysis. Indirect, unclear interpersonal communication patterns are identified in the course of therapy. These communication patterns are then altered, for instance, by role playing or asking the patient to try out different forms of communication during the session. Interpreting transference, pointing out resistance, and character change are more the focus of psychodynamically oriented psychotherapy. Hypnosis is a sleep-like state induced by a therapist, which has been of some use in uncovering psychodynamic processes and in behavioral modification such as stopping smoking. It is not part of interpersonal psychotherapy.

23. **(A)** Interpersonal psychotherapy focuses on the patient's role and communication style within important relationships and how that role may be causing or complicating the illness, such as depression. If one or two specific ways of communicating can be altered so that a relationship improves, the depressive illness also improves. This therapy also has the added benefit of durability; once a communication pattern is improved and the patient better understands how his or her role in a relationship may create distress, the depressive illness is not as likely to recur. Although other processes such as those in the remaining answers may be used, choice A best reflects the foundation of the therapy.

24. **(A)** It takes 4–5 days a week to successfully complete an analysis because it is difficult for patients to sustain a transference and keep their

defenses lowered with fewer sessions. There is no correlation between severity of mental illness and length of therapy. Psychoanalysis tends to be among the longest therapies and involves the process of free association in which the patient lies on a couch, facing away from the therapist, and says whatever comes to mind. Psychoanalysis is based on an expressive or exploratory model of therapy, as opposed to a supportive model aimed at stabilizing crisis and reestablishing a baseline level of function.

25.   **(A)** Psychoanalysis may accomplish many tasks, including changing maladaptive thoughts and behaviors and "solving" interpersonal problems, but these are the consequences of analysis, not the instrument of change. Altering cognitive errors is more in the domain of cognitive therapy. The major tool of psychoanalysis is the careful interpretations of the transference neurosis. Certainly, interpreting dreams can lead to deep insights into a patient's thoughts and feelings, but it is an adjunctive tool.

26.   **(A)** The term dynamic or *psychodynamic* refers to the notion that all mental phenomena are the result of a continual interaction of forces that oppose one another. Choices B, C, and D are related ideas; specifically, the notion that the psyche is organized into functional units called the id, ego, and superego was a construction formulated by Freud. Fun, interactive, and pleasant is close to a lay definition of *dynamo*.

27.   **(C)** Dreams provide information about psychic conflicts. Dreams can lead to a change in behavior, but they are not used per se in analysis to change behavior or cognitive errors. Dreams are used to uncover psychic conflicts, which, when interpreted appropriately (not subliminally), can lead to a productive change in behavior. According to the psychoanalytic theory, dreams represent the unconscious workings of the mind, not the conscious ones, and may be symbolic in content.

28.   **(B)** Far and away the most important factor in hypnosis is a patient who is highly responsive to suggestion. Some people are able to alter their subjective experience in response to suggestion

more than others; a patient can be taught self-hypnosis. Needless to say, a skillful hypnotist and induction technique are helpful. Neither a quiet room nor creative talent is a factor.

29.   **(E)** Hypnosis should not be used in psychotic disorders. Patients with schizophrenia often have cognitive disorders or paranoid symptoms that make the use of hypnosis problematic. Often, these patients do not remember the changes that were supposed to be induced through the hypnosis, and there is controversy over the extent to which patients with schizophrenia can be hypnotized. Hypnosis has been used successfully for the treatment of anxiety disorders and pain. There is also literature indicating its efficacy in the treatment of warts.

30.   **(D)** Family therapy is based on the idea that the interactional dynamics of the family can help to explain individual psychopathology. Individual psychotherapy can be very useful in conjunction with family therapy. Role playing can explore a patient's interpersonal relationships, personality makeup, and conflicts. However, this is not the basis for family therapy; it is the basis for psychodrama.

31.   **(A)** A dysfunctional marriage is a greater risk factor for depression than being single. Certainly, many people are content and single. The other three answers are not correlated risk factors for depression. Some studies have shown age greater than 45 to be a risk factor for depression in general. Others have shown age greater than 65.

32.   **(A)** Behavioral therapy helps patients who suffer from ADHD to derive satisfaction from learning and from ignoring disruptive behaviors. The other answers can also be very helpful; however, they are not examples of behavioral therapy.

33.   **(B)** A behavioral tool that is used quite effectively is a report card. This tool can function as a bridge between school and home. In addition, a report card can serve as a positive incentive to good behavior when the report is good and is therefore rewarded. The rewards can be adjusted for the degree of good behavior

obtained. So, a 40% increase in a desired behavior gets rewarded with a proportional prize. Methylphenidate is also effective in treating ADHD but is not a behavior therapy. Clozapine, a newer-generation antipsychotic, is not effective in treating the disorder. Interpretive strategies such as a well-timed interpretation of maladaptive behaviors and positively reframing a negative experience are not helpful behavioral tools.

34. **(C)** Motivation for change goes beyond a desire for removal of symptoms and includes a willingness to tolerate discomfort and to take risks in a search for understanding. Demographics do not play a role.

35. **(E)** Brief psychodynamic therapy identifies a single, focal area of conflict and spends the time of the therapy actively interpreting transferences as they pertain to this identified focal conflict. Interpretations of resistance certainly take place in brief psychodynamic therapy. However, the resistance is interpreted in light of the identified focal conflict. Many types of therapy correct cognitive errors and modify maladaptive behaviors, although cognitive therapy and behavioral therapy, respectively, are specifically concerned with these outcomes.

36. **(E)** The treatment of the devastating illness of schizophrenia needs to involve not only the patient but also the family who will care for the patient. This includes education of the patient and his family, medication of the patient, and family therapy to help the family accommodate the patient and his new illness. Recent evidence supports reducing high levels of expressed emotion in the family in order to decrease psychotic relapses. Psychoanalysis is not useful in the treatment of schizophrenia and is generally considered contraindicated in the treatment of patients with psychotic disorders.

37. **(B)** Psychoanalysis is usually not indicated in patients who have difficulty with reality testing. The introspection and self-examination required in psychoanalysis is usually overwhelming to psychotic patients and actually may cause more harm than good. All of the other treatments can be helpful.

38. **(C)** Patients who are suicidal characteristically have severe hopelessness and think about events in rigid, black-and-white ways. They see very few options and become overwhelmed with the hopelessness that is exacerbated by seeing "no way out." *Personalization* is a patient's tendency to relate events to himself without any reason for doing so.

39. **(B)** Cognitive therapy is the psychotherapy that would be most appropriate to help the patient solve problems more productively. *Behavioral therapy* is focused on behaviors, not on possible underlying factors that cause behaviors. *Interpersonal therapy* is aimed at understanding communication patterns and roles in relationships. *Hypnosis* is a sleeplike state induced by a therapist, which has been of some use in uncovering psychodynamic processes and in behavioral modification such as stopping smoking. In *paradoxical therapy*, developed by Bateson, the therapist suggests that the patient engage in the behavior with negative connotations (e.g., a phobia or compulsion).

40. **(D)** In *projective identification*, the patient attributes unacceptable thoughts or feelings to those around him; the patient also recognizes the feeling in himself. The unacceptable feeling in this case is the patient's anger resulting from his terminal diagnosis. It is common that the unacceptable feelings are experienced by the objects of the projective identification—in this case, the nurses, who have become angry with the patient. The remaining defense mechanisms may each play a role here, but we are given no direct clues to this. Denial occurs when a patient selectively ignores an unacceptable feeling or fact, as may occur in an alcoholic who refuses to believe he has a problem. Intellectualization occurs when a patient explains away through intellectual reasoning the emotional impact of some feature of his life. *Sublimation* is the channeling of unacceptable impulses into socially acceptable activities. *Reaction formation* is the endorsement of some

opposite view of an unacceptable feeling or impulse.

41. **(A)** In systematic desensitization, one response to some situation stimulus is substituted for another response. This is known as reciprocal inhibition. Most commonly, the former response is anxiety—usually enough to interfere with someone's ability to lead a fulfilling life—and the latter response is relaxation. This is accomplished by gradually exposing the patient to increasingly greater approximations of some situation that causes great concern—say air travel—and pairing that experience with a more pleasant response. The most effective way to conduct systematic desensitization is to gradually expose the patient to the very situations that cause him extreme concern, not some imagined facsimile. Systematic desensitization arises from the teaching of the behaviorists, who postulate that the behaviors are learned; the behaviorists are less concerned that some unconscious process might be at play as psychoanalytic theory proposes. The most common application of systematic desensitization is helping a patient deal with a phobia. Depression is more readily treated pharmacologically and/or with psychotherapy.

42. **(D)** Supportive psychotherapy attempts to fortify psychological defenses by providing empathetic reassurance as opposed to probing into a patient's psychological conflicts. Dynamic psychotherapy probes such conflicts to bring unconscious material into consciousness. Existential psychotherapy is based on existential philosophy and emphasizes personal feeling and experience over rational thinking. Biological psychiatry is a branch of psychiatry that specifically focuses on the genetic and the pharmacologic aspects of psychiatry. Cognitive-behavioral therapy, used often in mood and anxiety disorders, is a mix of behavioral therapy and cognitive psychology.

43. **(L)** *Biofeedback* is the process of giving a patient information on physiologic variables to alter those variables and ultimately the corresponding behavior. Patients with migraine headaches receive information on muscle tension or temperature. They use this information to decrease the intensity of the headaches by directly trying to relax and alter the known parameters. *Undoing* **(M)** is a concept described by Freud in which a patient with obsessive-compulsive disorder performs a compulsive act to prevent or undo the consequences from a feared impulse. *Negative reinforcement* **(N)** describes the delivery of an averse stimulus based on a given response. *Punishment* **(O)** is the administration of an unpleasant stimulus based on a given response; *reward* describes a pleasant stimulus delivered to a given response. In *operant conditioning* **(P)**, a response is rewarded or punished each time it occurs, so that over time the response increases or decreases in frequency. Friedrich Nietzsche was a nineteenth-century philosopher. Splitting **(Q)**, characteristic of patients with borderline personality disorder, occurs when an individual is unable to see others moderately; that is, people's actions are either all good or all bad.

44. **(I)** Transference and transference neurosis are synonyms. Transference can also be understood as a general phenomenon in which the person displaces onto all aspects of living the emotions and forgotten memories of one's past (particularly the earliest years of one's life).

45–47. **[45 (F), 46 (B), 47 (A)]** A patient with alcoholism who drinks alcohol while taking disulfiram will likely avoid this combination in the future. The goal of disulfiram therapy is to give patients negative associations with alcohol. Nevertheless, patients learning to not drink while on disulfiram still illustrates the principal of *conditioned avoidance*. The boy who receives a reward—a sweet—for something he is being trained to do more often is undergoing positive reinforcement; the boy who receives soap in his mouth for something he is being trained to do less often is undergoing punishment. *Desensitization* **(C)** refers to a behavioral modification technique of increasing exposure to an unpleasant or phobic stimulus with the goal of minimizing negative effects. *Avoidance* **(D)** is learned cessation of behavior. Extinction **(E)** is a learned response to removal of a stimulus. *Positive reinforcement* **(B)** is the process by which certain consequences of behavior raise the probability that the behavior will occur again.

Modeling (**J**) is a process by which behavior is changed simply by observation. *Flooding* (**G**) is an exposure technique that is commonly used in behavior therapy. The premise is confrontation with the feared symptom. Hypnosis (**I**) is a sleep-like state induced by a therapist, which has been of some use in uncovering psychodynamic processes and in behavioral modification such as stopping smoking.

48. (**A**) Certainly, Sigmund Freud is one of the most well-known figures of the twentieth century. He is generally credited with the modern form of psychoanalysis that is practiced today. However, Freud did not work in a vacuum; he was influenced by an array of people and ideas, including the internist Joseph Breuer and the neurologist Jean-Martin Charcot. Incidentally, Freud began his career as a neurologist. Just as there have been many changes in physics since Aristotle, there have been many changes in psychoanalysis since Freud.

49. (**B**) Franz Anton Mesmer is considered the father of modern hypnosis; the word *mesmerism* is derived from his name.

CHAPTER 6

Legal and Ethical Issues in Psychiatry and Medicine
Questions

DIRECTIONS (Questions 1 through 50): Each of the numbered items in this section is followed by answer choices. Select the ONE lettered answer or completion that is BEST in each case.

Questions 1 and 2

The case manager for an 18-year-old man that you are treating notifies you that your patient has been acting strangely lately. You learn from the case manager that the patient makes provocative sexual comments toward her on a daily basis. During your session, the patient expresses concern that his case manager is somehow conspiring against him and he plans to do something about it. On further questioning, he becomes increasingly anxious and abruptly storms out of your office. You hear him in the hallway, exclaiming, "That woman, I'm going to stab her and she won't bother me anymore."

1. Your first course of action should be which of the following?

    (A) Respect the patient's confidentiality and wait until your next scheduled appointment with him to discuss his feelings.

    (B) Contact the patient's family and let them know about his threats toward the case manager.

    (C) Inform the police of the content of your previous sessions and his recent threat toward the case manager.

    (D) Notify the case manager of the potential danger.

    (E) Attempt to contact the patient over the next several hours to discuss the intent of his parting comments.

2. The legal precedent that guides the appropriate course of action in this case is which of the following?

    (A) *Rogers v Commissioner of the Department of Mental Health*

    (B) *Tarasoff v Regents of University of California*

    (C) *Durham v United States*

    (D) *Zinerman v Burch*

    (E) *Kansas v Hendricks*

Questions 3 and 4

Two years ago, you were the examining pediatrician for a baby who was born with cerebral palsy. You had heard from your obstetrical colleague that the family was planning to sue, and today you are working in your office when a process server delivers papers notifying you that the family has brought an action against you.

3. In medical malpractice cases, the plaintiff must establish which of the following?

    (A) burden of proof beyond a reasonable doubt
    (B) clear and convincing evidence of wrong-doing
    (C) harm or damage
    (D) criminal intent
    (E) criminal mischief

4. In malpractice cases and others, as opposed to fact witnesses, expert medical witnesses have which of the following characteristics?

    (A) They are familiar with a particular body of evidence no more so than laypersons.
    (B) They are not allowed to charge a fee.
    (C) They can provide only factual information.
    (D) They can testify only for the defense.
    (E) They may provide opinion testimony.

Questions 5 and 6

An 80-year-old widow with a history significant for bipolar I disorder was recently diagnosed with end-stage hepatic cancer. She is concerned about the disposition of her estate and does not want her family to receive any of her money; she plans to donate her entire estate to the local humane society.

5. Which of the following is most important in establishing a legally valid will?

    (A) mens rea
    (B) informed consent
    (C) lack of mental illness
    (D) testamentary capacity
    (E) conservatorship of estate

6. The patient's family hires an attorney to challenge the integrity of her will. Which of the following items, if present, would undermine this patient's competence to make a will?

    (A) paranoid delusions regarding the patient's family
    (B) the presence of a diagnosable Axis I disorder
    (C) the patient's nondelusional explanation of why she wants to donate her estate to the local humane society
    (D) inability to read and write
    (E) refusal to undergo treatment with chemotherapy

Questions 7 and 8

A 23-year-old man with no prior psychiatric history is charged with murdering his next-door neighbor. His friends note that he became increasingly isolative and suspicious of others in the weeks prior to the crime. The examining psychiatrist found him to be having paranoid delusions regarding his neighbor and noted that his thought processes were too disorganized to complete the examination.

7. Which of the following legal standards is the current basis for establishing an insanity defense?

    (A) M'Naghten rule
    (B) American Law Institute test (Model Penal Code)
    (C) Durham rule
    (D) extreme emotional disturbance
    (E) irresistible impulse rule

8. Criminal responsibility requires demonstration of the criminal act along with which of the following elements?

    (A) actus reus
    (B) diminished mental capacity
    (C) mens rea
    (D) product test
    (E) "wild beast" test

Questions 9 and 10

An obese 54-year-old woman presents to the emergency department by ambulance complaining of severe substernal chest pain lasting 40 minutes, profuse sweating, and nausea. Her vital signs are blood pressure 195/96 mm Hg, heart rate 63/min, respiratory rate 18/min, temperature 98.8°F. An electrocardiogram reveals 3-mm ST-segment elevations in leads V_4, V_5, and V_6. Cardiac enzymes and laboratory workup are pending. You suspect a lateral wall myocardial infarction and recommend immediate thrombolytic therapy. The patient states, "You're crazy if you think I'm gonna let some intern care for me...my family will drive me across town to the private hospital." The patient then jumps from the gurney and begins walking toward the exit.

9. The appropriate next step is which of the following?

    (A) Sedate the patient and begin thrombolytic therapy.
    (B) Allow the patient to leave against medical advice.
    (C) Admit the patient to the cardiology service on a physician emergency certificate.
    (D) Detain the patient until the results of the cardiac enzymes are available.
    (E) Detain the patient until you can assess her ability to provide informed consent.

10. On further evaluation, the patient demonstrates a thorough understanding of the information you have given to her and appreciates the consequences of not being treated immediately. The appropriate next step is which of the following?

    (A) Sedate the patient and begin thrombolytic therapy.
    (B) Allow the patient to leave against medical advice.
    (C) Admit the patient to the cardiology service on a physician emergency certificate.
    (D) Detain the patient until the results of the cardiac enzymes are available.
    (E) Detain the patient until you can assess her ability to provide informed consent.

11. A 19-year-old man with a history significant for bipolar I disorder is charged with assaulting a police officer. The patient has been able to work with his attorney in preparation for his defense. Which of the following items would be consistent with the assertion that the patient is competent to stand trial?

    (A) comprehension of the court proceedings
    (B) ability to read and write
    (C) presence of a diagnosable mental illness
    (D) testamentary capacity
    (E) capability to provide informed consent

12. A 35-year-old man is admitted to the locked psychiatric unit of the emergency department after threatening to unload his 9-mm pistol into his "blood brother's" chest. Urine toxicology is negative for cocaine, phencyclidine (PCP), or opioids, and his blood alcohol level is 0.04. You learn from the patient's family that he has been threatening to assault his brother for several days and has even written notes about executing his plan. On Mental Status Examination (MSE), the patient's speech is loud, pressured, and very threatening toward the emergency department staff. Family history is significant for bipolar disorder. The patient states that he has not done anything wrong and wants to be released immediately. The next appropriate step is which of the following?

    (A) Notify the police about the patient's homicidal threats.
    (B) Warn the patient's "blood brother" about the threats.
    (C) Arrange for a police hold given the patient's potential for violence.
    (D) Involuntarily admit the patient to a locked psychiatric ward.
    (E) Medicate the patient with a mood stabilizer and arrange for outpatient follow-up.

Questions 13 and 14

You are the psychiatrist on duty one night when a man arrested by police for stabbing his lover is brought into the emergency room for evaluation. The man's behavior is wild and unpredictable; at one point he starts to pick up a chair and look menacingly at a nurse before being subdued by police officers. Detectives tell you that the man's only chance of staying out of a jail cell that night is to be admitted to the locked unit, but the man makes it clear that he does not want to stay in the hospital.

13. Criteria for involuntary admission to the hospital include which of the following?

    (A) medication noncompliance
    (B) inability to care for self
    (C) permission from the conservator of person
    (D) presence of at least one diagnosable mental disorder
    (E) clinical decompensation

You decide to admit the man who is released after a few days. Six months later, you receive a call from the man's attorney who says he would like you to testify at the upcoming trial about the man's mental state at the time of admission.

14. Which of the following is true of individuals found not guilty by reason of insanity?

    (A) have to serve their original criminal sentence once deemed sane
    (B) are barred from using the defense in the future
    (C) typically serve less time than those found guilty
    (D) generally spend at least the same amount of time or more than those found guilty
    (E) are immediately released without further psychiatric evaluation

Questions 15 and 16

A 9-year-old girl is brought to the pediatric emergency department by her parents for evaluation of a persistent cough. She is withdrawn and complains of a "scratchy throat." Vital signs are stable and the patient is afebrile. On examination, the lungs are clear to auscultation bilaterally and the posterior oropharynx is clear. There are multiple bruises on her buttocks and back. A chest x-ray demonstrates several rib fractures in different stages of healing. Her parents report that their daughter is quite active with her younger siblings and often gets into fights with them. The patient agrees with her parents.

15. The most likely diagnosis in this case is which of the following?

    (A) somatization disorder
    (B) sexual abuse
    (C) major depressive disorder (MDD)
    (D) age-appropriate "rough play"
    (E) physical abuse

16. The next appropriate step is which of the following?

    (A) discharge the patient with follow-up in 1 week to reevaluate her bruises
    (B) refer for family therapy to address the issue of rough play
    (C) treat the patient with penicillin 2.5 million units intramuscularly (IM)
    (D) notify Child Protective Services
    (E) confront the siblings about their behavior

Questions 17 and 18

A 17-year-old girl presents to your office complaining of a burning vaginal discharge. She informs you that she has been involved in a consensual sexual relationship with her boyfriend and is worried that she has contracted a sexually transmitted disease (STD). You start the patient on antibiotics. Three days later, you discover that the culture of her vaginal discharge grew *Neisseria gonorrhoea*.

17. A few days later, you receive a call from the patient's parents demanding to know why their daughter was seen in your office. Because the patient is a minor, the appropriate next step is which of the following?

(A) Explain to the parents that their daughter has contracted an STD and requires immediate antibiotic treatment.

(B) Maintain confidentiality by disclosing no information, but encourage the patient to discuss this issue with her parents.

(C) Ask the parents about their daughter's sexual history.

(D) Alert the parents that their daughter is at risk for human immunodeficiency virus (HIV) and should be tested.

(E) Find out the boyfriend's name and telephone number to confirm the history.

18. At the patient's next follow-up visit, she requests to be tested for HIV. She reports that her boyfriend recently tested negative, but given her promiscuity, she wonders if she has contracted HIV. Before administering the HIV test, you should do which of the following?

(A) Notify her parents about the HIV test.

(B) Directly inform the patient's boyfriend that he is at risk for HIV.

(C) Obtain a complete blood cell count to determine if the test is necessary.

(D) Explain how the test is performed and interpreted, along with information on confidentiality and how you will proceed if the result is positive.

(E) Perform a pregnancy test.

19. A 44-year-old man with insulin-dependent diabetes mellitus and end-stage renal failure has been on dialysis several years while awaiting a kidney transplant. He feels as though he has "waited long enough" and does not want to continue "living tied to a machine." After several family meetings and consultations with other physicians, he informs you that he no longer wishes to be dialyzed. You obtain a psychiatric consult that concludes no evidence of mood or thought disorder. The family is upset with the patient's decision and demands that you continue to administer dialysis until a transplant is available. The most appropriate next step is which of the following?

(A) Respect the patient's wishes and discontinue dialysis.

(B) Coerce the patient into continuing treatment.

(C) Continue dialysis until you convince the ethics committee to support the family's decision.

(D) Tell the patient you're sure a transplant will arrive soon and encourage him to remain in treatment.

(E) Place the patient on a physician's emergency certificate because he is a danger to himself.

20. A 40-year-old surgical attending is admitted to the medical unit after developing severe right flank pain. Further workup confirms a diagnosis of nephrolithiasis. One of the surgical residents asks you about the attending's diagnosis so that coverage can be arranged. The most appropriate next step is which of the following?

(A) Reveal only the estimated length of stay.

(B) Inform the chief surgical resident of the attending's condition and length of stay.

(C) Tell the surgical resident that you will not say anything, but she could take a look in the attending's chart.

(D) Tell the resident to address the questions directly to the attending.

(E) Arrange a conference between your medical attending and the surgical house staff.

21. A 43-year-old man is referred for continued treatment of depression after release from jail. The court mandated psychiatric treatment while he is on probation. The patient's probation officer calls you for information regarding his condition, progress, and treatment compliance. You should do which of the following?

   (A) Discuss the case with the probation officer because the treatment is court mandated.
   (B) Limit your discussion with the probation officer to only treatment compliance because the rest of the information is confidential.
   (C) Obtain a confidentiality waiver from the patient before speaking to the probation officer.
   (D) Ignore the request altogether because psychiatric treatment bears no relation to law enforcement.
   (E) Correspond with the probation officer only through written documents.

22. A 55-year-old woman is admitted for intravenous (IV) antibiotic treatment for acute hematogenous osteomyelitis. The nurse informs you that the patient was accidentally given the wrong antibiotic but has suffered no adverse reaction. Which of the following best applies in this case?

   (A) the "no harm, no disclosure" rule
   (B) informing the patient that she was given the wrong medication
   (C) first reporting the mistake to the hospital advisory committee
   (D) notifying the patient's family of the mistake
   (E) encouraging the patient to seek legal action because a critical mistake has occurred

23. A 38-year-old woman is admitted to the oncology unit with severe aplastic anemia. She appears pale and weak. Vital signs indicate a blood pressure of 110/75 mm Hg and a pulse of 90/min. Hematocrit is 18%. On MSE, cognition is intact and there is no evidence of a mood or psychotic disturbance. The patient states that she is a Jehovah's Witness. She refuses any blood transfusion on the basis of her religious beliefs. Which of the following best applies to your next step in the treatment of this patient?

   (A) administering packed red blood cells
   (B) persuading the patient that she must accept the transfusion
   (C) explaining the implications of nontreatment but respecting the patient's refusal for treatment
   (D) utilizing a "confrontation method" to secure lifesaving treatment
   (E) referring the patient for involuntary psychiatric treatment based on her life-threatening decision

24. The parents of a newborn with Down syndrome find their daughter to be lethargic and minimally responsive. Medical evaluation is significant for the following cerebrospinal fluid findings: opening pressure of 100 mm Hg, white blood cell count of $5000/\mu L$ (predominantly neutrophils), protein >40 mg/dL, glucose content <40 mg/dL, and Gram stain positive for bacteria. You suspect group B streptococcal meningitis and recommend IV antibiotic therapy. The parents feel as though their Down child will ultimately have a poor quality of life and request that treatment be withheld. You should do which of the following?

   (A) Respect the parents' wishes because they are the primary decision makers.
   (B) Refer the case to the ethics committee for review at their next scheduled meeting.
   (C) Inform the parents that after reviewing the laboratory data you realize the patient has viral meningitis and care will be mostly supportive.
   (D) Start ampicillin and cefotaxime against the parents' wishes.
   (E) Repeat the lumbar puncture to verify the diagnosis.

25. You are called by a local news station to offer a specific psychiatric diagnosis on a prominent politician. There is considerable information in the print and television media that suggests the politician has bipolar I disorder. Which of the following best applies?

    (A) Stating your opinion publicly is legitimate as long as the politician is not your private patient.
    (B) Offering a psychiatric diagnosis in such instances is unethical.
    (C) Comment in written form only.
    (D) Agree to an "off-the-record" or anonymous interview.
    (E) State your diagnosis but indicate that other problems may account for the symptoms.

26. An 84-year-old widowed man with severe dementia, for whom you have been the primary care physician for years, is diagnosed with hepatocellular carcinoma. The patient does not have an advance directive and never designated a power of attorney. Psychiatric consultation concludes that the patient is unable to make an informed decision regarding treatment options, and you turn to his family for guidance. The patient's oldest son is adamant that his father receive chemotherapy, while the two younger daughters feel that he should not suffer the adverse effects of chemotherapy "especially because he's so demented." Which of the following is the next appropriate step?

    (A) Ask the patient which family member he would like to designate power of attorney.
    (B) Let the patient decide whether or not to proceed with treatment.

    (C) Abide by the son's wishes because he is the oldest.
    (D) Abide by the daughters' wishes because the patient's quality of life is already poor.
    (E) Seek the hospital ethics committee's opinion.

Questions 27 and 28

A 25-year-old woman is referred to you for evaluation of insomnia, frequent crying spells, and weight loss. She informs you that her symptoms began several weeks ago after she lost her job and that she now experiences bouts of helplessness and hopelessness. On MSE, she describes her mood as "depressed" and notes that she occasionally has thoughts of taking an overdose of aspirin.

27. The most significant predictor for suicidal behavior is which of the following?

    (A) prior serious suicide attempt
    (B) current alcohol use
    (C) current diagnosis of MDD
    (D) physical pain
    (E) recent loss of a family member

28. Which category of mental disorders is most common in individuals who have completed suicide?

    (A) affective disorders
    (B) psychotic disorders
    (C) alcohol-related disorders
    (D) anxiety disorders
    (E) toxic metabolic states

Questions 29 and 30

You have been treating a patient for a minor phobia. At the end of a suggested course of treatment, he has been cured of his phobia. He proceeds to tell you that he finds you attractive and would like to have dinner with you the following Saturday night.

29. Which of the following statements is most accurate in regard to sexual relations with psychiatric patients?

    (A) Sexual relations with a former patient is unethical.
    (B) Sexual relations with a former patient is permissible as long as the physician does not exploit his or her past position of authority.
    (C) Sexual relations with a current or former patient is ethical.
    (D) Terminating the physician-patient relationship is not required prior to dating a patient.
    (E) Sexual relations between consenting adults is not bound by any professional code of ethics.

30. Which of the following would be true if the patient had been one of your medical or surgical patients?

    (A) Sexual relations with a former patient is unethical.
    (B) Sexual relations with a former patient is permitted as long as the physician does not exploit his or her past position of authority.
    (C) Sexual relations with a current or former patient is ethical.
    (D) Terminating the physician-patient relationship is not required prior to dating a patient.
    (E) Sexual relations between consenting adults is not bound by any professional code of ethics.

31. A 52-year-old man, for whom you have been the primary care physician for the last 20 years, was recently diagnosed with amyotrophic lateral sclerosis. The disease has rapidly progressed and he has experienced multiple respiratory complications that likely will require a tracheotomy. Severe muscle weakness and atrophy are apparent in all limbs. The patient states that there is no meaning in continuing without his physical capacities. He asks for your help in ending his life in a humane and dignified manner. MSE is at baseline and there is no evidence of any psychiatric disorder. You discuss the patient's request with his family and they unanimously support his desire to "end the suffering." The most appropriate course of action would be which of the following?

    (A) Respect the patient's wishes by helping him end his life in a painless and respectful manner.
    (B) Refuse to participate in assisting the patient with suicide and focus on responding to the patient's end-of-life issues.
    (C) Provide the patient with plenty of medication refills to provide a lethal dose.
    (D) Provide the patient with information regarding how to effectively end his life.
    (E) Ignore the patient's request.

32. You are asked to see an incarcerated man for evaluation. He is serving a sentence for murder and often has trouble with guards, who punished his behavior with solitary confinement. Antisocial personality disorder is estimated to exist in what percentage of the male prison population?

    (A) 80–100%
    (B) 55–75%
    (C) 30–50%
    (D) 10–20%
    (E) <10%

Questions 33 and 34

You receive a subpoena from an attorney representing a party that has filed a lawsuit against one of your patients. The subpoena pertains to releasing the medical records of your patient.

33. Which of the following is the appropriate next step?

(A) Contact the attorney who obtained the subpoena to discuss the process of releasing the medical information.

(B) Release the medical records upon receiving the subpoena.

(C) Sign a release of information form and turn over the records.

(D) Not release the information and contact your patient regarding the subpoena.

(E) Release the medical records directly to the presiding judge.

34. A court hearing has been organized by your patient's attorney to quash the subpoena you have been issued. At the hearing, the judge rules that you should release the medical records even though your patient has not consented to the release of information. Which of the following statements is most accurate regarding the release of this patient's records?

(A) Disclosing this patient's medical records is unjustifiable.

(B) Releasing a patient's medical records is always unethical regardless of court orders.

(C) It would be appropriate to release this patient's records.

(D) Disclosing a patient's medical records when there is potential harm to the therapeutic alliance is unethical.

(E) Work out a plan of legal action with your patient.

35. A 12-year-old boy has a 1-year history of vandalism, violating parental curfews, starting fights, and stealing. Which of the following personality disorders is this patient most likely to develop?

(A) borderline personality disorder

(B) narcissistic personality disorder

(C) oppositional defiant disorder

(D) antisocial personality disorder

(E) paranoid personality disorder

36. A 28-year-old woman with dysthymic disorder has been seeing you in weekly psychotherapy and has failed to pay her bill for 2 months. The appropriate next step is which of the following?

(A) Contract with a billing collector to demand immediate payment.

(B) Terminate the treatment.

(C) Contact the patient's family to determine if the patient is financially stable.

(D) Inquire as to the reasons she has been avoiding payment at the patient's next visit.

(E) Inform the patient that you will not see her if she doesn't pay for her treatment.

37. A wealthy 46-year-old male banker is in psychotherapy with you for treatment of a single episode of depression. After significant improvement in his symptoms, he offers you the opportunity to take part in one of his financial ventures. The investment appears to be sound. The most appropriate comment to make to the banker is which of the following?

(A) "Thanks for thinking about me . . . I'd be honored to invest with you."

(B) "Because your depression is improved, it would be appropriate for us to be business partners."

(C) "I can invest with you only when our treatment is nearing its end."

(D) "It is probably a bad idea; I'm already committed in other investments."

(E) "I have to decline; it potentially may interfere with our treatment relationship."

38. A 23-year-old Caucasian Catholic woman with a history of schizophrenia presents to your office after arguing with her husband. She is unemployed and has been staying home taking care of the couple's children. She notes feeling sad and reports thoughts of killing herself. She has a past history of an overdose attempt with aspirin. Which of the following places this patient in a high-risk category for suicide?

    (A) age
    (B) past history of suicide attempt
    (C) gender
    (D) marital status
    (E) terminal medical illness

Questions 39 and 40

A 36-year-old man with a history of bipolar I disorder is brought to the emergency department by police after stabbing a patron in a barroom brawl. His blood alcohol level was 0.320 upon arrival, and the patient required intramuscular (IM) droperidol (Inapsine) for agitation. The patient has no recollection of the event, and the victim died 2 hours later. The patient has a history of assault while psychotic and is currently in weekly psychotherapy. His lawyer has chosen to assert an insanity plea in defense of the patient.

39. Which factor may undermine this patient's assertion of the insanity defense?

    (A) voluntary intoxication
    (B) mental disease or defect
    (C) inability to recall the event
    (D) involuntary intoxication
    (E) prior conviction of a violent crime

40. A psychiatrist called as an expert witness is primarily responsible for which of the following?

    (A) obtaining a not guilty by reason of insanity verdict
    (B) rendering an opinion based on reasonable medical certainty
    (C) establishing reasonable doubt
    (D) evaluation, diagnosis, and initiation of treatment of the accused
    (E) countering evidence of criminal responsibility

Questions 41 and 42

A 48-year-old man is involuntarily admitted to the hospital after an acute manic episode. The patient is pressured, demanding, and increasingly talkative on the unit. He becomes intrusive, not able to be redirected, and demands immediate release. You explain to him that you feel he is gravely disabled and unable to care for himself. He respectfully disagrees with you and demands "due process."

41. The patient's request for a hearing is based on which of the following legal principles?

    (A) parens patriae
    (B) actus reus
    (C) habeas corpus
    (D) rights under the Fourth Amendment
    (E) mens rea

42. The court agrees that the patient is severely disabled and in need of acute medical management. You load the patient with divalproex sodium 20 mg/kg, and 3 days later his symptoms of mania are markedly diminished. The patient requests immediate discharge and agrees to follow up with a partial hospital program. You feel that he would benefit from further inpatient treatment but is no longer gravely disabled or a threat for self-harm. The next appropriate step is which of the following?

    (A) file for another court hearing to detain the patient further
    (B) ignore the patient's request because he has been committed by the court
    (C) release the patient to the partial hospital program
    (D) persuade the patient to stay for a few more days
    (E) appease the patient by increasing smoking privileges

Questions 43 and 44

You are treating a woman on the medical unit who suffers from dementia. In your opinion, she requires a central line for fluids and medication, but you are not sure if she can fully comprehend the risks and benefits of the procedure. You call the family for a meeting and request a psychiatric consult.

43. Which of the following is most important in discussing informed consent?

    (A) raising alternative treatment options
    (B) involving family members in this discussion
    (C) petitioning a court to establish the patient's competence
    (D) capacity to read and write
    (E) absence of mental illness

44. Which of the following best characterizes the intent of a living will?

    (A) establishing personal preferences regarding end-of-life issues
    (B) requesting physician-assisted suicide if the patient were to become terminally ill
    (C) arranging for funeral services and distributing the estate to loved ones
    (D) preventing patients from changing their minds about life support as they become ill
    (E) absolving personal responsibility

45. A 28-year-old man involved in a motor vehicle accident brings a lawsuit against the driver. Emergency department records do not show any physical injuries, but the patient is claiming to suffer from posttraumatic stress disorder (PTSD). You are asked to evaluate the patient's symptoms. He complains of distressing dreams of the accident, having flashbacks while awake, and avoiding the intersection where the accident occurred. His symptoms have lasted for 3 months. Past psychiatric history is significant for major depression, impulsivity, and violent behavior. He has been incarcerated numerous times, showing a blatant disregard for the law. On MSE, the patient is likable and cooperative. His mood is reported as being depressed and he currently denies any hallucinations or delusions. Which of the following items from your evaluation of the patient raises your suspicion regarding a diagnosis of malingering?

    (A) history of major depression
    (B) lack of physical injuries

    (C) flashbacks while awake
    (D) antisocial personality disorder
    (E) duration of symptoms

Questions 46 and 47

A 35-year-old woman is referred by her plastic surgeon for a psychiatric evaluation in preparation for sexual reassignment surgery. The patient recalls dressing in her brother's clothes since she was 4 years old and has always preferred opposite-gender playmates. She insists that she is "a man trapped inside of a woman's body." She has fully assumed the male gender role for the last 15 years. On MSE, there is no evidence of psychosis, delusions, or cognitive impairment. She does report a mildly dysphoric mood, which she attributes to her lack of male genitalia. Complete blood count, serum electrolytes, folate, vitamin B_{12} level, and liver function tests are within normal limits; rapid plasma reagin/Venereal Disease Research Laboratory (RPR/VDRL) are nonreactive. Karyotype analysis demonstrates XX genotype.

46. Which of the following is the most appropriate diagnosis in this case?

    (A) homosexuality
    (B) transvestite fetishism
    (C) frotteurism
    (D) schizophrenia
    (E) gender identity disorder

47. The plastic surgeon and patient decide to proceed with the surgery. Which of the following is most important in obtaining informed consent?

    (A) contingency analysis
    (B) discussing potential complications of the procedure
    (C) establishing the lack of any mental illness
    (D) seeking approval from family members
    (E) exploring the patient's dreams and desires

48. One of your patients consistently misses appointments without giving you advance notice. After numerous failed attempts at resolving this issue with the patient, you realize that the patient's behavior is not changing and you decide to discharge the patient from your care. Which of the following most appropriately describes the discharge process?

    (A) Write a letter to the patient notifying her that she has been discharged due to her failure to comply with treatment.
    (B) Notify your staff that the patient is not to be given further appointments.
    (C) Contact the patient's family/friends to request their help in improving the patient's attendance.
    (D) Write a letter to the patient stating that she will be discharged in 60 days.
    (E) Notify the patient's insurance company that she is discharged from your care.

49. You are asked by the court to provide a forensic evaluation for a child custody case. Which of the following is the most important factor in determining which parent should get custody?

    (A) Who is the biologic parent?
    (B) Who can provide for the best interests of the child?
    (C) Who is most financially stable?
    (D) Who has the highest level of education?
    (E) Who is in the best mental and physical health?

50. You discover that one of the physicians in your hospital is abusing narcotics. The appropriate course of action is which of the following?

    (A) Notify the local police.
    (B) Contact the Drug Enforcement Administration to rescind his license.
    (C) Do nothing so as to avoid personal liability.
    (D) Admonish him for using but do not report.
    (E) Notify the hospital's committee for impaired physicians.

Answers and Explanations

1. **(D)** A physician or therapist has a duty to protect identifiable victims from imminent danger. This obligation may be fulfilled by directly contacting the party at risk, notifying the police, or taking other appropriate measures to protect the victim. Contacting the patient's family fails to protect the intended victim. Although notification of the police is an acceptable intervention in this case, disclosing unrelated confidential information about the patient is inappropriate. When notifying third parties, care should be taken to release only information necessary to protect the potential victim. The remaining choices fail to protect the potential victim.

2. **(B)** *Tarasoff v Regents of University of California* is the landmark legal precedent establishing liability to third parties. It states "when a psychotherapist determines...that his patient presents a serious danger of violence to another he incurs an obligation to use reasonable care to protect the intended victim against such danger." Therefore, the physician may ethically break confidentiality in cases involving imminent harm to others. In the *Tarasoff* case, a student at the University of California (Prosenjit Poddar) expressed intentions to kill a fellow student (Tatiana Tarasoff) to his therapist. Poddar tragically followed through on his threat and murdered the young woman at her home. *Tarasoff v Regents of University of California* holds legal precedent only in the state of California; however, the case has been adopted by physicians/therapists as the standard of care and has led to nationwide legislative changes. There have been two rulings regarding the *Tarasoff* case. The original decision,

Tarasoff I (1974), established a "duty to warn." The California Supreme Court revised its previous holding in *Tarasoff II* (1976) with a "duty to protect." In *Rogers v Commissioner of the Department of Mental Health,* the court expounded opinions regarding the treatment of involuntarily committed patients. *Durham v United States* held that an individual "is not criminally responsible if the unlawful act was the product of mental disease or mental defect." The holding of this case has become known as the "product test" for determining an insanity defense and ultimately was replaced by the American Law Institute standard. *Zinerman v Burch* and *Kansas v Hendricks* involve court decisions regarding civil commitment.

3. **(C)** The 4 Ds of establishing medical malpractice cases involve proving that a *d*ereliction of *d*uty *d*irectly causes *d*amage. The plaintiff must establish the presence of a fiduciary relationship (a duty), negligence (dereliction of duty), and damages directly caused by that negligence. Typically, the burden of proof in medical malpractice cases (civil cases) is by a preponderance of the evidence (greater than 50%). Proof beyond a reasonable doubt refers to criminal cases; clear and convincing evidence is reserved for special cases decided by the court. Neither criminal intent nor criminal mischief is required to prove medical malpractice.

4. **(E)** An expert medical witness may be called to testify in both civil and criminal trials. Expert witnesses have a familiarity with a body of knowledge that exceeds that held by laypersons and are often called to provide opinion testimony, making choices A and C incorrect.

Choices B and D are incorrect because expert witnesses commonly charge a fee for their services and provide testimony for either defense or plaintiff.

5. **(D)** *Testamentary capacity* refers to the level of competence required to make a legally valid will. Case law and statutes differ across states. However, the central elements of testamentary capacity include: (1) comprehension of the act of writing/signing a will, (2) knowledge of potential heirs, (3) understanding the extent of one's assets, (4) lack of undue influence, and (5) the absence of delusions compromising rational thought. *Mens rea* refers to criminal intent and has nothing to do with drafting a will. *Informed consent* is the process of obtaining permission for medical treatment. Important elements include the ability to make a voluntary decision regarding treatment, explanation of risks and benefits, and competency to make an informed decision. The presence or absence of a mental illness does not necessarily impair an individual's competency to make a will. Therefore, the lack of mental illness is incorrect. *Conservatorship* of estate refers to an individual's ability to manage his or her finances.

6. **(A)** Paranoid delusions regarding the patient's family may significantly undermine this patient's assertion that she was competent to make a will. The absence of delusions, which may compromise rational decision making, is one of several criteria required for testamentary capacity. The presence of a diagnosable Axis I disorder, the inability to read and write, and refusal to undergo treatment with chemotherapy do not automatically undermine a patient's competence to make a will as long as the criteria for testamentary capacity are met. An explanation of why the patient wants to donate her estate to the local humane society does not undermine the patient's competence to make a will unless such an explanation demonstrates that the patient is unable to meet any of the specified criteria.

7. **(B)** The American Law Institute test is the modern standard for the insanity defense. It holds that a person with a mental disease or defect should not be held criminally responsible for an act if the person (1) could not appreciate the wrongfulness of the conduct and (2) could not conform the conduct to the requirements of the law. The American Law Institute test expanded upon the 1843 M'Naghten rule, which held that an individual was not guilty by reason of insanity if, as a result of a mental defect, the person did not know the nature of what he or she was doing or did not know that what he or she was doing was wrong ("right-wrong test"). The Durham rule arose from a 1954 District of Columbia case in which the court held that "an accused is not criminally responsible if his unlawful act was the product of a mental disease or mental defect." This is also known as the "product test." Extreme emotional disturbance and the irresistible impulse rule are not modern standards for proving an insanity defense. *Extreme emotional disturbance* is an affirmative defense used to render the accused less culpable for the crime (i.e., reduce the charge from murder to manslaughter). The *irresistible impulse rule*, established in England in 1922, states that an individual is not responsible for a criminal act if he was unable to resist that act due to a mental illness.

8. **(C)** Criminal responsibility requires (1) criminal intent (mens rea) and (2) a criminal act (actus reus). Diminished mental capacity serves to avoid criminal responsibility; certainly, it is not required to prove criminal responsibility. The product test and the wild beast test are antiquated standards of the insanity defense.

9. **(E)** Before discharging or transferring the patient, it is important to determine whether she can make an informed decision regarding her care. Informed consent requires that the patient (1) comprehend the issues and/or choices furnished by the physician, (2) appreciate the consequences of making a certain decision, and (3) arrive at a voluntary decision after weighing the facts. At this point in the vignette, there is not enough information to establish the patient's ability to make an informed decision regarding her care. Exceptions to informed consent include incompetence, emergency situations (e.g., comatose,

unresponsive patient), a competent patient's waiver of informed consent, and therapeutic privilege. The other choices are incorrect because this patient's ability to make an informed decision has not been assessed.

10. **(B)** A competent patient has the right to refuse treatment, even if the consequences are life-threatening. In the extension of this vignette, the patient has adequately demonstrated the elements of an informed decision. The other choices are incorrect because they would prevent a competent patient from making an informed decision in her treatment.

11. **(A)** In *Dusky v United States,* the Supreme Court ruled that competency to stand trial requires the ability to (1) rationally consult with one's attorney and (2) understand the proceedings in both factual and rational terms. Illiteracy does not constitute grounds for incompetency. A person can suffer from a mental illness and be competent to stand trial. Testamentary capacity refers to the level of competence required to make a valid will. Informed consent is important in making decisions related to medical treatments but has little bearing on one's competency to stand trial.

12. **(D)** Involuntary commitment is used when a physician believes that an individual is a threat to self or others or is gravely disabled. Medicating the patient and arranging for outpatient treatment when the patient is actively homicidal is an improper course of action. Notification of the police or warning the patient's blood brother is not immediately necessary because this patient is well-contained in a locked unit. Arranging a police hold is incorrect. Police holds are issued when an individual who is arrested requires a psychiatric evaluation. If the arrested individual does not require inpatient psychiatric care, he is released back into the custody of the police.

13. **(B)** Involuntary admission to the hospital is justified when the patient is judged to be (1) a danger to self or others or (2) gravely disabled. The criteria for involuntary commitment derive from the doctrines of *police power* (state as

protector of public safety) and *parens patriae* (the state as parent for those unable to care for themselves), respectively. State laws differ on the length of time a person can be committed to the hospital on the basis of either criteria. Permission from the conservator of person is not required for involuntary commitment. The other choices may be important factors, but are not requisite elements for involuntary hospitalization.

14. **(D)** Contrary to popular opinion, the insanity defense (1) is seldom asserted, (2) is usually unsuccessful, and (3) typically leads to a greater number of years of incarceration. Individuals found not guilty have no obligation to serve a criminal sentence. There is no limit to the number of times one may assert the insanity defense. Releasing an individual found not guilty by reason of insanity without an appropriate psychiatric evaluation and treatment is unethical and fails to protect society.

15. **(E)** Typical signs of physical abuse include burns with peculiar patterns (e.g., cigarette marks, geometric designs, bilateral immersion patterns), bruises in low-trauma areas (e.g., buttocks, genital areas, or back), retinal hemorrhages, and multiple fractures at different stages of healing. Although there is a high rate of comorbidity between physical and sexual abuse, there is no evidence to suggest sexual abuse in this particular case. Sexual or physical abuse may predispose an individual to the development of other psychiatric disorders such as depression, PTSD, and borderline personality disorder. Although the differential in this case should include depression and somatization disorder, history and mental status do not provide sufficient evidence to diagnose either. Age-appropriate "rough play" is not relevant.

16. **(D)** Each state requires mandatory reporting of abuse or neglect to Child Protective Services. In cases in which there is a reasonable suspicion of abuse, a report should be filed even if the patient and family deny the allegations. In cases of suspected abuse, steps to ensure the safety of the minor should be taken immediately. Discharging the patient with follow-up in 1 week to reevaluate her bruises disregards her

safety and potentially subjects the minor to continued abuse. Considering the extent of physical injuries, it is unlikely that they were inflicted by the patient's younger siblings. Consequently, confronting the siblings about their behavior serves no purpose.

17. **(B)** Confidentiality in the treatment of minors should be maintained unless specifically prohibited by state law (e.g., in cases of abortion) or when the parents' involvement is necessary to make complicated or life-threatening treatment decisions. The other choices all constitute violations of confidentiality to your patient.

18. **(D)** Informed consent for HIV testing involves a thorough explanation of the test's interpretation, information regarding confidentiality, and further evaluation needed if the test is positive. The patient should be aware of the risk of false positives and negatives, and the need for confirmatory testing if the test result is positive. Choices A and B are incorrect because they violate patient confidentiality. When a patient tests positive for HIV, state laws may require notification of the sexual partner (this is usually done without revealing the patient's identity). There is no reason to first perform a complete blood count or a pregnancy test before administering an HIV test.

19. **(A)** The patient's desire to stop dialysis should be respected because competent adults are able to determine which treatment to accept or deny. The American Medical Association (AMA) Code of Ethics notes that there is no ethical distinction between withdrawing and withholding medical treatment. The remaining choices undermine the patient's right to make an informed decision.

20. **(D)** Physician-patient confidentiality should be maintained except in certain cases (i.e., duty to protect others, mandatory reporting, or emergencies). The remaining choices violate physician-patient confidentiality.

21. **(C)** Confidentiality between patient and physician should be respected even in cases of court-mandated treatment. In such cases, issues around disclosure to a probation officer can be used to explore the patient's attitudes toward probation and incarceration. Obtaining a confidentiality waiver from the patient should be done in a thoughtful manner and is essential before releasing any information to the probation officer. Ignoring the probation officer's request is inappropriate in such circumstances. The other choices are incorrect because they violate physician-patient confidentiality.

22. **(B)** The patient should immediately be informed that she was accidentally given the improper medication. The physician should also evaluate for potential adverse reactions. The fact that the patient did not suffer harm is no reason to conceal the medication error. Although many hospitals require documentation of such errors or reporting of them to the appropriate person or committee, this should not be the first course of action. Evaluating the patient for any adverse reaction and explaining the mistake is the appropriate first step. Notifying the patient's family of the mistake is a breach of confidentiality and inappropriate. Encouraging the patient to seek legal action is both alarmist and inappropriate in such a case.

23. **(C)** Explaining the implications of nontreatment but respecting the patient's refusal for treatment is the most appropriate course of action. This allows the patient to make an informed decision with regard to her treatment. The elements integral to informed consent include (1) competency to make a decision; (2) an adequate explanation of the risks, benefits, rationale for treatment, and alternative treatments (including no treatment at all); and (3) a voluntary decision. In this vignette, there is no evidence that the patient suffers from a condition that might impair her competency. Further, her stated religious belief is consistent with a Jehovah's Witness's refusal of human blood products. Administering packed red blood cells infringes on the patient's right to refuse a blood transfusion and consequently is incorrect. Strongly persuading the patient to arrive at a decision for treatment or utilizing a confrontational method to secure lifesaving treatment is coercive in nature and could prevent the patient from making a voluntary decision. It is inappropriate

to involuntarily hospitalize this patient if she has arrived at her decision in compliance with the elements of informed consent.

24. **(D)** According to the AMA Code of Medical Ethics, treatment decisions must be made in the best interest of the child or neonate regardless of the desires of the parents. Treatment can be withheld or withdrawn only in cases in which the risks far outweigh the benefits, there is low potential for success, or when treatment extends the child's suffering without potential for a joyful existence. The lumbar puncture results unequivocally demonstrate bacterial meningitis. In this particular case, the neonate suffers from a serious, but treatable, central nervous system infection and treatment should not be withheld. Withholding treatment until the next regularly scheduled ethics meeting would likely result in the neonate's demise.

25. **(B)** It is unethical to offer specific psychiatric diagnoses for individuals that you have not personally examined. Moreover, commenting on an individual that you have evaluated would be a breach of confidentiality.

26. **(E)** Family and/or close associates should be consulted to aid in reaching treatment decisions if there is no advance directive or designated power of attorney. Consultation with the ethics committee should be sought when the patient's prior wishes are unclear or family members are unable to agree on treatment options. Ethics committee consultations are also useful when the power of attorney's decision is unreasonable or contrary to the patient's prior wishes. It would be inappropriate to allow a severely demented patient to designate a power of attorney or make treatment decisions. Choosing sides in a family conflict would be arbitrary; consultation with the hospital ethics committee would help clarify issues in a complicated case such as this.

27. **(A)** The most significant predictor of suicidal behavior is a prior serious suicide attempt. The other choices are all associated risk factors for suicidal behavior but are not the most significant predictor of it.

28. **(A)** Affective disorders (e.g., MDD, bipolar I/II disorder) account for 40–70% of completed suicides. Alcohol-related disorders account for 20–30% of completed suicides. Psychotic and anxiety disorders are less frequently associated with completed suicides, as are toxic metabolic states. However patients with schizophrenia are at high risk for suicide.

29. **(A)** Sexual or romantic relationships between current and former psychiatric patients are considered unethical, making the other choices incorrect.

30. **(B)** The AMA Code of Medical Ethics cautions that sexual and/or romantic relations with former patients may be influenced by the previous physician-patient relationship; care should be taken to not exploit the power derived from the professional relationship. Sexual relations with current patients is unethical and constitutes sexual misconduct. At the very least, current physician-patient relationships should be terminated prior to initiating any romantic or sexual relationships.

31. **(B)** According to the AMA Code of Medical Ethics, "physician-assisted suicide is fundamentally incompatible with the physician's role as healer," and the physician should aggressively respond to a patient's end-of-life needs rather than assist in suicide. *Physician-assisted suicide* is defined as the act of facilitating a patient's death by "providing the necessary means and/or information to enable the patient to perform the life-ending act." Simply ignoring the patient's request is inappropriate because it fails to recognize and address potential end-of-life issues. End-of-life issues that should be addressed with the patient include adequate pain control, emotional/family support, comfort care, respect of patient autonomy, and appropriate multidisciplinary referrals (hospice, counseling, religious issues). The remaining choices are consistent with the definition of physician-assisted suicide and are therefore unethical.

32. **(C)** The rate of antisocial personality disorder in the male prison population has been estimated at 30–50%.

33. **(D)** When a physician is served a subpoena to release medical information, the appropriate first step is to contact the patient to find out if he or she consents to the release. Discussing the implications of the lawsuit with your patient and clarifying whether the patient has the proper legal counsel for the lawsuit also are important. Contacting the attorney of the party requesting the subpoena and releasing the medical records without consent from the patient constitute unethical breaches of physician-patient confidentiality. The confidentiality privilege belongs to the patient, not the physician. Releasing the medical information directly to the judge at this stage makes no sense and would likewise be a breach of confidentiality.

34. **(C)** Turning over medical records to comply with a direct court order is ethical. Working out a plan of legal action is not the role of the physician, but rather the patient's attorney. The other choices are incorrect because there are cases in which disclosing the patient's medical records without consent is ethically permissible (e.g., in certain criminal proceedings, malpractice cases initiated by the patient, contestation of a will).

35. **(D)** Antisocial personality disorder is an Axis II psychiatric disorder (i.e., personality disorder) characterized by a pervasive disregard for the rights of others, which often develops out of the symptoms described in this patient. Behaviors associated with antisocial personality disorder include repeated unlawful acts, lying, stealing, contempt for the safety of others, and lack of remorse for having hurt or mistreated others. A diagnosis of antisocial personality disorder requires evidence of conduct disorder with onset before 18 years of age. Conduct disorder describes the clinical picture of the patient presented in the vignette; further, it is not classified as a personality disorder. Oppositional defiant disorder is an Axis I disorder characterized by a pattern of hostile, defiant, or negative behaviors, generally of less severity than that of conduct disorder. Narcissistic and paranoid personality disorders might develop in this patient but are not as likely to occur as antisocial personality disorder.

36. **(D)** Inquiring about possible reasons the patient may be avoiding payment may help uncover important treatment issues. Such inquiry often leads to how the patient feels about the therapy and/or the therapist. These feelings can be utilized to address factors related to her symptoms. Exploring such issues should be done in a sensitive manner to avoid alienating the patient. Requesting that the billing collector demand immediate payment and terminating treatment would be far too aggressive at this point. Contacting the patient's family violates physician-patient confidentiality. At this point, informing the patient that you will not see her if she doesn't immediately pay her bill may be perceived as confrontational and threatens the therapeutic alliance.

37. **(E)** Becoming involved in the business venture of a psychotherapy patient could have significant adverse effects on the patient's transference (feelings and memories experienced by the patient that are aroused by the therapist) as well as on the physician's countertransference (feelings aroused in the physician while working with the patient); therefore, it should be avoided. Anger, distrust, and guilt are some of the feelings that may occur if a business venture such as the one described were to fail. Further, a physician's business involvement with a patient might affect the neutral stance essential to effective psychotherapy. A central problem is that involvement in a business venture might interfere with treatment. This is best explained to the patient honestly.

38. **(B)** Suicide risk factors include: advancing age (>40); gender (M > F); marital status (separated or divorced > married); past history of suicide attempt or threat; race (Native Americans/Alaskan natives > Whites > Blacks/Hispanics); religion (Catholics are lowest risk); employment status (unemployed or retired > employed); support system (living alone > living with others); and health status (serious medical condition or terminal illness > good health).

39. **(A)** An individual who commits a crime while voluntarily intoxicated cannot assert an insanity

defense because the basis of such behavior stems from a rational decision to drink. Involuntary intoxication may be used effectively as an insanity defense if the individual had no choice in becoming intoxicated (e.g., the person was drugged). A mental disease or defect or inability to recall the event might be used to enhance an insanity defense, not undermine it. Prior conviction of a crime in itself should have no bearing on an insanity defense. However, if prior violent behavior has been associated with mental illness and the inability to appreciate the criminality of one's conduct or conform to the law, this might be used to strengthen an insanity defense.

40. **(B)** Medical expert witnesses are called to present their professional opinions based on reasonable medical certainty. Expert witnesses are expected to perform an impartial evaluation and testify as to their findings; it is not the responsibility of the expert to ensure a particular outcome for either side. Unlike the traditional physician-patient relationship, the expert witness does not typically initiate treatment of patients and has limits on confidentiality.

41. **(C)** *Habeas corpus* refers to the U.S. Constitution's Fourth Amendment's clause that the state shall not "deprive any person of life, liberty, or property, without due process of law." Under habeas corpus, citizens have the right to petition the court when detained to decide whether they are being held lawfully. Parens patriae refers to the state's function as parent for those unable to care for themselves. This is often used for justification of involuntary commitment. Establishing criminal responsibility requires the presence of both actus reus and mens rea. *Actus reus* refers to the voluntary act of committing a crime, and *mens rea* refers to criminal intent. They are both incorrect because they have nothing to do with the patient's right to due process. The Fourth Amendment is incorrect; it protects citizens from unreasonable searches and seizures.

42. **(C)** It would be unethical to involuntarily detain a patient in treatment if he or she is no longer deemed to be gravely disabled or a threat to self or others. In this case, the patient should be promptly discharged to the partial hospital program. Ignoring the patient's request because the court has committed him is incorrect. Filing for another court hearing is appropriate only if the patient is still gravely disabled or a danger to self or others. Persuading the patient to stay a few more days even though he wishes to leave the hospital and no longer meets criteria for involuntary commitment is inappropriate. Appeasing the patient by increasing smoking privileges fails to address the key issue in this question.

43. **(A)** The key elements to informed consent include competency to make a decision; a voluntary choice; and an adequate explanation of the rationale, risks, benefits, and alternative treatment options. The remaining choices are not necessary for informed consent.

44. **(A)** Living wills, or advance directives, preserve patient autonomy by establishing personal preferences regarding end-of-life issues. If patients lose capacity in the future, advance directives outline what procedures they do or do not desire without relying on physician or family member opinions. The remaining choices are not characteristics of a living will.

45. **(D)** Malingering is characterized by intentional feigning of symptoms for secondary gain (i.e., financial remuneration, disability benefits, avoiding criminal prosecution or military duty). A diagnosis of malingering should be suspected when there is the presence of one or more of the following factors: (1) litigation (especially when the patient is referred by a lawyer), (2) discrepancy between objective findings and the patient's complaints, (3) a diagnosis of antisocial personality disorder, and (4) a failure to comply with the evaluation and recommended treatments. A past history of major depression does not raise one's suspicion of malingering. The lack of physical injuries or the presence of flashbacks in a claim of PTSD is not sufficient to raise suspicions of malingering. PTSD occurs in individuals exposed to actual or threatened death or injury and consequently may have no physical injuries. Classic symptoms of PTSD include flashbacks, distressing dreams, intrusive

memories, avoidance of trauma-related stimuli, and increased autonomic activity. The duration of symptoms in this case has no bearing on a diagnosis of malingering.

46. **(E)** Gender identity disorder is characterized by a persistent desire/claim to be the opposite sex, a desire to participate in games/play of the opposite gender, preference for opposite-gender playmates, wearing cross-gender clothing, and the desire to change one's physical characteristics to conform with his or her gender identification. Generally, homosexuals lack the desire to assume the opposite gender role. Rather, they are attracted to members of the same gender. Transvestite fetishism is characterized by cross-dressing behaviors for sexual excitement without an underlying desire to assume the opposite gender identity. Frotteurism is the act of rubbing or touching nonconsenting individuals for sexual excitement. Psychotic disorders such as schizophrenia are associated with disorganized speech/behavior, hallucinations, delusions, or impaired reality testing. In this case, the patient's desire to become a male is not delusional in nature. She acknowledges that she is genetically a female but identifies herself as the opposite gender without evidence of psychosis.

47. **(B)** Elements essential to informed consent include (1) voluntary decision making, (2) explanation of risks and benefits of treatment, (3) discussion of alternative treatment options (including consequences of withholding treatment), (4) ability to understand/appreciate the information presented, and (5) absence of any condition that would impair an individual's competency to make a decision. Contingency analysis is not relevant to informed consent. The presence of a mental illness does not necessarily preclude one from making an informed decision. The severity of impairment caused by a mental illness is vital in determining whether the patient is capable of providing informed consent. Although the patient may desire to discuss the issue with members of her family, the physician is not obliged to take into consideration their opinions in seeking an informed decision. Exploring a patient's dreams and desires, while perhaps useful in understanding possible reasons behind any decision, is not an essential element in determining informed consent.

48. **(D)** According to the AMA Code of Medical Ethics, physicians are obligated to provide continuity of care for their patients. When discharging a patient from your care, advance notice of the pending discharge must be given with sufficient time to obtain another physician. Contacting the patient's family breaches confidentiality and is not the appropriate procedure for discharging the patient. Notifying the insurance company fails to inform the patient of her discharge and does not provide her time to obtain a new physician. The remaining choices fail to provide the patient with sufficient notice to obtain proper medical follow-up.

49. **(B)** The prevailing concept in determining child custody is based on which individual(s) can provide for the best interests of the child. Factors that can be used to determine the best interests of the child include assessing the individual's biologic relation, financial stability, level of education, and health; however, it is the aggregate best interest, rather than any single factor, that determines what is in the best interest of the child.

50. **(E)** Physicians are ethically obliged to report impaired colleagues. Reporting procedures vary from state to state. However, the AMA Code of Medical Ethics suggests initial reporting to a hospital's in-house impaired physician program. If no such program exists, the chief of staff or clinical service director should be notified. For physicians without hospital privileges, an impaired physicians program run by a medical society or the state board licensing committee should be made aware of the impaired physician. The other choices do not meet the AMA guidelines and fail to initiate proper treatment and supervision of the impaired physician.

CHAPTER 7

Differential Diagnosis and Management
Questions

Questions 1 and 2

A 37-year-old man presents to your office complaining of auditory hallucinations that have worsened over the last several months. He notes that the Devil has been telling him that he is "no good," and that he will not "amount to anything." During the last several months, the patient also reports feeling "depressed" and has been sleeping poorly. He has no desire to get out of bed and has lost interest in even watching sports (normally one of his favorite activities). The patient states that even when his mood is improved, he still cannot "get the voices out of my head." He denies using any drugs or alcohol.

1. Which diagnosis best accounts for this patient's symptoms?

    (A) major depression
    (B) schizophrenia
    (C) schizoaffective disorder
    (D) bipolar II disorder
    (E) schizoid personality disorder

2. What medication combination could be used to adequately treat this patient's symptoms?

    (A) mirtazapine (Remeron) and citalopram (Celexa)
    (B) fluoxetine (Prozac) and diazepam (Valium)
    (C) ziprasidone (Geodon) and sertraline (Zoloft)
    (D) haloperidol (Haldol) and perphenazine (Trilafon)
    (E) divalproex sodium and lorazepam (Ativan)

Questions 3 and 4

A 20-year-old single woman presents to your office complaining of "episodes of complete terror." She states that "totally out of nowhere" she became extremely anxious, experienced heart palpitations, felt short of breath, began sweating profusely, and believed that she was going to die. She reports that these episodes last approximately 10 minutes and that they have occurred several times over the last 3 months. She constantly worries that they will occur again.

3. What general medical condition should be considered in the differential diagnosis for this patient's cluster of symptoms?

    (A) hypothyroidism
    (B) systemic lupus erythematosus (SLE)
    (C) pheochromocytoma
    (D) folate deficiency
    (E) hypertension

4. Which of the following is the most likely diagnosis for this patient's symptoms?

(A) generalized anxiety disorder (GAD)
(B) social phobia
(C) panic disorder
(D) obsessive-compulsive disorder (OCD)
(E) agoraphobia

Questions 5 and 6

A 64-year-old woman is brought to the emergency department by her neighbor, who says "my friend isn't acting right." The patient requires the support of a nurse while walking to an examination table. Examination reveals that she cannot correctly identify the season or the town she is in. She does not recognize her neighbor. She is inattentive and seemingly apathetic to the activity around her. She dozes off repeatedly during the interview, but each time is arousable and resumes answering questions. Her answers are illogical and inconsistent.

Vital signs are within normal limits and she is neither tremulous nor diaphoretic. Neurologic examination finds bilateral sixth nerve palsy and horizontal nystagmus. Urine toxicology screen and blood alcohol level are negative.

5. What is the most likely diagnosis?

(A) subdural hematoma
(B) alcohol withdrawal
(C) Wernicke encephalopathy
(D) folic acid deficiency
(E) normal pressure hydrocephalus (NPH)

6. What is the most important first step in managing this patient?

(A) administration of a benzodiazepine
(B) computed tomography (CT) scan of the head
(C) administration of folic acid
(D) administration of thiamine
(E) intravenous (IV) fluids and observation

Questions 7 and 8

A 52-year-old man with no psychiatric history is brought in by the police to the emergency department after threatening a neighbor with a knife. He says that people in his neighborhood have organized against him in an effort to ruin his life. According to the patient, people are tape-recording his telephone conversations and videotaping him with cameras concealed in his house, and have recently recruited the police in their efforts. Although he is intensely distraught over this invasion of his privacy, he is performing well at his job, exercising daily, and eating and sleeping well. He is well-groomed and well-related in his conversation. His thinking seems otherwise logical.

7. What is the most appropriate treatment?

(A) fluoxetine
(B) alprazolam (Xanax)
(C) olanzapine (Zyprexa)
(D) electroconvulsive therapy (ECT)
(E) lithium

8. Which statement regarding this illness is true?

(A) Auditory hallucinations are common.
(B) The delusions are usually bizarre.
(C) Negative symptoms predominate.
(D) The delusion is plausible but unlikely.
(E) Persecutory delusions are relatively rare.

Questions 9 and 10

A 29-year-old man with a history of chronic paranoid schizophrenia comes to the emergency department with a temperature of 102.9°F, labile blood pressure rising to 210/110 mm Hg, a pulse of 110/min, and a respiratory rate of 22 breaths/min. This patient's medications include haloperidol, benztropine (Cogentin), and clonazepam (Klonopin). He cannot correctly identify the day, date, or year, and believes himself to be in a city from which he moved 10 years ago. A family member indicates that 3 days ago he was healthy and completely oriented and that he has no significant medical or surgical history.

9. Physical examination reveals that he is in acute distress with hypertonicity. Laboratory examination reveals a creatine phosphokinase (CPK) of 45,000 Iμ/L, a white blood cell count of 14,000/μL and no left shift, a sodium of 145 mEq/L, and a creatinine of 2.5 mg/dL. Lumbar puncture produces clear fluid with a

slightly elevated protein count. What is the most likely diagnosis?

- (A) anticholinergic syndrome
- (B) malignant hyperthermia
- (C) central nervous system (CNS) infection
- (D) prolonged immobilization
- (E) neuroleptic malignant syndrome (NMS)

10. With appropriate treatment, the patient recovers completely and returns home. In a month's time, he comes to the emergency department stating that the "voices in the walls" are telling him to kill himself. He has taken no medications since he left the hospital. His vital signs are stable and a medical workup is negative. Initial therapy may include which of the following?

- (A) ECT
- (B) haloperidol depot injections
- (C) olanzapine
- (D) safety monitoring only
- (E) physical restraints

pt already getting "x" so continue him only

Questions 11 and 12

A 39-year-old woman comes to the emergency department and complains that since her boyfriend broke up with her 3 months ago, she has been sleeping and eating poorly, has lost all interest in her work, and feels guilty that she drove her boyfriend away. In the past month, she has begun to feel hopeless, helpless, and that "life may not be worth it." In the past 2 weeks, she has developed a belief that a rare disease is rotting her heart, and in the past week, a voice in her ear tells her she is no good and that she should take an overdose of a heart medication she is prescribed.

11. What is the most appropriate treatment?

- (A) medication and discharge to a close family member
- (B) referral to an outpatient psychiatrist
- (C) admission to a psychiatric unit
- (D) admission to a medical unit
- (E) restraints and medication in the emergency department

12. What medication(s) would be most appropriate?

- (A) tricyclic antidepressant (TCA) only
- (B) lithium and a selective serotonin reuptake inhibitor (SSRI)
- (C) an SSRI and a neuroleptic
- (D) a benzodiazepine only
- (E) lithium only

Questions 13 and 14

A 21-year-old man is brought to the emergency department by police after an episode in which he ransacked the office where he works looking for "evidence." He started this job 2 months ago after graduating from college. He lives with four roommates and he believes they are jealous of him because of his job and have been poisoning his food. His family reveals that once before when he went away to college he went through a period of "acting crazy" but got better without treatment and has done well since. In the emergency department, he is shouting that he has been up for a week writing a "classic" book about accounting and someone at the office stole it from him. He needs to be physically restrained by emergency department security. Physical examination and complete laboratory workup and toxicology screen prove to be negative.

13. Initial medications should include which of the following?

- (A) lithium
- (B) a neuroleptic and a benzodiazepine
- (C) an SSRI
- (D) carbamazepine (Tegretol)
- (E) buspirone (BuSpar)

Bz for agitation;

14. Three months later, the patient sees his doctor for follow-up. He is taking lithium and haloperidol. He is doing well, except he complains of muscle stiffness. His lithium level is 0.8 mEq/L. A reasonable intervention is which of the following?

- (A) increase the lithium dose
- (B) decrease the lithium dose
- (C) start baclofen (Lioresal)
- (D) decrease the haloperidol dose
- (E) increase the haloperidol dose

Not Li toxicity that occurs 1–1.5; so from haldol;

Questions 15 and 16

A 29-year-old woman tells her doctor that about 3 weeks ago a child she was caring for ran into the street and was killed by a bus. Since then, she cannot get the image of the accident out of her mind. Even in sleep, she dreams about it. She used to take a bus to work but she now drives because she cannot bear to be near buses. In the past week, she has begun missing work because she is uncomfortable leaving her house. She feels guilty, believing the accident was her fault.

15. What is the most likely diagnosis?

    (A) posttraumatic stress disorder (PTSD)
    (B) acute stress disorder
    (C) major depressive disorder (MDD)
    (D) panic disorder with agoraphobia
    (E) adjustment disorder

16. The patient decides against any medication and follows up with psychotherapy. A year later, although she is no longer having distressful symptoms relating to the accident, she complains she feels sad and tearful most of the time, is having trouble eating, has lost interest in gardening, and wakes up at 4 AM every morning, unable to get back to sleep. What is the most likely diagnosis?

    (A) PTSD
    (B) acute stress disorder
    (C) MDD
    (D) panic disorder with agoraphobia
    (E) adjustment disorder

17. A patient is admitted to a psychiatric hospital. Her medications include an SSRI and a benzodiazepine, which are both discontinued on admission. A neuroleptic and a mood stabilizer are started. Two days after admission, she calls the nursing staff to her bed. She is extremely frightened and complains excitedly that she cannot stop looking up. On examination, her eyes are noted to be deviated upward bilaterally. This specific reaction is called which of the following?

    (A) torticollis
    (B) trismus
    (C) oculogyric crisis
    (D) retrocollis
    (E) NMS

Questions 18 and 19

A 59-year-old woman with a long history of GAD tells her primary care doctor that in a crowded supermarket 2 days previously she felt dizzy, with associated heart palpitations, pressure on her chest, and a frightening sense of doom. Shortly thereafter, she fell unconscious and woke up minutes later with a crowd around her. She felt somewhat better and rejected others' advice that an ambulance be called. She quickly made her way home.

18. What is the most appropriate next step?

    (A) short-acting benzodiazepines
    (B) an SSRI
    (C) cognitive-behavioral therapy
    (D) electrocardiogram (ECG)
    (E) reassurance that her condition is benign

19. What is the most likely diagnosis?

    (A) cardiovascular disease
    (B) panic attack
    (C) GAD
    (D) acute stress disorder
    (E) anxiety disorder due to cardiovascular disease

20. A 41-year-old woman you have been following for depression comes for a follow-up visit. She has taken increasing doses of an SSRI over the past 10 weeks, is now at the recommended maximum dose, and has shown little, if any, improvement. She is having no side effects to the medication. What is the appropriate next step in her treatment?

    (A) Add lithium.
    (B) Stop the SSRI and try a second antidepressant.
    (C) Add a second antidepressant.

(D) Continue at the current dose and follow up in 2 weeks.

(E) Discontinue all antidepressant treatment.

Questions 21 and 22

A 19-year-old college junior goes to the university health care office because she has stopped menstruating. Physical examination reveals a lean, athletic woman in no apparent distress, but is notable for poor dentition and erosion of the enamel of her teeth. With respect to her body habitus, age, and height, her weight is below average but within normal limits. She admits to being "a little weird" about her weight and exercises vigorously in response to "pigging out."

21. Associated laboratory and physical examination findings of this patient might include which of the following?

(A) low serum amylase
(B) salivary gland atrophy
(C) hyperkalemia
(D) hypermagnesemia
(E) normal thyroid function

22. Which of the following statements regarding the treatment of this patient is true?

(A) A reasonable intervention is to prescribe an SSRI, with follow-up in 1 month.
(B) Anorexia nervosa tends to be more responsive to pharmacotherapy than is bulimia nervosa.
(C) Hospitalization is typically indicated.
(D) Treatment is necessary because she is at risk for seizures.
(E) Cognitive-behavioral therapy is of little value.

Questions 23 and 24

A 19-year-old man with no previous psychiatric history is noted by his college roommate to be acting bizarrely for the past month and a half, talking to people who are not there, walking around the dormitory room naked, and accusing the roommate of calling the Federal Bureau of Investigation (FBI) to have him monitored. The patient's vital signs are all within normal limits and the neurologic examination shows no deficits or abnormalities.

23. The most important first test is which of the following?

(A) a noncontrast CT scan of the brain
(B) a toxicology screen
(C) an erythrocyte sedimentation rate (ESR)
(D) a complete blood count (CBC)
(E) liver function tests

24. If this test were negative, the most likely diagnosis would be which of the following?

(A) major depression with psychotic features
(B) delusional disorder
(C) schizophreniform disorder
(D) chronic paranoid schizophrenia
(E) substance-induced psychosis

Questions 25 and 26

You have been asked by the surgery team to evaluate a 35-year-old man who had surgery to repair his fractured right wrist 24 hours ago and is now complaining of anxiety. The patient has been in the hospital for 2 days. His heart rate is 120/min, and his blood pressure is 160/106 mm Hg. He is afebrile and reports that he has never suffered anything like this before. He is not in any pain and has no previous psychiatric history. His medication includes only acetaminophen for pain control. You note that he is diaphoretic and tremulous.

25. The most appropriate single-agent therapy is which of the following?

(A) clonidine (Catapres)
(B) methadone
(C) lorazepam
(D) carbamazepine
(E) naltrexone (ReVia)

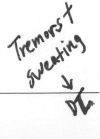

26. Without this treatment, he is at risk for developing which of the following?

(A) fatty liver
(B) abdominal pain
(C) seizures
(D) muscle cramps
(E) appendicitis

Questions 27 and 28

You are working in the psychiatric emergency department of a large metropolitan hospital. A 20-year-old man with unknown psychiatric history is brought in by the police after being found stumbling naked around a local college campus. He is markedly agitated, pacing, and appears to be responding to internal stimuli. On examination, you note that he is tachycardic with a heart rate in the 110s, he has tics or spasms in his face, and he has vertical nystagmus.

27. The test most likely to be diagnostic is which of the following?

(A) a noncontrast head CT
(B) a magnetic resonance image (MRI) of the brain
(C) an electroencephalogram (EEG)
(D) a CBC
(E) a toxicology screen

28. The most appropriate treatment is which of the following?

(A) placing the patient in a low-stimulus environment
(B) phenytoin (Dilantin)
(C) methylphenidate (Ritalin)
(D) benztropine
(E) propranolol (Inderal)

29. A 40-year-old divorced woman is brought in to the emergency department after being found sleeping in a pile of leaves. Initially, she is difficult to arouse and has trouble answering your questions, but she appears to be in no respiratory distress. You also notice that her pupils are pinpoint. After a few hours, she becomes more interactive and is complaining of diffuse, crampy abdominal pain and symptoms of "the flu." Her pupils are now slightly dilated, and she is yawning. Her vital signs are a temperature of 99.3°F, a heart rate of 99, and blood pressure of 142/90 mm Hg. After the second interview, your diagnosis is which of the following?

(A) cannabis abuse
(B) opiate withdrawal
(C) cocaine withdrawal
(D) cocaine intoxication
(E) opiate intoxication

Questions 30 and 31

A 70-year-old widow is admitted for an evaluation of depression and anxiety. She tells you that for the past 15 years her family doctor has prescribed "some pills" that have helped her sleep and feel less nervous. She says that she ran out of them yesterday and since that time has felt increasingly anxious and jittery. She also notes that she's now having tremors in her hands that have not been there before.

30. Your initial concern would be greatest if you found that the medication was which of the following?

(A) nortriptyline (Pamelor)
(B) triazolam (Halcion)
(C) thioridazine (Mellaril)
(D) fluphenazine (Prolixin)
(E) imipramine (Tofranil)

31. The most worrisome side effect of abruptly stopping this medication is which of the following?

(A) autonomic hyperactivity
(B) seizures
(C) hallucinations
(D) worsening anxiety
(E) vomiting

Questions 32 and 33

A 73-year-old man is admitted to the hospital for community-acquired pneumonia and dehydration. On day 2 of hospitalization, you are asked to evaluate the patient for depression; the staff has noted that he seems very withdrawn. He is not eating or sleeping well. Last night, the nursing staff reports, he was angry and requested to leave the hospital. You talk with the patient's family and find that the patient has no previous psychiatric history. Prior to the onset of this illness 5 days ago, he had no depressive symptoms and no difficulties with cognition. On examination, his vital signs are temperature 98.2°F, heart rate 87, blood pressure 130/86 mm Hg, and a peripheral oxygen saturation of 95% on room air. He is drowsy and oriented only to person. His Mini-Mental Status Examination (MMSE) score is 24/30.

32. The most likely diagnosis is which of the following?

    (A) MDD
    (B) anxiety disorder
    (C) dementia
    (D) delirium
    (E) factitious disorder

33. The medical team asks for medication recommendations if the patient becomes agitated. You recommend which of the following?

    (A) lorazepam
    (B) benztropine
    (C) thioridazine
    (D) diphenhydramine
    (E) haloperidol

Questions 34 and 35

A 75-year-old widow is brought to the hospital by her son, who says that his mother has been having progressive difficulty with her memory since her husband died 3 years ago. The memory difficulties, however, have worsened in the last week. Prior to a week ago, the patient and her family noted that she had difficulty remembering new names, often could not remember where she had left her purse, and was having more problems paying her bills. One week ago, however, her family noted that she was having difficulty dressing and feeding herself. On examination, her vital signs are significant for a blood pressure of 170/100 mm Hg, a heart rate of 80, a temperature of 98.8°F, and a peripheral oxygen saturation of 99% on room air. She is alert, pleasant, and oriented to person, place, and time. She scores a 24/30 on the MMSE.

34. The next step in the diagnosis is which of the following?

    (A) physical examination
    (B) noncontrast head CT
    (C) lipid profile
    (D) carotid ultrasound
    (E) transesophageal echocardiogram

35. The most concerning part of the history and examination is which of the following?

    (A) history of progressive memory difficulties
    (B) recent sudden decline in function
    (C) hypertension
    (D) fact that she is fully oriented
    (E) low score on the MMSE

Questions 36 and 37

A 65-year-old woman with a past medical history of non-insulin-dependent diabetes mellitus and depression is admitted with increasingly depressed mood over the last month. She is unable to complete her crossword puzzles because of difficulty concentrating. She has difficulty falling asleep and also wakes up in the middle of the night. She denies suicidal ideation, but does feel guilty that she is depressed. Prior to this episode, she was doing well and was actively engaged in community volunteer groups. In the last month, she has lost 13 lb due to poor intake. When you ask why she is not eating, she tells you that she is worried that she will become infected with bacteria. She has been to her primary physician for an evaluation, but she says everything was normal. Her husband confirms that the patient has been very worried about "getting a disease" to the point where she will eat only food in sealed containers. He also confides in you that she has been worried that she might have cancer and despite reassurances from her primary care physician, she continues to voice her concerns to her husband that "my intestines are not working."

36. The diagnosis that best describes her illness is which of the following?

    (A) somatization disorder
    (B) MDD without psychotic features
    (C) dysthymia
    (D) MDD with psychotic features
    (E) OCD

37. Which of the following is the treatment of choice?

    (A) sertraline
    (B) sertraline and perphenazine
    (C) lithium and sertraline
    (D) divalproex sodium
    (E) nortriptyline and lorazepam

Questions 38 and 39

An 18-year-old man is brought to the psychiatric emergency department by his parents for evaluation of his behavior. Three months ago, the patient started classes at the state university in a different city, but he comes home each weekend. His parents have noticed that over the past 2 months the patient has become increasingly withdrawn and does not seem to be taking care of himself. The parents were called by the patient's roommate who says that the patient has not been going to classes for the last 2 months, has not been eating or bathing, and has been talking about how people in his classes are trying to kill him. On examination, the patient's vital signs are all within normal parameters. He is pacing and appears to be responding to internal stimuli. His mood is euthymic and his affect is flat. He denies any drug use and is not on any medication. He is fully oriented. He says that he hears a number of people talking to him, "maybe in my head." They seem to be saying bad things about him. He looks frightened and asks, "What is happening to me?"

38. If this condition had been occurring for less than 1 month, your diagnosis would be which of the following?

    (A) delusional disorder
    (B) chronic undifferentiated schizophrenia
    (C) brief psychotic disorder
    (D) schizophreniform disorder
    (E) substance-induced psychotic disorder

39. The most helpful laboratory test to make this diagnosis is which of the following?

    (A) toxicology screen
    (B) EEG
    (C) noncontrast head CT
    (D) CBC
    (E) electrolytes

Questions 40 through 41

A 35-year-old woman with no previous personal or family psychiatric history is brought to the emergency department by her husband, who reports that his wife was attempting to kill herself by cutting her wrists. Her husband tells you that 6 months ago the patient's grandmother died. Since that time, her husband thinks the patient has been becoming more depressed. She has difficulty falling asleep and has lost 15 lb in 2 months. She was recently fired from her job as a paralegal because she was unable to concentrate.

She feels guilty that she cannot feel better and endorses feelings of hopelessness and worthlessness. She believes that her only way out of this is to kill herself.

40. You choose to treat her with which of the following?

   (A) flumazenil (Romazicon)
   (B) fluoxetine
   (C) fluphenazine
   (D) triazolam
   (E) phenelzine (Nardil)

41. A common side effect of this class of medication that may mimic a symptom of depression is which of the following?

   (A) insomnia
   (B) nausea
   (C) constipation
   (D) akathisia
   (E) diarrhea

mnemonic "J H E D G E"

Questions 42 and 43

A 25-year-old man is brought to the emergency department by his fiancé, who says that over the last week the patient has been increasingly angry. He has been yelling about minor things like taking out the trash. His behavior has become so erratic that his boss is going to fire him unless he gets some help. He has not slept more than 3 hours a night for the past week, instead staying up buying over $50,000 worth of stocks. On examination, his vital signs are within normal limits. His speech is rapid, and you are having great difficulty following his conversation because he jumps from topic to topic. He reports increased energy, but also endorses a depressed, anxious mood and suicidal ideation.

42. The most helpful test in this person would be which of the following?

   (A) an ESR
   (B) a noncontrast head CT
   (C) a Venereal Disease Research Laboratory (VDRL) test
   (D) a toxicology screen
   (E) serum electrolytes

43. You choose to begin treatment with which of the following?

   (A) divalproex sodium only
   (B) haloperidol only
   (C) fluoxetine
   (D) divalproex sodium and lorazepam
   (E) lorazepam only

Li + anticonvulsants → mania; Haloperidol for psychosis

Questions 44 and 45

You are asked to see an 18-year-old woman with no previous psychiatric or medical history because the head of her college is concerned about her and worried that she may be depressed. The patient tells you that despite being far away from her home for the first time, she was enjoying school and her new friends until 2 months ago, when she learned that her parents were getting divorced. Since that time, her grades have gone from As and Bs to Bs and Cs because she is worried about her parents and her sister at home. She says she feels "bummed out" most of the time, and her friends note that she seems unhappy and occasionally becomes tearful when talking about her family. She denies difficulty sleeping or changes in appetite or weight and continues to enjoy daily trips to the gym to work out.

44. The diagnosis that best captures her symptoms is which of the following?

   (A) GAD
   (B) acute stress disorder
   (C) MDD
   (D) bereavement
   (E) adjustment disorder with depressed mood

45. For treatment, which of the following would you recommend?

   (A) risperidone (Risperdal)
   (B) fluoxetine
   (C) psychotherapy
   (D) nortriptyline
   (E) alprazolam

Questions 46 and 47

A 26-year-old woman with no previous psychiatric history is referred to you by her primary care physician for evaluation of an episode of anxiety. She tells you that approximately 2 months ago she began having episodes lasting 10 or 15 minutes during which, she says, "I feel like I'm going to die." During these episodes, her heart races, she feels as though she cannot catch her breath, she is dizzy and worried she may pass out, and has tingling and tremors in her hands. She is concerned because she is now having problems leaving her house because she is worried these episodes will occur and make it impossible for her to get home. She cannot identify any triggers leading to the episodes. She is not on any medication and has no medical problems.

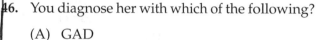

46. You diagnose her with which of the following?

    (A) GAD
    (B) panic disorder with agoraphobia
    (C) separation anxiety disorder
    (D) social phobia
    (E) panic disorder without agoraphobia

47. You initiate treatment with which of the following?

    (A) sertraline
    (B) alprazolam
    (C) lithium
    (D) propranolol
    (E) tranylcypromine (Parnate)

Questions 48 and 49

A 36-year-old woman with no former psychiatric history is referred to you by a dermatologist for evaluation of her chronically chapped hands. She says she has been seeing her dermatologist for about 5 years for this problem and treated with a variety of topical agents with limited success. Over the past 3 weeks, her hands have become worse, to the point where they are always cracked and bleeding. Reluctantly, she confides in you that she has had a fear of germs, but since her colleague has been sick, she has been washing her hands at least 40 times a day because she is afraid of contracting the disease. She also refuses to

touch anything that might infect her without using a handkerchief. She also admits to being very tidy at home as well. She tells you that she spends about $2^1/_2$ hours in the morning getting showered. She realizes her fears of contamination are irrational, but every time she tries to stop she becomes increasingly anxious.

48. You discuss which of the following diagnoses with the patient?

    (A) MDD
    (B) GAD
    (C) OCD
    (D) panic disorder
    (E) somatization disorder

49. Which of the following treatments do you recommend for the patient?

    (A) cognitive-behavioral therapy
    (B) risperidone
    (C) ECT
    (D) lithium
    (E) psychodynamic psychotherapy

50. A 47-year-old secretary comes to your office complaining, "I'm always worried." She says that she worries about her job, her kids, her housework, and her husband. She is seeking help now because she has been having an increasingly difficult time concentrating at work and has been more irritable with people around her. Her sleep has been "okay," but she does not feel rested when she gets up in the morning. She has been more aware of these feelings over the last 2 years and they occur almost every day. She denies any discrete episodes of increased anxiety. You discuss which of the following diagnoses with the patient?

    (A) GAD
    (B) OCD
    (C) social phobia disorder
    (D) panic disorder
    (E) schizophrenia

51. A 28-year-old woman with no previous psychiatric or medical history is admitted to the neurology service for evaluation of acute onset of numbness and weakness of the right side of her face and right arm and leg. Physical examination shows symmetrical 2/4 reflexes in all distributions, downgoing plantar reflexes bilaterally, and 2/5 strength in the right upper and lower extremity in all muscle groups. No atrophy or fasciculations are noted. Her gait is ataxic and staggering with extreme exaggerated movements of her arms; however, she does not fall when ambulating without assistance. Extensive neurologic workup is negative. Given the severity of her deficits, she seems unconcerned by her level of disability. The diagnosis that best captures the patient's symptoms is which of the following?

(A) factitious disorder
(B) undiagnosed neurologic disease
(C) conversion disorder
(D) malingering
(E) somatization disorder

52. A 54-year-old woman with a past medical history of hypothyroidism is admitted with a septic right knee. The surgery team asks you to evaluate the patient because they found that the fluid aspirate from the knee was growing a pathogen found primarily in the human mouth. They suspect the patient was injecting saliva into her knee. You evaluate the patient and find her to be pleasant and cooperative. She tells you that she has had a very tough time lately because her husband has recently been sick. Fortunately, she is a nurse and has been able to care for him at home. Lately, she admits to feeling overwhelmed and not appreciated. She has no idea what has caused the problem with her knee. You talk to the family and they tell you she is in no financial difficulty and she continues to enjoy work as a nurse. After working with you for a few weeks, she admits to injecting her knee but she cannot understand why she did. You tell the surgery team that you have diagnosed her with which of the following?

(A) malingering
(B) somatization disorder
(C) hypochondriasis
(D) conversion disorder
(E) factitious disorder

Questions 53 and 54

An 18-year-old woman in her first year in college comes to see you for evaluation of depression. Her roommates also encouraged her to see someone. She reports difficulty falling asleep and early morning awakenings, poor concentration, fatigue, and anxiety over the past month since she arrived for the fall semester. She tells you that her parents are very strict and she is worried that she will not get straight As. On examination, she is a calm, thin woman dressed in a very baggy jogging suit. You comment on her thinness, and she tells you she prides herself on her appearance and tries to stay slim by exercising about 4 hours a day along with a good diet. She denies problems with eating too much or too little and says just diet and exercise help her to control her weight. Despite your concerns about her thinness, she tells you she would like to lose a few more pounds. She tells you she has not had a regular menstrual period for over a year. Before you proceed with therapy, you discuss the need for further testing today.

53. The test that would help most in making the diagnosis would be which of the following?

(A) serum potassium level
(B) weight and height
(C) ECG
(D) serum amylase
(E) serum magnesium level

54. Even before this test is completed, your working diagnosis is which of the following?

(A) bulimia nervosa
(B) body dysmorphic disorder
(C) MDD
(D) anxiety disorder
(E) anorexia nervosa

Questions 55 and 56

A 5-year-old boy is referred to you by his pediatrician for evaluation of aggressive behavior. A pediatric neurologist's extensive workup was negative. Interview with parents and the patient reveals a restless boy who is able to engage in conversation. He tells you he gets angry and frustrated in school and thinks it is boring. His parents report that he has never been a strong student. He is currently repeating kindergarten due to poor performance and difficulty socializing with other children. His mother tells you that she still has to help him pick out his clothes for school and get dressed. Aggressive outbursts at school seem to occur at times when he does not understand the schoolwork. His family history is positive for two paternal uncles with learning disabilities.

55. You recommend that which of the following tests be done first in the evaluation?

    (A) Kohs Block Test
    (B) Minnesota Multiphasic Personality Inventory-2 (MMPI-2)
    (C) Wechsler Intelligence Scale for Children (WISC)
    (D) Peabody Vocabulary Test
    (E) Goodenough Draw-a-Person Test

56. A score of 69 on this test is consistent with which of the following?

    (A) borderline intellectual functioning
    (B) mild mental retardation
    (C) moderate mental retardation
    (D) severe mental retardation
    (E) profound mental retardation

Questions 57 and 58

A 12-year-old boy is brought in by his mother for evaluation of hyperactivity. She has been told by teachers and has observed herself that her son has marked difficulty sitting still and concentrating. On examination, you note a well-developed boy who is highly distractible, walking around the room playing indiscriminately with toys for a few seconds, then moving to the windows and the chairs. His mother has a hard time getting him to sit down so that you may talk with him. When he does sit down, he

swings his legs and has poor eye contact. He frequently clears his throat, sniffs, and blinks his eyes. Further examination reveals that he suffers from frequent episodes of counting numbers in his head that do not stop until he does it six times. He is very fussy about his clothes, requiring them to feel just right. He often feels the need to touch smooth surfaces to see how they feel. He admits these habits are bothersome but he cannot stop them because when he does he gets very anxious. His mother reports that his father has a number of mannerisms similar to her son's, such as clearing his throat and blinking his eyes, but they are noticeable only when he is under stress.

57. The most likely primary diagnosis is which of the following?

    (A) Tourette disorder
    (B) attention deficit disorder (ADD)
    (C) OCD
    (D) normal 12-year-old behavior
    (E) childhood schizophrenia

primary Dx is Tourette by ADD or OCD might be comorbid conditions.

58. You decide to treat the patient with pimozide (Orap). Prior to starting this medication and while on therapy, you will need to monitor which of the following?

    (A) liver function
    (B) CBC
    (C) serum dopamine levels
    (D) blood urea nitrogen (BUN)
    (E) ECG

59. A 17-year-old boy with a history of attention deficit hyperactivity disorder (ADHD) presents with odd behavior, confusion, a blood pressure of 128/85 mm Hg, and a heart rate of 68. His parents reported that at times they have observed him repetitively touching his stomach and rapidly blinking his eyes. On examination, he appears dazed and unable to concentrate. The most likely diagnosis is which of the following?

    (A) somatization disorder
    (B) hypoglycemia
    (C) amphetamine toxicosis

(D) epilepsy

(E) MDD

60. A 50-year-old man with a long history of IV drug use is brought to the hospital by police after a local homeless shelter worker noted him to be confused and "walking funny." While at the shelter, he became very suspicious of the workers and accused them of taking his belongings. On examination, you observe that he has a left pupil that accommodates but does not react, depressed deep tendon reflexes in all distributions, and loss of position sense at the great toes bilaterally. Although the patient was treated with antipsychotic medications in the past, he denies currently taking any medication. Which of the following items best accounts for all of this patient's neurologic symptoms?

(A) Wernicke encephalopathy

(B) Korsakoff psychosis

(C) NMS

(D) neuroleptic-induced dyskinesia

(E) neurosyphilis

61. A 57-year-old woman with no previous psychiatric history complains of increasing anxiety over the last 2 months. Today, she reports, it became "very bad." She also notes that with these periods of anxiety she gets a pounding headache and once fainted. She continues to feel "shaky." When you check her vital signs, her heart rate is 170 and her blood pressure is 230/130 mm Hg. She is diaphoretic and tremulous. Which of the following conditions is most likely given this patient's physiologic symptoms?

(A) hypothyroidism

(B) hypercalcemia

(C) pheochromocytoma

(D) acute alcohol intoxication

(E) posterior circulation stroke

DIRECTIONS (Questions 62 through 73): Each set of items in this section consists of a list of lettered headings followed by several numbered words or phrases. For each numbered word or phrase, select the ONE lettered option that is most closely associated with it. Each lettered option may be selected once, more than once, or not at all.

Questions 62 through 67

(A) SLE

(B) human immunodeficiency virus (HIV)

(C) hepatic encephalopathy

(D) conversion disorder

(E) pheochromocytoma

(F) somatization disorder

(G) hypoglycemia

(H) hyperthyroidism

62. You are asked to see a 55-year-old man who was admitted to the hospital today. Initially, he was cooperative, but now he is very agitated and wants to leave. His wife reports that he has periods during which he becomes very upset. She also tells you that he's a completely different person from a year ago and is becoming very forgetful. On examination, you observe that he has significant memory impairment, asterixis, palmar erythema, and a large ecchymotic area on his right scapula.

Liver DS ecchymosis since their ↓ plts;

63. A 52-year-old man with a long history of IV drug use is brought to the emergency department for evaluation after a worker at a homeless shelter found the patient having a difficult time trying to figure out how to use his eating utensils. The worker, who has known the patient for the last 10 years, says that she has seen a drastic change in the patient over the last year. He previously was jovial and interactive with the staff, but now seems disengaged and subdued. She also says that he has been increasingly forgetful. She is concerned about other health issues as she says he has lost at least 40 lb in the last 6 months and has complained about feeling weak and losing his balance. On examination, he is withdrawn and on MMSE he scores a 20/30.

64. A 33-year-old woman is brought to the emergency department by her husband, who tells you that in the last week his wife has been increasingly tearful and easily upset. Over the last few months, she has been increasingly irritable and has a hard time sitting still. Additionally, she had told him she was having some difficulty doing her usual tasks like paying her bills and balancing her checkbook. She has occasional "hot flashes." On examination, she is alert and oriented, but continuously changes position in her seat and gets up frequently. Her speech is normal for rate, volume, and production. She has difficulty with simple arithmetic and short-term memory. Her deep tendon reflexes are brisk symmetrically throughout. She has a fine resting tremor of her hands and has difficulty rising from a seated position.

hyperthyroidism hot Flashes + Diff rising from a seated position

65. A 33-year-old woman presents with a 1-year history of headaches. She was diagnosed with tension headaches by a neurologist after an extensive evaluation that was negative. Her headaches are worsening and now she also reports blurry vision. Despite a repeat negative neurologic evaluation, the patient is concerned that she has not been treated appropriately. She volunteers that she has been sick most of her life. The real trouble began for her at age 16 when she had surgery for presumed endometriosis, which has left her unable to have sexual relations. Since the surgery, she has intermittent abdominal cramping, bloating, and diarrhea. Three months ago, she saw a rheumatologist for knee, back, and eye pain.

66. A 30-year-old woman is brought to the hospital by her fiancé. He says that over the last 2 weeks, she has been "a totally different person." She has not been eating or sleeping and has been irritable and angry. Earlier in the month, she complained of headaches, pain in her hands and feet, and a fever. On examination, she looks tired; she is fully oriented but has difficulty relating the events of the last month. Occasionally, she seems to become confused.

67. You are asked to evaluate a 42-year-old woman in the emergency department because she appears confused and will not allow any blood

to be drawn. She is not oriented to time or place. She knows she takes medications for "a condition," but cannot elaborate further. The only set of vital signs that were taken show a heart rate of 140 and a blood pressure of 172/98 mm Hg. Physical examination is remarkable for a fine tremor of her hands bilaterally and diaphoresis. Five minutes after you leave the room, a nurse calls to tell you that the patient has just had a seizure.

Questions 68 through 73

(A) cocaine withdrawal
(B) phencyclidine (PCP) intoxication
(C) cannabis abuse
(D) opiate intoxication
(E) 3,4-methylenedioxy-methamphetamine (MDMA) intoxication
(F) alcohol withdrawal
(G) opiate withdrawal
(H) alcohol intoxication

68. A 35-year-old woman with no significant past medical or psychiatric history is brought to the hospital by police after crashing her car. You notice that she is slurring her speech, her gait is unsteady, and she demands her car keys so she can drive home. On cognitive examination, she has difficulty paying attention, and tests of her memory show difficulty on immediate recall. Her vital signs are all within normal limits. The physical and neurologic examination is unremarkable.

69. A 25-year-old graduate student is brought to the emergency department by his roommate, who says that since a big party this weekend he has been acting unusual. This morning he has been walking around the room "in a trance" and has not been eating or going to class. He is quite disheveled, and periodically makes odd facial grimaces. Examination shows mild increased muscle tone, vertical nystagmus, and a large laceration on his upper arm that the patient reports is not painful. Vital signs are remarkable for a blood pressure of 145/95 mm Hg and a heart rate of 105/min. Just after you leave the room, he starts screaming at someone and throwing chairs.

Dr. Newmark → PCP pain threshold is ↑ so don't feel laceration.

70. A 32-year-old woman with a history of poly-substance abuse refers herself to the hospital because she is feeling depressed and intensely suicidal and is worried she may hurt herself. While in the emergency department, she asks for something to eat and then falls asleep for the next 4 hours. Upon awakening, the patient is no longer suicidal but does report intense, unpleasant dreams.

Cocaine with hungry than sleep long time;

71. A 17-year-old boy is brought to the emergency department by his parents. They are concerned because he was previously an A student and is now failing all of his classes. They are worried because the patient's uncle was diagnosed with schizophrenia at about the same age. You find the patient difficult to engage in conversation but otherwise without evidence of psychosis. He tells you he has been "partying" more in the past few months but denies drug use. He has marked conjunctival injection. He also asks if he will be able to leave soon because he is very hungry. His only complaint is a dry mouth.

72. A 46-year-old woman complains of diffuse muscle pain and vague abdominal cramps. She continuously yawns, blows her nose, and has "goose bumps."

73. A 16-year-old boy is brought to the emergency department by friends after being out all night partying. The patient is found to be diaphoretic and exquisitely sensitive to tactile sensations. Vital signs are heart rate 98, blood pressure 200/100 mm Hg, and temperature of 103°F. The patient is also noted to be wearing a pacifier.

DIRECTIONS (Questions 74 through 81): Each of the numbered items in this section is followed by answer choices. Select the ONE lettered answer or completion that is BEST in each case.

74. A 56-year-old man presents to your office at the request of his wife, who says that he drinks too much. What would be the most important strategy in evaluating this patient for alcoholism?

(A) Quantify the average amount he drinks.
(B) Ascertain how often he drinks.
(C) Ask him how frequently he gets drunk.
(D) Ask him what his family and friends say about his drinking.
(E) Perform a complete laboratory investigation.

75. You are the consulting doctor for a corporate employee assistance program. A 53-year-old man is referred to you because he has difficulty concentrating and is falling behind in his work. He tells you that he feels restless and has not been able to get a good night's sleep recently. "I can't shake this feeling," he tells you. The symptoms have been present for about a year but have worsened as the company took on a new client that has been very demanding of the man's time. Which of the following is the most likely diagnosis?

(A) panic disorder
(B) GAD
(C) MDD
(D) separation anxiety
(E) dependent personality disorder

Questions 76 and 77

You are interviewing a 54-year-old married woman who has been urged to "see a shrink" by her family. She describes symptoms of feeling ineffectual, believing that the world is always hostile to her, and knowing that things will never change.

76. This triad of symptoms is associated with which of the following disorders?

(A) depressive disorders
(B) GAD
(C) panic disorder
(D) schizophrenia
(E) dissociative disorder

77. Which of the following treatments would best target these symptoms?

    (A) behavioral therapy
    (B) paradoxical therapy
    (C) interpersonal therapy
    (D) couples therapy
    (E) cognitive therapy

Questions 78 and 79

You are seeing an 18-year-old White man who is brought in by police after being found passed out on the street. He regains consciousness long enough to answer "yes" when you ask him whether he uses drugs, and then refuses to answer your questions about which drugs.

78. In general, more severe drug withdrawal syndromes are seen with which of the following?

    (A) drugs with short half-lives
    (B) drugs with long half-lives
    (C) drugs that are more lipophilic
    (D) drugs that are less lipophilic
    (E) IV drugs

79. In general, drugs of abuse are more addictive if they have which of the following characteristics?

    (A) cross the blood-brain barrier
    (B) have antidepressant effects
    (C) have a shorter onset of action
    (D) have a longer onset of action
    (E) can be smoked

Questions 80 and 81

A 52-year-old man is admitted to the hospital requesting alcohol detoxification. You request some of his old charts and find that he has been admitted for similar reasons at least six times in the past 10 years. On neurologic examination, the patient is found to have nystagmus, confusion, and ataxia.

80. The most likely diagnosis is which of the following?

    (A) Wernicke encephalopathy
    (B) alcoholic cerebellar degeneration

    (C) subacute combined degeneration
    (D) alcoholic peripheral neuropathy
    (E) Ménière disease

81. In Korsakoff dementia (alcohol-induced persisting amnestic disorder), which of the following is true?

    (A) the treatment is vitamin B_{12}
    (B) one often sees focal neurologic signs
    (C) lesions are seen in the mammillary bodies and thalamus
    (D) confabulation is a rare finding
    (E) Lewy bodies are often found

82. A 27-year-old man complains that he has felt "down in the dumps" for months and is feeling guilty because he has been having an extramarital affair. In recent weeks, he has started to believe that his wife is poisoning his food and the rest of his family is involved in an elaborate plot to drive him from the house. Assuming his thinking is delusional, how would his delusions be best characterized?

    (A) ego-syntonic
    (B) bizarre
    (C) somatic
    (D) mood congruent
    (E) mood incongruent

83. What diagnosis would these delusions most likely accompany?

    (A) schizophrenia
    (B) mania
    (C) MDD
    (D) dysthymia
    (E) adjustment disorder

    In recent wks major Dep since it usually takes 2 wks

84. A 45-year-old man is in the emergency department because of a diabetic foot ulcer. In gathering a history, the physician learns that this man lives alone and works nights as a security guard. He says he has no friends but that this does not bother him. He has never been hospitalized or received any psychiatric help. His affect is flat. Although he answers questions and seems to trust the judgment of the doctors,

he has little interest in the interview. He exhibits no signs or symptoms of psychosis or depression. What is the most likely diagnosis?

(A) schizotypal personality disorder
(B) schizoid personality disorder
(C) paranoid personality disorder
(D) MDD
(E) schizophrenia

85. The identified patient is a 30-year-old separated female brought into the emergency room by her identical twin sister. The patient's history is notable for a prior episode of depression 5 years ago successfully treated with venlafaxine. The patient has been staying with her sister since her separation 1 month ago. For the past 2 weeks, she has been pacing around the house, not sleeping more than 2–3 hours per night. Despite her feeling "sad" immediately after the separation, the patient now feels "wonderful, like I can accomplish anything!" In fact, she has been attempting to remodel her sister's bathroom, even though she has no training or experience. Her sister has been extremely concerned about her, but she has been unable to talk to her about is as, "I can't get a word in edgewise, and she doesn't always make sense." The patient is only taking oral contraceptives and omeprazole for acid reflux. Her sister is concerned that she, herself, may eventually develop this illness. What is her approximate risk of developing this disease?

(A) 40–50%
(B) 50–60%
(C) 60–70%
(D) 70–80%
(E) 80–90%

86. A 19-year-old man is admitted to a psychiatric hospital for the first time and discharged with a diagnosis of schizophrenia. When he returns to the hospital a month later for follow-up, the patient's speech is logical and he is able to sit and talk with the interviewer becoming relatively engaged in the examination. He says that he has been hearing voices since his discharge and he believes his every word is being recorded by a tape recorder inside his mouth. What is the most likely type of schizophrenia in this patient?

(A) paranoid
(B) disorganized
(C) catatonic
(D) undifferentiated
(E) residual

87. A 33-year-old woman with a history of paranoid schizophrenia tells you she has been hearing voices. What is the most important information to obtain regarding her auditory hallucinations?

(A) whether the voices come from inside or outside her head
(B) how loud the voices are
(C) how long she has been hearing voices
(D) what the voices are saying
(E) whether she recognizes the voices

88. A 38-year-old man complains that for the past 2 years he has required several naps over the course of the day; he finds the naps quite refreshing, but sees his doctor because lately, as he is waking up, he feels momentarily "paralyzed." What is the most likely diagnosis?

(A) cataplexy
(B) hypnagogic hallucinations
(C) idiopathic hypersomnolence
(D) narcolepsy
(E) advanced sleep wave syndrome

✓ 89. A 65-year-old woman is admitted to the hospital for cellulitis and you are asked to evaluate her because the intern on duty suspects that she is in delirium tremens. Which of the following statements should you keep in mind while evaluating her?

(A) Delirium tremens is expected to occur 2 or more weeks after the last drink.

(B) Her symptoms might be confused by a comorbid diagnosis of dementia.

(C) Auditory hallucinations are common.

(D) It is important to look for signs of autonomic instability.

(E) As many as half of patients in alcohol withdrawal experience delirium tremens.

DT only 5% of pt but 20% mortality; Hall are rare; DT 3Days from last Drink;

DIRECTIONS (Questions 90 through 101): Each of the numbered items in this section is followed by answer choices. Select the ONE lettered answer or completion that is BEST in each case. For each description, choose the axis used.

Questions 90–101

(A) Axis I
(B) Axis II
(C) Axis III
(D) Axis IV
(E) Axis V

90. A 32-year-old woman has been sleeping on the street for 6 months.
✓

91. A 57-year-old man who comes to see you for a consultation has diabetes that is difficult to control.
✓

92. A 12-year-old boy has an intelligence quotient (IQ) of 72.
✓

93. A 34-year-old woman has just gone through a divorce.
✓

94. A 45-year-old woman carries a diagnosis of borderline personality disorder.
✓

95. A 32-year-old man carries a diagnosis of schizophrenia.
✓

96. A 46-year-old man is diagnosed with MDD.
✓

97. A 43-year-old woman has just been diagnosed with late-stage breast cancer.
✓

98. A 34-year-old woman carries a diagnosis of bipolar I disorder.
✓

99. A 32-year-old man who suffers from paranoid delusions is given a diagnosis of paranoid personality disorder.

100. A 78-year-old man is being seen after the death of his wife.

101. An 18-year-old man has a history of heroin dependence.

Recall Lloyd corrected the resident → Drugabuse is axis I; Any substance abuse;

MR and PD → axis II

Answers and Explanations

1. **(C)** The most likely diagnosis in this case is schizoaffective disorder. The patient has prominent psychotic symptoms, including auditory hallucinations and paranoid ideation, but also has concurrent mood symptoms, including depressed mood, decreased sleep, anhedonia, and decreased motivation. Also important, the patient's hallucinations have occurred in the absence of mood symptoms, and his mood symptoms appear to have been present for a substantial portion of the total duration of his illness. The presence of prominent psychotic symptoms in the absence of mood symptoms makes major depression unlikely. A diagnosis of schizophrenia alone would not adequately account for this patient's mood symptoms. Bipolar II disorder is not a valid choice since there is no clear history of a hypomanic episode. Schizoid personality disorder is unlikely because that diagnosis would not account for the patient's psychotic and mood symptoms.

2. **(C)** In schizoaffective disorder, it is important to treat both the mood and psychotic symptoms. Because the patient's symptoms mainly consist of depression and psychosis, a combination of an antipsychotic and antidepressant medication would be a reasonable approach. Mirtazapine, citalopram, fluoxetine, and sertraline are antidepressant medications, while ziprasidone, haloperidol, and perphenazine are antipsychotic medications. Lorazepam and diazepam are benzodiazepines. Divalproex sodium is the only mood stabilizer listed.

3. **(C)** Hyperthyroidism, hyperparathyroidism, pheochromocytoma, cardiac arrhythmias, and substance abuse should all be considered in the differential diagnosis of panic disorder. *Pheochromocytomas* can produce similar symptoms to panic disorder, such as flushing, sweating, trembling, and tachycardia. Cardiac arrhythmias should obviously be considered in a patient complaining of palpitations. Substance abuse with caffeine, cocaine, or amphetamines can cause symptoms similar to a panic attack as can withdrawal from alcohol, barbiturates, or benzodiazepines. Hypertension, folate deficiency, hypothyroidism, and lupus are not generally thought of as causing an anxiety-like syndrome.

4. **(C)** The most likely diagnosis in this case is panic disorder. This patient reports some classic symptoms of a panic attack, namely an intense fear in a very short amount of time, associated with palpitations, sweating, shortness of breath, and a feeling of being unable to breathe. The patient has also related past multiple episodes and that she spends a lot of time worrying she will have another episode. These symptoms fit criteria for a panic disorder and not GAD, social phobia, or OCD. *Agoraphobia* is the fear of crowded spaces.

5. **(C)** This patient presents with the signs of Wernicke encephalopathy, which results from thiamine (vitamin B_1) deficiency. It is characterized by bilateral abducens nerve palsy, horizontal nystagmus, ataxia, and a global confusion accompanied by apathy. Each of the other choices are possible and should be actively ruled out. Alcohol withdrawal usually presents with unstable vital signs, tremulousness, and agitation. Folic acid deficiency presents with diarrhea, cheilosis, and glossitis;

neurologic abnormalities are usually not seen. NPH is associated with the classic triad of dementia, incontinence, and gait disturbance.

6. **(D)** If Wernicke is suspected, emergent administration of IV thiamine is essential, because many sequelae of thiamine deficiency are reversible with this treatment; mistaken administration of thiamine is rarely harmful. A CT scan of the head should be ordered immediately in this case; optimally, the IV thiamine would be started as the CT was being arranged. The remaining choices do not address the urgent need to replete thiamine.

7. **(C)** This patient is clearly psychotic and the delusion has progressed sufficiently far as to render the patient potentially dangerous to others. Therefore, most clinicians would prefer to address his delusional thinking with an antipsychotic, in this case olanzapine, a newer atypical antipsychotic. Although alprazolam, a short-acting benzodiazepine might provide temporary relief from the stress of the delusion, it would provide little long-term benefit. ECT, lithium, and SSRIs have been shown to be helpful in some cases of delusional disorder, but they would not be a first choice in this patient with severe psychosis.

8. **(D)** Although tactile and olfactory hallucinations may be present, the presence of auditory hallucinations would suggest a diagnosis such as schizophrenia. In delusional disorder, the delusions are not bizarre (logically impossible); usually, they have some internal logic and could conceivably be possible. As in this case, negative symptoms are not generally a part of the presentation. The most common delusions are of the persecutory type.

9. **(E)** NMS is characterized by severe ("lead pipe") rigidity, change in mental status, autonomic instability, elevated CPK, and elevated white blood count; a slight elevation in cerebrospinal fluid protein count is possible. NMS may be induced by any neuroleptic including the newer atypicals. No one symptom is necessary for the diagnosis; instead, a constellation of symptoms and their severity, in a setting of neuroleptic exposure, makes the diagnosis more or less likely. Anticholinergic syndrome, resulting from overdosing on anticholinergic medications, does not produce rigidity and an elevated CPK. Malignant hyperthermia, an acute muscular pathologic process, resembles NMS, but follows the administration of inhaled anesthetic agents, as in general surgery. A diagnosis of CNS infection would be better supported by findings on the lumbar puncture and CT or MRI scan; an elevated CPK would be possible if the CNS infection caused seizures. Prolonged immobilization could result in an elevated CPK, but would not account for the other findings.

10. **(C)** Command auditory hallucinations are a psychiatric emergency and most clinicians would agree that this patient should be restarted on a neuroleptic. Because they are long-acting (i.e., hard to stop), depot injections of a neuroleptic are not a first choice. Because the patient is not violent, physical restraints should be avoided. ECT has some efficacy in treatment-resistant schizophrenia but is not a first-line therapy.

11. **(C)** Command auditory hallucinations to perform suicidal attempts such as overdosing on medications are a psychiatric emergency and in virtually all cases require a psychiatric admission. We are given no clues that there is a necessity to admit the patient to a medical unit; however, she will need a complete medical workup to rule out organic causes of depression. This can usually be accomplished on a psychiatric unit. We are given no indication, such as violent behavior, that this patient needs to be restrained.

12. **(C)** This patient requires an antidepressant. Treating her depression is likely to relieve her psychotic symptoms as well, but the antidepressant cannot be expected to start taking effect for at least a week and likely longer. In fact, either an antidepressant or an antipsychotic would not treat this condition as well as both together. Therefore, many clinicians would add a neuroleptic, a class of drugs that is relatively quick acting, to treat her auditory hallucinations. A TCA would not be the first

choice. First, there is a suggestion that this patient has some cardiac history and the tricyclics can have a proarrhythmia effect. Second, unlike SSRIs, tricyclics can be lethal in overdose and this patient has risk factors for overdose. Lithium does have some antidepressant effects but in the absence of convincing evidence that this patient has a bipolar disorder lithium is not used. (If this patient has only a partial response to the SSRI, lithium may at some point in the future be added for augmentation.) Although a benzodiazepine may help this patient's irritability, as a sole agent it is a poor choice for treating her depression and psychosis.

13. **(B)** Initial medications in this case are aimed at the target symptoms of agitation, delusional thinking, and disruptive behavior and could reasonably include a neuroleptic and a benzodiazepine. Although he clearly needs a mood stabilizer such as lithium or carbamazepine as well, these are not expected to start showing an effect for at least a week and are not the critical medications to start emergently. SSRIs must be used with extreme caution in bipolar illness because they can incite or exacerbate mania. Buspirone is an anxiolytic used mostly in GAD. It is of extremely limited use in bipolar disorder and does not adequately address the target symptoms seen in this case.

14. **(D)** When the patient returns for his first follow-up visit, his lithium level is therapeutic at 0.8 mEq/L and is not in need of adjustment. However, his muscle stiffness is a parkinsonian side effect of haloperidol. This is normally treated by lowering the dose of the neuroleptic or with anticholinergic medication not with a muscle relaxant such as baclofen. The patient would have to be followed closely for reemergence of psychotic symptoms.

15. **(B)** *Acute stress disorder* is a reaction that causes clinically significant disruption or distress in a patient who witnesses or somehow participates in a traumatic event. The event must be quite horrible, invoking in the patient intense fear, and usually involving death or threatened death. The typical symptoms include hyperarousal states, dissociative states, and intrusive reexperiencing of the event (e.g., flashbacks and avoidance behaviors). PTSD is similar in most respects to acute distress disorder, but in PTSD the symptoms persist for at least 4 weeks following the trauma; a shorter duration suggests a diagnosis of acute distress disorder. The patient does not appear to be suffering from any of the typical criteria for MDD or adjustment disorder, except for guilt. Although she is suffering from agoraphobia, a symptom consistent with an acute stress reaction, there is no evidence of panic disorder.

16. **(C)** Although MDD, panic disorder with agoraphobia, and adjustment disorder are all in the differential diagnosis at the initial presentation and should be carefully considered, MDD does not emerge as a clear diagnosis until this question's additional information is presented. At this time, the principal symptoms of the acute stress disorder have remitted, and the classic symptoms of depression—feelings of sadness, loss of interest, a change in sleep habits, tearfulness, and change in appetite are apparent. These outweigh the earlier working diagnoses.

17. **(C)** *Oculogyric crisis* is a specific example of an acute dystonic reaction in which there is spasm of the muscles of extraocular motion. *Torticollis* and *retrocollis* refer to muscle spasms that cause abnormal positioning of the head. *Trismus* is a spasm of the jaw muscles. NMS, also a reaction to neuroleptic medications, is characterized by dystonia, autonomic instability, and usually some degree of delirium.

18. **(D)** Benzodiazepines, SSRIs, and cognitive-behavioral therapy each have a place in treatment of the anxiety disorders. In this case, however, these should not be considered until an organic cause is ruled out.

19. **(A)** Regardless of a patient's past psychiatric diagnosis, organic causes of physical signs and symptoms must always be ruled out. The anxiety disorders, although intensely distressing and uncomfortable to patients, rarely, if ever, result in unconsciousness. Many aspects of the

patient's story seem to be related to anxiety and could in fact occur during a panic attack, but this patient's presentation is more consistent with ischemic heart disease and should prompt a cardiac workup.

20. **(B)** Most clinicians agree that after 10 weeks at a reasonable dose, if one SSRI is not working, it is time to stop the medication and try a new one. Monoamine oxidase inhibitors (MAOIs), however, require a 2-week washout period before initiation. Lithium is usually used only as augmentation to antidepressant medication when at least a partial response is obtained from the antidepressant. In the absence of evidence that the depression has remitted, there is no advantage gained in discontinuing all medications.

21. **(E)** Despite the tremendous toll binge eating and purging takes on the body, thyroid function tends to remain intact. However, each of the other choices offers the opposite trend in what one tends to find in bulimia. Laboratory abnormalities include hypokalemic, hypochloremic alkalosis; high serum amylase; and hypomagnesemia. The salivary and parotid glands and the pancreas tend to enlarge.

22. **(D)** The fluid shifts and electrolyte imbalances introduced by excessive vomiting may cause seizures. Hospitalization is only required if patients become severely underweight or physically compromised. Medications have been of limited success in the treatment of anorexia. However, many studies have documented the benefits of SSRIs and TCAs in controlling bulimic behaviors. Simply prescribing an SSRI to this patient, however, would be a woefully inadequate intervention. Typically, bulimic patients are steered toward a combination of pharmacotherapy and some form of talk therapy (e.g., cognitive-behavioral therapy, group therapy).

23. **(B)** The key points in this case presentation are the absence of a previous psychiatric history and the duration of symptoms. Before diagnosing a mental illness, it is necessary to rule out the effects of a substance. A urine toxicology screen usually includes opiates, cocaine,

and PCP. Amphetamines, cocaine, and PCP intoxication can mimic symptoms of schizophrenia. Although a CT scan is helpful to rule out a mass lesion or bleeding, it is not likely in this age group nor is it likely, given the nonfocal neurologic examination, to provide further information influencing treatment. Liver function tests, CBC, and ESR are unlikely to aid in the diagnosis.

24. **(C)** Delusions, hallucinations, and disorganized behavior are some of the hallmark symptoms of schizophrenia. Because the symptoms have been present for more than 1 month but less than 6 months and there is no previous psychiatric history, the most appropriate diagnosis is schizophreniform disorder. There is no history suggestive of a mood disorder and thus major depression with psychotic features is not correct. The toxicology screen is negative, so the diagnosis of substance-induced mood disorder is less likely. Delusional disorder usually manifests in a person who is functional in society, with the exception of a circumscribed delusion, which can be of the jealous, erotomanic, grandiose, persecutory, or somatic type. The patient is also suffering hallucinations, which in combination with delusions exclude the diagnosis of delusional disorder.

25. **(C)** Benzodiazepines are the treatment of choice for alcohol withdrawal. Any benzodiazepine can be used—the choice depends on the desired route of delivery or the presence of liver dysfunction. With abnormal liver function tests, lorazepam or oxazepam (Serax) would be chosen because they are primarily metabolized and eliminated renally instead of through the liver as are the other benzodiazepines. Additionally, lorazepam may be chosen because it can be given IV, intramuscularly (IM), or by mouth (PO). Methadone or clonidine may be used for opiate withdrawal. Carbamazepine in conjunction with propranolol has been advocated in some settings for alcohol withdrawal, but carbamazepine is not used as single-agent therapy. Naltrexone has been used to help maintain abstinence from alcohol but has no efficacy in withdrawal.

26. **(C)** Alcohol withdrawal can be life-threatening. Tremors begin about 6–8 hours after cessation, followed within 8–12 hours by psychotic and perceptual abnormalities (hallucinosis). Seizures may follow anywhere from 12 to 72 hours after cessation. Delirium tremens (DTs) may occur any time in the first week of abstinence. Untreated DTs have a mortality rate of approximately 20%. Fatty liver is a long-term consequence of alcohol abuse. Abdominal pain and muscle cramps can be symptoms of opiate withdrawal.

27. **(E)** A toxicology screen is the best way to diagnose this condition. Often, a urine toxicology screen include opiates, cocaine, and PCP, but this varies depending on individual institutions. There is no indication for an EEG at this time because no seizure history is elicited and the patient does not appear postictal. Although structural brain lesions can cause psychotic symptoms, substance-induced symptoms are more common in this age group. A nonfocal neurologic examination would further decrease the likelihood that imaging studies would alter the diagnosis or treatment plan in this case.

28. **(A)** Unless the patient is extremely agitated and at risk for hurting himself or others, the best choice for treatment would be to place him in a quiet, dark (low stimulation) room. If the patient is violent and/or psychotic, a combination of neuroleptics and benzodiazepines could be used to keep the patient safe. Methylphenidate is a stimulant; benztropine, used to prevent extrapyramidal symptoms associated with neuroleptic use, might worsen the patient's delirium. Because the patient is not suffering a seizure or at risk for seizures, phenytoin is not indicated.

29. **(B)** The first part of the vignette illustrates some of the features of opiate intoxication, namely pupillary constriction, drowsiness, impaired attention and memory, and slurred speech. In the second interaction, the patient shows signs and symptoms of opiate withdrawal. Yawning, muscle aches, diarrhea, lacrimation or rhinorrhea, and fever are all typical of opiate withdrawal. Additionally, mildly elevated vital signs may occur; however, tachycardia and hypertension should always signal possible alcohol withdrawal. Pharmacologic management of withdrawal can include clonidine, a centrally acting alpha-2-agonist; buprenorphine, a mixed opiate agonist/antagonist; and methadone, a synthetic long-acting opiate. Lorazepam can be used to treat elevated vital signs.

30. **(B)** Your concern is greatest with sudden discontinuation of any sedative, hypnotic, or anxiolytic agent, which can cause seizures. Triazolam is a short-acting benzodiazepine. Thioridazine and fluphenazine are neuroleptics, and nortriptyline and imipramine are TCAs. Neither TCAs nor neuroleptics cause life-threatening withdrawal symptoms.

31. **(B)** As with the sudden discontinuation of alcohol, benzodiazepine or barbiturate withdrawal can be life-threatening. Withdrawal symptoms include tremors; anxiety; auditory, visual, and tactile hallucinations; autonomic hyperactivity; and seizures. The onset of symptoms depends on the half-life of the medication, the dose, and duration of use. The most concerning discontinuation side effect is seizures.

32. **(D)** The patient is exhibiting typical signs of delirium, including impaired consciousness and difficulty with cognition, manifested as drowsiness and disorientation. Classically, these symptoms may fluctuate during the day. Patients who meet criteria for delirium may appear depressed with a decreased level of arousal or may appear overly active and energetic, with the depressed type occurring more commonly. Patients also show cognitive and memory impairments, which may be manifested as disorientation or decreased capacity to register, retain, and recall information. An MMSE during periods of delirium may be misleadingly low, suggesting a dementing or pseudodementing process. In this setting, it is important to gather information from the people who know the patient to evaluate for a possible coexisting depression or dementia. Risk factors for delirium are extremes of age, prior history of delirium, alcohol dependence, sensory

impairment (auditory or visual), and preexisting brain damage. There is a broad etiologic differential for delirium. In this case, causative factors may be infection, hypoxia, metabolic abnormalities, and current medications.

33. **(E)** Haloperidol is the drug of choice for managing the agitated or confused patient with delirium. Thioridazine, benztropine, and diphenhydramine all have anticholinergic properties that may exacerbate delirium. Lorazepam, especially in older patients, may have a paradoxical effect and exacerbate agitation and confusion. Haloperidol in low doses, such as 0.5 mg every 8 hours, helps to manage the agitated patient. It has the advantage of IM, IV, or PO administration.

34. **(A)** The most important next step is to perform a physical examination. Particular attention should be concentrated on the neurologic examination looking for any evidence of focal deficit suggesting an acute neurologic event that may have led to the sudden decline. The remainder of the test may be helpful in assessing the etiology of the deficit.

35. **(C)** A sudden decline in an otherwise slowly progressive course should alert the clinician to evaluate for an underlying cause. In this case, the patient is hypertensive, which increases the risk for stroke and therefore vascular dementia. Further workup for reversible causes of dementia should include a CBC with differential; electrolytes; BUN; creatinine; B_{12}; folate; VDRL; calcium, magnesium, and phosphorus; urinalysis; ESR; urine toxicology screen; thyroid studies; liver function tests; ECG; and chest x-ray. If focal neurologic deficits are found on the neurologic examination, a noncontrast head CT could be helpful in the assessment. The differential diagnosis of dementia includes pseudodementia (depression) and delirium. Depressed individuals may show evidence of cognitive impairment that can appear identical to dementia, which makes obtaining a history from those who know the patient crucial. Similarly, delirium may also present with cognitive deficits. In delirious states, these tend to fluctuate over time and may be associated with periods of agitation and confusion. Alzheimer dementia is the most common form of dementia, followed by vascular dementia. Together, these account for between 70% and 80% of all dementias.

36. **(D)** This patient is exhibiting signs and symptoms consistent with MDD with psychotic features. For more than 2 weeks, the patient has displayed depressed mood, loss of interest in pleasurable activities, weight loss, inability to concentrate, poor sleep, and guilt about her current depressive state. She is also suffering delusional-type concerns about bodily functioning and possible infection. If the patient were complaining of contamination fears and performing multiple compulsive tasks to rid herself of the pathogens, a diagnosis of OCD with comorbid depression could be considered. Somatization disorder is characterized by more somatic complaints as well as at least one neurologic and pain symptom. Dysthymia presents with a chronic moderate level of depressive symptoms, but this patient is describing an episodic decompensation over the last month.

37. **(B)** Because of the delusional quality to her presentation, it is reasonable to treat this patient with a neuroleptic such as perphenazine for a few days prior to beginning a trial of an antidepressant. Antidepressants alone or with benzodiazepines would not help with the delusional aspects of her symptoms. Similarly, lithium and divalproex sodium are used as mood stabilizers in bipolar depression or mania but not commonly in the treatment of unipolar depression.

38. **(C)** Brief psychotic disorder is diagnosed when symptoms have been persistent for more than 1 day but less than 1 month. *Delusional disorder* is a rare condition in which the primary symptoms are delusions that are usually nonbizarre; that is, they could occur. Delusional disorder is further classified into subtypes, including grandiose, jealous, persecutory, somatic, erotomanic, and unspecified. There are no symptoms of a mood disorder and the other associated symptoms of schizophrenia are not present.

39. **(A)** The most helpful test is a urine toxicology screen. Intoxication with a variety of substances including cocaine, PCP, or amphetamines may mimic the symptoms of schizophrenia, and thus it is necessary to rule out these intoxication syndromes. A CT scan helps to rule out a mass lesion or a bleed, but in this age group and with a nonfocal neurologic examination, it is unlikely to contribute to the diagnosis and treatment. Because the patient does not present with signs or symptoms of a seizure disorder, an EEG is unlikely to provide information that will impact the diagnosis in this case. There is no diagnostic finding on CBC or electrolytes specific for any of the psychotic disorders.

40. **(B)** There are two choices for antidepressants in this group. Phenelzine, an MAOI, is not the first choice of antidepressant because the SSRIs have a more favorable side effect profile, are safer in overdose, and have similar efficacy in the treatment of MDD. Fluoxetine, therefore, is the best choice at this time. Triazolam is a benzodiazepine, flumazenil is an opioid antagonist, and fluphenazine is an antipsychotic.

41. **(A)** SSRIs have a number of side effects, including diarrhea, constipation, insomnia, nausea, headache, sexual dysfunction, and agitation. The side effect shared by the symptoms of depression is insomnia. Constipation and akathisia are also common side effects of antipsychotics.

42. **(D)** It is essential to evaluate whether the behavioral disturbance is caused by an exogenous substance. The symptoms of bipolar illness can be mimicked by intoxication with a number of substances, including amphetamines and cocaine. A CT scan, VDRL, ESR, and electrolytes may all be appropriate to evaluate initially but are unlikely to change the diagnosis, and therefore are of limited utility in making the diagnosis of bipolar illness.

43. **(D)** Given the severity of this patient's symptoms, it is likely that he will require the use of both lorazepam and valproic acid to control his illness. Divalproex sodium can be loaded rapidly to achieve therapeutic blood levels in

3–5 days. Prior to the onset of mood-stabilizing properties, a benzodiazepine such as lorazepam can be useful in keeping the patient calm. An SSRI such as fluoxetine is not indicated in bipolar disorder and can precipitate or worsen mania.

44. **(E)** Adjustment disorder is characterized by the onset of emotional or behavioral disturbances within 3 months of a significant life event that may manifest as marked change in an individual's ability to function in school, work, or interpersonal relationships. The disturbances are not so severe, however, as to suggest the diagnosis of another disorder such as MDD. The differential diagnosis for adjustment disorder includes mood disorders such as MDD and anxiety disorders such as PTSD, GAD, and acute stress disorder. In this case, the patient may be suffering from depressed mood but does not have other neurovegetative signs of depression. Acute stress disorder is usually diagnosed when an individual who has experienced an extreme stressor has dissociative experiences and anxiety after the stressful experience. This patient is not describing these symptoms. Similarly, PTSD usually requires exposure to or witnessing of a life-threatening event, with episodes of reexperiencing the event and making efforts to avoid settings that may remind the patient of that experience. In this case, the patient has experienced a significant stressor, but it is not a life-threatening event that is usually required for the diagnosis of acute stress response or PTSD. *Bereavement* is the normal response to the loss or death of an individual close to the patient.

45. **(C)** The diagnosis of adjustment disorder does not usually require pharmacotherapeutic intervention, but instead may respond to supportive individual or group psychotherapy. Risperidone is an atypical antipsychotic. Fluoxetine is an SSRI, nortriptyline is a TCA, and alprazolam is a benzodiazepine.

46. **(B)** This patient is describing symptoms associated with panic disorder. This disorder occurs in late adolescence or the early twenties and is more common in women than men. People typically describe feelings of fear, dread, or

intense discomfort associated with a variety of somatic symptoms, including tachycardia, chest pain, shortness of breath, tremulousness, diaphoresis, nausea, fear of dying, paresthesias, light headedness, and hot or cold flashes. The diagnosis of agoraphobia is made when fears of having an attack or being unable to leave a place where they are having an attack force patients to remain in familiar places. The medical workup for panic disorder includes CBC, electrolytes, fasting glucose, calcium, liver function tests, BUN, creatinine, urinalysis, toxicology screen, ECG, and thyroid function studies. A careful substance abuse and caffeine intake history should also be taken. Social phobia or social anxiety disorder occurs in the context of public appearances or performances. Individuals may experience anxiety and fear. These feelings cause great distress and may cause people to limit or avoid these settings. This disorder differs from panic disorder by having an identifiable trigger. Separation anxiety disorder is commonly diagnosed in young children when separated from their primary caregiver. GAD occurs in individuals experiencing continued anxiety and worry for periods greater than 6 months, occurring throughout the day. Unlike panic disorder, there do not seem to be discrete episodes.

47. **(A)** A variety of medications, including SSRIs (sertraline), TCAs, MAOIs (tranylcypromine), and benzodiazepines (alprazolam) have been used to treat panic disorder. Although all have shown some efficacy in the treatment of panic, SSRIs are usually the first agent of choice because they are generally well-tolerated, with fewer side effects than TCAs or MAOIs, and lack the dependency potential of benzodiazepines. Common side effects include sexual dysfunction, gastrointestinal disturbances, and insomnia. Lithium is used in the treatment of bipolar disorder, and propranolol is used for social phobia.

48. **(C)** The patient has OCD in which she suffers from recurrent, intrusive, unwanted thoughts or images (obsessions) and either repetitive behavior or mental acts (compulsions) that are performed in response to these obsessions.

Patients realize that the obsessions and compulsions are intrusive, unreasonable, and unwanted and cause marked impairment in their lives. Many patients with OCD may hide their symptoms and may first come to the attention of other medical specialists. Somatization disorder presents with numerous somatic complaints that cannot be fully explained by the results of medical investigations. GAD is an appropriate diagnosis in people who have worries and concerns that are not limited to any particular aspect of their lives, with the anxiety significantly impairing their ability to function. Panic disorder occurs as recurrent, discrete episodes of extreme anxiety and fear that occur unexpectedly and remit spontaneously.

49. **(A)** A common intervention for OCD is cognitive-behavioral therapy, during which the patient is exposed to the threat or fear (obsession) with the response (hand washing) prevented for progressively longer periods of time until the behavior is extinguished. SSRIs have been successful in treatment of OCD. Risperidone is an atypical neuroleptic that is used to treat psychotic disorders. Lithium is used in the treatment of bipolar disorder and has not been shown to be effective in the treatment of OCD. Psychodynamic psychotherapy is intensive, long-term therapy that may be helpful for people who wish to better understand the nature of their relationship with others.

50. **(A)** Symptoms of excessive worry and anxiety occurring for over 6 months without discrete episodes are best characterized by the diagnosis of GAD. Other symptoms of GAD include sleep difficulties, irritability, and difficulty concentrating. Patients with GAD may also suffer from muscle tension, fatigue, and restlessness. Although this patient does admit to anxiety, it does not occur in episodic fashion or in response to public performances, as with panic disorder or social phobia. Similarly, although the symptoms of anxiety and worry are in excess of what would be expected, they do not reach the magnitude characteristic for OCD, nor are any compulsions elicited. There is no evidence of psychosis or a thought disorder in this patient.

51. **(C)** The diagnosis of conversion disorder is most likely given that the primary symptoms are neurologic and exhaustive workup is negative for evidence of pathology that accounts for the deficits. Neurologic deficits in conversion disorder involve either motor or sensory modalities and are felt to be a result of psychological stressors. Had the symptoms been intentionally produced, the diagnosis of factitious disorder or malingering would be appropriate. If the primary incentive for the behavior was to assume the sick role, the diagnosis would be factitious disorder. If the symptoms are feigned or exaggerated for another reason, such as to gain monetary reimbursement, the diagnosis would be malingering. Somatization disorder is not appropriate in this case because the number and types of complaints do not extend past the neurologic complaints. An undiagnosed neurologic condition is a possibility, but given the extensive workup, it is less likely. It is important to note that as many as 50% of those diagnosed with conversion disorder are eventually diagnosed with a neurologic condition that could have produced the initial symptoms.

52. **(E)** Factitious disorder is an appropriate diagnosis when physical or psychological symptoms are intentionally produced in order to assume the sick role. It must be clear that these symptoms are not intentionally produced for other reasons, such as avoiding work, gaining monetary compensation, or avoiding legal issues. If any of these reasons are present, the diagnosis is malingering. Somatization disorder presents with complaints of pain, gastrointestinal symptoms, sexual dysfunction, and pseudoneurologic symptoms. The diagnosis of hypochondriasis is incorrect because this patient is not preoccupied with the idea of having a severe disease that is unrecognized despite repeated reassurances by medical personnel. Classically, people with factitious disorder are more likely to be female and to have experience in health care. Often, these patients will have numerous admissions to many different hospitals with a variety of symptoms. The psychological factors underlying this disorder are not well understood. No effective form of psychotherapy or pharmacotherapy has been identified for the treatment of factitious disorder.

53. **(B)** Obtaining height and weight is crucial for establishing the diagnosis of anorexia nervosa. Patients with anorexia nervosa are unable to achieve or maintain greater than 85% of expected body weight for height and frame structure. Additionally, they have continued concerns about thinness and body image despite being underweight. In contrast, most patients with bulimia nervosa are of normal height and weight or are slightly overweight. Some people with bulimia nervosa engage in recurrent binge eating with compensatory purging (e.g., via vomiting or laxatives) or other behaviors to control weight in the absence of binge eating. Both disorders occur more commonly in women than men. Anorexia tends to begin in the teens to twenties, whereas bulimia's onset is somewhat later in the twenties. Patients with anorexia have a higher risk of comorbid disorders, including depression and anxiety.

54. **(E)** Patients with eating disorders may have a variety of medical complications including (1) amenorrhea secondary to starvation and alterations in hormonal regulation, (2) electrolyte abnormalities (low serum magnesium and potassium) due to purging, (3) elevated amylase, and (4) loss of cardiac muscle with resulting conduction abnormalities detected by ECG. Body dysmorphic disorder is a somatoform disorder with a preoccupation of physical imperfection. Anorexia and bulimia are considered eating disorders and not somatoform disorders.

55. **(C)** Given the patient's history of angry, aggressive outbursts around not understanding schoolwork and difficulties with socialization and caring for himself along with a family history of learning disabilities, you suspect the diagnosis of mental retardation. A diagnosis of mental retardation includes subnormal functioning with an IQ of less than 70. Either the WISC or the Stanford-Binet Intelligence Scale is an adequate instrument for estimating IQ. The MMPI-2 is frequently used to assess personality

[handwritten marginalia: prof less 20) 20 interval OCEP / mild 20–70)) 10 interval DIFF / Mod + severe]

structure, and the Goodenough Draw-a-Person Test and Kohs Block Test assess visual-motor coordination. The Peabody-Vocabulary Test is used when patients suffer from a language barrier.

56. **(B)** Mental retardation is classified according to severity based on IQ scores: mild mental retardation, 50–70; moderate, 35–49; severe, 20–34; and profound, less than 20. *Borderline intellectual functioning* is a term no longer in use, but referred to IQ scores in the 71–84 range.

57. **(A)** Tourette disorder is a syndrome of multiple motor and vocal tics that occur daily for at least 1 year, with the onset before age 18. Tourette occurs more commonly in men than women and is associated with attention deficits and obsessive and compulsive behaviors. Currently, it is unclear whether obsessive-compulsive behaviors and ADD behaviors are separate entities from Tourette or if these behaviors are always comorbid. This patient demonstrates none of the psychoses that characterize childhood schizophrenia.

58. **(E)** Prior to induction of therapy with pimozide, and while in active treatment, ECGs should be performed to evaluate the QT interval. Pimozide has been associated with QT prolongation and an increased risk of ventricular arrhythmias.

59. **(D)** Epilepsy is a complex set of disorders that may initially come to the attention of a psychiatrist because of unusual behaviors. Complex partial seizures, in particular, may be associated with a wide range of symptoms, including sensory auras and automatic behaviors. Prior to the seizure, the patient may notice a bad smell, an unusual taste, or gastrointestinal symptoms. During the event, the patient may look dazed or frightened and may exhibit a number of automatisms such as lip smacking, eye blinking, and fumbling with his or her clothes. Additionally, there is impairment of consciousness. Complex partial seizures are usually associated with temporal lobe epilepsy but can also be derived from lesions elsewhere in the brain. In this case, another diagnosis to rule out is amphetamine

intoxication. Amphetamines are commonly used to treat ADHD and may be drugs of abuse in this age group. Intoxication with amphetamines may present as seizures and can be easily ruled out by a urine toxicology screen.

60. **(E)** Although syphilitic infections have been on the decline since World War I, they must still be considered in the differential for a wide variety of psychiatric disorders, especially when combined with neurologic abnormalities. In this case, two forms of neurosyphilis (tabes dorsalis and general paresis) are combined in one patient. The taboparetic form occurs in about 20% of patients with neurosyphilis. Patients demonstrate sensory ataxia with a wide-based gait, a positive Romberg sign, and a loss of vibratory and proprioceptive senses initially in the lower extremities. Deep tendon reflexes are decreased and pupil abnormalities are common, although the full Argyll-Robertson pupil is infrequent. General paresis is usually associated with a dementing process along with neurologic symptoms such as pupil abnormalities, tremors, dyscoordination, and spasticity in the lower extremities. Testing for neurosyphilis should include a blood test for VDRL and fluorescent treponemal antibody absorption test (FTA-ABS). Consideration should also be given to performing a lumbar puncture to test cerebrospinal fluid for evidence of treponemal infection. Although this patient has some symptoms of Wernicke encephalopathy and Korsakoff psychosis, neither diagnosis alone would account for this patient's constellation of neuropsychiatric symptoms. Finally, a diagnosis of NMS should not be entertained because he is currently not taking an antipsychotic medication.

61. **(C)** Pheochromocytoma is a tumor of the chromaffin cells, usually occurring in the adrenal medulla. Symptoms may differ according to the predominant catecholamine released. As norepinephrine-secreting tumors are the most common, baseline hypertension with paroxysmal exacerbations are frequent. Anxiety, fear, and palpitations may accompany exacerbations of hypertension. Because this may mimic

symptoms of a panic attack or GAD, it is essential to consider this in the differential diagnosis when patients present with anxiety.

62. **(C)** Hepatic encephalopathy can present in many ways and may have a fluctuating course making it difficult to diagnose without peripheral stigmata. Neurologically, the patient may exhibit asterixis, which, although characteristic for hepatic encephalopathy, is not specific for the disorder. Patients may suffer 6- to 9-Hz tremors, mildly increased deep tendon reflexes, and an altered sensorium. Typical psychiatric symptoms may include changes in personality, abrupt mood swings, and changes in cognitive ability. In an acute decompensation, depression, catatonia, psychosis, and delirium may develop. Physical stigmata reflecting changes in liver function can include ecchymosis, peripheral edema, ascites formation, palmar erythema, and spider angiomas.

63. **(B)** HIV may produce a spectrum of neuropsychiatric manifestations as a result of opportunistic infections, neoplasms, or direct invasion of the CNS by the virus. HIV-associated dementia is one of the most common manifestations of primary CNS invasion. It may present in a variety of ways, including motor abnormalities, cognitive decline, or behavioral changes. This case presentation describes typical behavioral change, apathy, and social withdrawal. HIV dementia may also have neurologic abnormalities such as weakness, imbalance, or ataxia. Occasionally, patients present with irritability and apathy. Cognitively, this patient has been described as increasingly forgetful, and the results of the MMSE support the diagnosis of dementia. Criteria for dementia include the presence of multiple cognitive deficits, including aphasia, apraxia, agnosia, or disturbance in executive function.

64. **(H)** Hyperthyroidism may present with symptoms consistent with a variety of psychiatric disorders, including depression, anxiety, psychosis, mania, and, at an extreme, delirium. This case illustrates a more moderate presentation of hyperthyroidism with some depressive, hypomanic, and cognitive features.

Hyperthyroidism may cause mild cognitive deficits in calculation and recent memory. Neurologically, patients may show a fine 8- to 12-Hz tremor, lid lag, brisk deep tendon reflexes, proximal myopathy with muscle wasting, and myalgias. Patients may report hot flashes and/or increased sensitivity to heat.

65. **(F)** Somatization disorder is characterized by a variety of somatic complaints that cannot be verified by laboratory and physical findings. The disorder has its onset before age 30 and is more common in women than in men. Diagnosis is based on the occurrence of four pain symptoms, two gastrointestinal symptoms, one sexual symptom, and one pseudoneurologic symptom. It is important to determine that these symptoms are not intentionally produced or feigned for other purposes. Similarly, it is important to ensure that the patient has received the appropriate medical workup because a number of disease processes may present with a constellation of symptoms.

66. **(A)** Neuropsychiatric complications occur in up to 60% of patients with SLE. Although neuropsychiatric conditions may arise at any time during the course of the disease, they are most frequent during acute exacerbations or late in the disease process. Of the psychiatric manifestations, organic mental syndromes, including "lupus psychosis," schizophrenia-like syndromes, and affective disorders are the most common. Organic mental syndromes include psychotic symptoms, delirium, personality changes, anxiety, and emotional lability. Patients may also exhibit cognitive impairment on neuropsychological testing. Most of the reactions are short, lasting hours to days, and are associated with flares of the illness. Affective illnesses and schizophrenia-like syndromes are less common. Neurologically, patients can present with seizures, stroke, cranial nerve abnormalities, and headache.

67. **(G)** This patient is exhibiting signs and symptoms consistent with a delirium secondary to hypoglycemia. In this case, a psychiatric consultation was likely requested to evaluate the acute confusional state and to evaluate the

refusal to provide blood. Signs of hypo-glycemia manifested by this patient include tachycardia, tremor, hypertension, and, finally, seizure. Delirious states should receive immediate workup for an organic etiology because delirium carries a high rate of morbidity and mortality. The standard workup consists of a CBC with differential, electrolytes, BUN, creatinine, VDRL, vitamin B_{12}, folate, urinalysis, thyroid-stimulating hormone (TSH), calcium, magnesium, phosphorus, glucose, urine toxicology screen, liver function tests, peripheral oxygen saturation, chest x-ray, ECG, and mental status and physical examination.

68. **(H)** Alcohol intoxication and dependence are the most common substance abuse-related problems. This case exhibits some of the common signs of alcohol intoxication: impaired judgment, slurred speech, lack of coordination, unsteady gait, and impaired attention. Other signs can include nystagmus, stupor, and coma. This patient's vital signs are stable, and there is no mention in the case of diaphoresis or tremor. The presence of any of these would arouse suspicion for alcohol withdrawal.

69. **(B)** PCP intoxication can be quite striking in its similarities to schizophrenia, especially with regard to psychosis. In any case in which a substance-induced state may mimic psychiatric disorders, a toxicology screen should be obtained. This case highlights aspects of PCP intoxication, including nystagmus, hypertension, tachycardia, a decreased responsiveness to pain, and muscular rigidity. Violence or aggressive tendencies may be apparent with or without psychotic symptoms. No clear psychotic symptoms are occurring in this patient. Most patients recover in a few days from PCP-induced psychosis, but others may remain psychotic for periods up to 1 month.

70. **(A)** This case is typical for cocaine withdrawal or "crashing." After cessation or reduction of cocaine use, patients frequently report an intensely dysphoric mood, which may be associated with suicidal ideation. Additionally, patients are fatigued, with increased appetite, insomnia or hypersomnia, unpleasant dreams,

and psychomotor agitation or retardation. The time frame for withdrawal can last hours to weeks depending on the pattern of use and the amount used.

71. **(C)** Although it is concerning that this patient has a family history of schizophrenia, the more likely cause of his failure at school is cannabis abuse. The findings of conjunctival injection, increased appetite, and dry mouth are consistent with this diagnosis. Mild tachycardia can also be associated with cannabis abuse. Behavioral abnormalities such as impaired coordination, poor judgment, social withdrawal, euphoria, or anxiety may also be present. At this point, there is no evidence of psychosis, but with a family history one would want to monitor closely for any prodromal symptoms of schizophrenia.

72. **(G)** This patient is exhibiting the classic signs of opiate withdrawal: piloerection, diaphoresis, abdominal cramps, yawning, lacrimation, and muscle aches. Other signs that may be suggestive of withdrawal include dysphoric mood, insomnia, fever, and nausea, vomiting, or both. Shorter-acting opiates tend to produce withdrawal symptoms more quickly and more intensely than longer-acting agents.

73. **(E)** MDMA, or ecstasy, has stimulant properties and its biologic effects include enhanced perception/sensation, increased heart rate, hypertension, dilated pupils, trismus (tightness of jaw muscles), bruxism (grinding of teeth), hyperthermia, and diaphoresis. Drug paraphernalia associated with MDMA use includes pacifiers, Popsicle sticks, and candy necklaces to help alleviate MDMA-induced bruxism.

74. **(D)** Because the defense mechanism of denial is active in alcoholism, the best approach in evaluating a patient is to explore how alcohol affects his life, rather than direct questions about drinking behavior. Hearing about his drinking from his friends and family may provide a more accurate description of a patient's alcoholism than the alcoholic would provide of himself. Although laboratory work might

provide clues to the presence of alcoholism, it cannot be relied on to make the diagnosis.

75. **(B)** GAD is defined by excessive anxiety or worry occurring for at least 6 months. Associated symptoms include feeling restless, fatigued, or irritable; muscle tension; difficulty with concentration; and sleep disturbance. Patients with panic disorder are usually more disabled by their symptoms and seek help much earlier than patients with GAD. Although depression and dysthymia share some symptoms with GAD, the depressive symptoms are more severe in the mood disorders than with the anxiety disorders. The onset of anxiety with panic disorder is more sudden and more intense, with the fear of choking or dying more common. Separation anxiety requires the onset of symptoms before the age of 18, and dependent personality disorder represents a pervasive need to be taken care of, leading to submissive, clinging behavior that begins in early childhood.

76. **(A)** These symptoms are known as *Beck's triad*. Beck, who developed the Beck Depression Inventory, is a seminal thinker with respect to cognitive therapy. His triad of symptoms has been very helpful in the diagnosis and treatment of MDD. This particular triad is not characteristically seen in other disorders.

77. **(E)** Cognitive therapy can help to alter these negative ways of perceiving the self and the environment. In paradoxical therapy, developed by Bateson, the therapist suggests that the patient engage in the behavior with negative connotations (e.g., a phobia or compulsion). Behavioral therapy is focused on behaviors, not on possible underlying factors that cause behaviors such as cognitive errors. Couples therapy would be less efficacious than cognitive therapy given this patient's symptoms. The major focus of interpersonal psychotherapy is communication analysis and one's role in relationships.

78. **(A)** This is a general rule that almost always applies, at least in the cases in which a drug has a withdrawal syndrome. Lipophilia generally is related to half-life in the sense that body stores of the drug are available for a "self-taper," but is not directly related to severity of withdrawal. Route can have some effect on withdrawal severity, because IV drugs can be shorter acting, but is not necessarily directly related; some IV drugs can still have long half-lives.

79. **(C)** The shorter the onset of action, the quicker the "high" and the quicker the addiction potential; hence, users simply like, and get addicted to, such drugs more easily.

80. **(A)** This is a classic presentation of Wernicke encephalitis: **A**taxia, **C**onfusion, and **E**ye movement findings (mnemonic: **ACE**). The other responses describe similar but distinct syndromes. Alcoholic cerebellar degeneration is a disorder of the cerebellar vermis in which patients have difficulty with gait and stance but characteristically do not have arm ataxia or nystagmus. Subacute combined degeneration results from B_{12} deficiency, which leads to demyelination and axonal degeneration of the peripheral nerves, posterior and lateral columns of the spinal cord, and the cerebrum. Patients have cognitive impairment, diminished position and vibration sensation, and abnormal gait. Alcoholic peripheral neuropathy is a sensory peripheral neuropathy in which alcohol may directly cause axonal damage, although malnutrition may also play a role. Ménière disease is a vestibular disorder in which distention of the endolymphatic sac causes intermittent vertigo, tinnitus, and hearing loss.

81. **(C)** Pathologic lesions in Korsakoff are found in the mammillary bodies and thalamus. Confabulation is a common finding. Treatment is with thiamine, not vitamin B_{12}. The neurologic findings are ataxia and nystagmus. Lewy body disease, which presents as a dementia similar to Alzheimer disease, involves deposition of inclusion bodies in the cerebral cortex.

82. **(D)** *Mood-congruent delusions* are compatible and consistent with the state of mind of the patient. In this case, the patient feels guilty and presumably believes he deserves punishment. His delusions express these thoughts. If he described delusions of grandiosity, that would be an example of a mood-incongruent delusion.

Bizarre delusions describe a circumstance that is virtually impossible to be true, for example, a schizophrenic patient believing a computer chip is implanted in his brain. The delusions in this question, however unlikely, are in some sense conceivable. *Somatic delusions* focus on bodily functions and integrity. *Ego-syntonic delusions* are experienced by the sufferer as acceptable; for example, the manic patient believing he is the greatest actor in the world. This patient's delusions are ego-dystonic, that is, experienced as unacceptable and unpleasant. Often, the nature of the delusion and its relation to mood state provide clues to a diagnosis. Delusions arising out of a severe depression, as in this case, are frequently mood congruent.

83. **(C)** The delusions of schizophrenic patients can be bizarre and are often unrelated to mood state. Mania produces delusions that are grandiose, usually related to a sense of inflated self-esteem. The presence of delusions rules out dysthymia and adjustment disorder because these affective illnesses do not reach an intensity that includes delusional thinking.

84. **(B)** Patients with schizoid personality disorder are typically socially isolated and be distinctly inept at forming and carrying on interpersonal relationships. They often come to the attention of physicians as a result of some other issue, as seen in this case. Their apparent apathy and indifference may resemble the negative symptoms of schizophrenia, and indeed, that is in the differential here; but it would be difficult to make a diagnosis of schizophrenia without evidence of psychosis. This patient lacks the actively odd and peculiar mannerisms or eccentric way of thinking seen in schizotypal personality disorder. He exhibits none of the mistrust and suspiciousness seen in paranoid personality disorder. Although he may be depressed, we are given no direct evidence of this.

85. **(E)** Bipolar disorder has one of the largest genetic components of all the mental illnesses. Having a monozygotic twin with bipolar disorder increases the risk of developing bipolar disorder to 80–90%.

86. **(A)** Schizophrenia is commonly classified according to types, which try to capture descriptively the symptoms that predominate the clinical picture. In the *paranoid type*, the patient is preoccupied with delusions, typically persecutory in nature, and often has auditory hallucinations. Speech and behavior appear relatively organized. The *disorganized type* is characterized by disorganized speech and behavior as well as flat or inappropriate affect. In *catatonic type*, motor activity is retarded to the point of immobility, or excessive, yet purposeless and unrelated to external events. A diagnosis of *undifferentiated type* means that the patient meets criteria for schizophrenia, but does not meet criteria for paranoid, disorganized, or catatonic types. The *residual type* describes an absence of positive symptoms and a preponderance of negative symptoms.

87. **(D)** The most important aspect of voices heard by a patient with schizophrenia is the nature of what the voices are saying. Command auditory hallucinations telling a patient to harm or kill him or herself or someone else is almost always a psychiatric emergency, and the patient requires hospitalization to be safe or to keep someone else safe. The only possible exception is the case in which an experienced clinician knows the patient well and believes the situation to be safe; even then, hospitalization is probably necessary. All of the other choices in this question speak to important characteristics of auditory hallucinations and should be evaluated but the presence of command auditory hallucinations requires immediate attention.

88. **(D)** *Narcolepsy* is characterized by persistent daytime hypersomnolence that is temporarily relieved by brief naps. Narcolepsy is often accompanied by phenomena commonly associated with REM sleep, including *hypnagogic hallucinations* (vivid hallucinations upon waking up), *cataplexy* (a sudden dramatic loss of muscle tone, usually following an intense emotional reaction), and *sleep paralysis* (a loss of voluntary muscle tone at the beginning or end of sleep, seen in this case). *Idiopathic hypersomnolence* is also characterized by persistent

sleepiness but can be distinguished from narcolepsy by the fact that the naps accompanying it are often long and unrefreshing.

89. **(D)** *Delirium tremens*, an acute confusional state induced by severe alcoholic withdrawal, occurs in 3–5% of patients withdrawing from alcohol. Although it may be seen in patients with dementia, as well as in those without, any delirium, including delirium tremens, differs from dementia in that one finds a relatively acute onset. The patient with dementia, by history, has a slow (months to years) decline, whereas the patient in an alcohol withdrawal delirium is expected to manifest symptoms in a matter of days, if not hours. Although auditory hallucinations are possible, visual hallucinations (e.g., little scary creatures lurking about the room) are far more common. Delirium tremens usually occurs 3–7 days after the patient's last drink. Autonomic instability, particularly fever and elevated pulse and blood pressure, are common signs of alcohol withdrawal and often provide a key clue to the fact that the patient is in withdrawal and in need of emergent treatment, namely, administration of benzodiazepines.

90–101. [90 (D), 91 (C), 92 (B), 93 (D), 94 (B), 95 (A), 96 (A), 97 (C), 98 (A), 99 (B), 100 (D), 101 (A)] Although this set of questions is unlikely to show up on the United States Medical Licensing Examination (USMLE) Step 2, it is useful to be able to distinguish the various axes of the *Diagnostic and Statistical Manual of Mental Disorders* (DSM's) multiaxial classification system from one another, particularly on the wards when it is necessary to write notes. The system is used to break out and describe the diagnoses of a given patient and what contributes to each. *Axis I* includes all mental illness diagnoses, including substance abuse and developmental disorders, except personality disorders and mental retardation, which are coded on *Axis II*. *Axis III* includes general medical conditions, and *Axis IV* includes psychosocial and environmental factors that may be contributing to the mental illness. The Global Assessment of Functioning, a scale of 0–100 that the assessor uses to rate the level of daily functioning, is coded on *Axis V*.

CHAPTER 8

Practice Test 1
Questions

DIRECTIONS (Questions 1 through 89): Each of the numbered items or incomplete statements in this section is followed by answer choices. Select the ONE lettered answer or completion that is BEST in each case.

Questions 1 and 2

A 29-year old man with a history of bipolar disorder presents to the psychiatric emergency department saying that he is the king of "Pumbar" and needs everyone's allegiance for the upcoming war with the Martians. In the past few days, he has slept a total of 3 hours but says that he is not tired. He has spent all of his money soliciting phone sex. Now, he is agitated, demanding, and threatening.

1. What is the best treatment for this patient in the acute setting?

    (A) hydroxyzine (Atarax)
    (B) lithium
    (C) divalproex sodium (Depakote)
    (D) haloperidol (Haldol)
    (E) carbamazepine (Tegretol)

2. After treating the patient acutely, a medication is needed to control his bipolar disorder. You find that he has a history of agranulocytosis. Which of the following is the best choice for a mood stabilizer?

    (A) lithium
    (B) carbamazepine
    (C) divalproex sodium
    (D) antipsychotic medication
    (E) lorazepam (Ativan)

Questions 3 and 4

A 44-year-old woman presents to her primary care doctor with multiple complaints, including weakness in her lower extremities, bloating, headaches, intermittent loss of appetite, and back pain. A careful review of symptoms reveals many other vague symptoms. Her complaints date back to adolescence and she has seen many doctors. Thorough workups, including an exploratory laparotomy, have failed to uncover any clear, organic cause.

3. What is the best approach to this patient?

    (A) Tell her any physical workup is unnecessary.
    (B) Tell her to come back in 1 month and, if the symptoms are still present, you will initiate a physical workup.
    (C) Tactfully ask her why she is inventing symptoms.
    (D) Assess her for other psychiatric illnesses.
    (E) Initiate a physical workup and arrange for follow-up in a year's time.

4. Which statement regarding this patient's diagnosis is correct?

    (A) It has a good prognosis.
    (B) It is most common in high socioeconomic groups.
    (C) Women are overwhelmingly more likely to receive this diagnosis than are men.
    (D) Conversion symptoms are uncommon.
    (E) Regularly scheduled, frequent visits with a primary care doctor will exacerbate symptoms.

Questions 5 and 6

A 25-year-old man is a concern to his neighbors. He dresses in odd, outdated clothes; seems to utter his own language; and although he tends to keep to himself, he has told neighborhood children that witches who live down the road have it in for him.

5. Which of the following statements about the personality disorder from which this patient is most likely suffering is true?

    (A) Auditory hallucinations are common.
    (B) Visual hallucinations are common.
    (C) This diagnosis may be confused with schizophrenia in remission.
    (D) This diagnosis is found overwhelmingly in men.
    (E) Onset of symptoms is usually in the second or third decade of life.

6. The patient's brother brings him to a doctor after the death of their mother. Since then, the patient's paranoia has caused him to question his neighbors' activities. He moved into a hotel he could not afford to get away from the "spies" living next to him. What is an appropriate intervention?

    (A) no treatment
    (B) psychoanalysis
    (C) benzodiazepines
    (D) a neuroleptic
    (E) a selective serotonin reuptake inhibitor (SSRI)

Questions 7 and 8

A 25-year-old female college graduate is brought to her doctor by her mother. Described as "odd" since she lost her job a year ago, the patient has complained of hearing voices and believes that her body is a receiving antenna for a foreign spy operation. Her mother notes she has been isolating herself in her room. She is alert and oriented but suspicious and guarded on examination. Her affect is flat and her speech reveals loose associations. A complete medical workup is negative.

7. Which of the following symptoms is considered a "negative symptom" with regard to her illness?

    (A) auditory hallucinations
    (B) delusions
    (C) paranoia
    (D) flat affect
    (E) loose associations

8. The patient is started on medication and many of her symptoms improve. She begins a new job and does well. One year later, she is brought to her doctor floridly psychotic, actively hearing voices, and extremely paranoid. She thinks her boss is trying to kill her. She has an upper respiratory viral illness that she believes to be the work of a foreign government. She discontinued her medication 4 weeks ago because she felt too sedated. In the past year, her cigarette smoking habit has decreased to one pack per day. What is the most likely cause of her exacerbation?

    (A) stress from work
    (B) a reaction to the viral illness
    (C) medication noncompliance
    (D) medication side effects
    (E) decreased cigarette smoking

Questions 9 and 10

A 44-year-old man complains to his doctor that he is always tired and is having difficulty getting out of bed in the morning. Upon questioning, he reveals he has three or four drinks each night and perhaps more on the weekends, but denies he has any problem with alcohol.

9. A diagnosis of alcohol dependence is made and the patient comes to your office in acute alcohol withdrawal. He has a withdrawal seizure. What might be found on laboratory investigation?

    (A) thrombocytosis
    (B) elevated or depressed liver enzymes
    (C) decreased prothrombin time
    (D) hypermagnesemia
    (E) a high blood alcohol level

guarded - schizophrenia)

When in alcohol withdrawal your BAL reduces)

10. Which of the following statements regarding this patient is true?

(A) Cerebellar degeneration is uncommon.
(B) He is at risk for developing a peripheral neuropathy.
(C) Alcoholic "fatty liver" is irreversible.
(D) He is at decreased or normal risk for heart disease.
(E) Immune function should remain relatively intact.

Questions 11 and 12

A 28-year-old woman is brought to the emergency department for active suicidal ideation with a plan to overdose on acetaminophen. She has no history of a psychiatric illness but endorses many criteria for major depressive disorder (MDD), including poor sleep for the past 2 weeks. She recently lost her job and fears that she may not be able to pay her rent. You speak to a friend, who reports that the patient has been abusing alcohol. Attempts to obtain additional collateral information have been unsuccessful. You believe the patient requires inpatient evaluation but her health maintenance organization (HMO) denies authorization for inpatient care, alternatively authorizing eight outpatient visits with a psychiatrist. You speak to the weekend on-call physician-reviewer and report that the patient remains unsafe and wishes to be discharged. Upon learning that the patient does not have a history of psychiatric illness, the reviewer fails to authorize inpatient care, despite your assessment.

11. Which of the following is the most appropriate intervention?

(A) Begin antidepressant therapy and arrange for outpatient follow-up the next day.
(B) Admit the patient on an emergency certificate to an inpatient facility on the basis of danger to self.
(C) Administer an antipsychotic medication and reevaluate the patient in 1 hour.
(D) Explain to the patient that her HMO did not authorize hospitalization and discharge her with follow-up care.
(E) Prescribe a medication to help her sleep, discharge her, and arrange for follow-up care.

12. A 67-year-old woman with a history of depression presents to your office for evaluation. Her symptoms of poor appetite, insomnia, and feelings of hopelessness have worsened recently. She has been on SSRIs, which you learn have failed in several previous trials. She has not tried a tricyclic antidepressant (TCA). The pharmacology of TCAs involves which of the following?

(A) 5-hydroxytryptamine-2a (5-HT_{2a}) antagonism
(B) 5-HT_{2a} agonism
(C) dopamine blockade
(D) inhibition of norepinephrine and serotonin reuptake
(E) inhibition of dopamine reuptake

Questions 13 and 14

A 29-year-old woman presents to the emergency department with her 3-year-old child reporting that the child suffered a seizure while at home. Hospital records verify that this is the third emergency department visit in as many weeks for the same presentation. Neurologic workup for seizure disorder was negative. Initiation of an anticonvulsant has been ineffective.

13. Which of the following statements is likely to be true?

(A) The child suffers from a conversion disorder.
(B) The child is experiencing separation anxiety.
(C) The child's history is falsified.
(D) The child does not have a therapeutic level of anticonvulsant.
(E) The child suffers from a seizure disorder.

14. The mother is most likely to suffer from which of the following?

(A) schizophrenia
(B) bipolar disorder
(C) depression
(D) epilepsy
(E) posttraumatic stress disorder (PTSD)

emergency certification → crisis center

Questions 15 and 16

A 26-year-old man is being evaluated in the emergency department for sudden onset of chest pressure and dyspnea. This is his third emergency department visit for similar symptoms for which he reports "I feel like I'm going to die." An electrocardiogram (ECG) and stress test were normal. The patient denies risk factors for heart disease and does not have a family history of heart disease. Urine toxicology was negative.

15. Which of the following is the most likely diagnosis?

    (A) delirium
    (B) panic disorder
    (C) acute stress reaction
    (D) acute myocardial infarction
    (E) hypochondriasis

16. Which of the following medications is most useful in the initial treatment of this disorder?

    (A) sertraline (Zoloft)
    (B) propranolol
    (C) clonidine (Catapres)
    (D) haloperidol
    (E) lithium

17. A woman being treated for major depression is brought to the emergency department after being found unconscious by a neighbor. The neighbor said that over the past few days the woman had been complaining of severe headaches. She also said the woman enjoys red wine. The woman's blood pressure is recorded as 220/110 mm Hg. This emergency is best managed by intravenous (IV) administration of which of the following?

    (A) an alpha-blocking agent
    (B) a beta-blocker
    (C) dantrolene sodium (Dantrium)
    (D) bromocriptine (Parlodel)
    (E) a calcium channel blocker

Questions 18 and 19

A 28-year-old man recently began taking clozapine (Clozaril) to treat symptoms of schizophrenia. He does not suffer from any medical illness.

18. Which of the following adverse effects is associated with this medication?

    (A) bradycardia
    (B) hypertension
    (C) weight loss
    (D) galactorrhea
    (E) seizures

19. Which of the following hematologic disorders associated with this medication can be life-threatening?

    (A) a decreased granulocyte count
    (B) leukocytosis
    (C) thrombocytopenia
    (D) pancytopenia
    (E) microcytic anemia

20. A 35-year-old patient exhibits odd beliefs and thinking, paranoid behavior, and has no close friends. Which of the following diagnoses is the most appropriate to consider?

    (A) schizoid personality disorder
    (B) avoidant personality disorder
    (C) paranoid personality disorder
    (D) narcissistic personality disorder
    (E) schizotypal personality disorder

21. A 28-year-old woman demonstrates a pervasive pattern of unstable relationships, poor self-image, impulsiveness, and irritability. Which of the following is the most appropriate diagnosis to consider?

    (A) histrionic personality disorder
    (B) borderline personality disorder
    (C) antisocial personality disorder
    (D) dependent personality disorder
    (E) schizoid personality disorder

Questions 22 and 23

A 30-year-old woman is brought to the emergency department by the police after being arrested for breach of the peace. The woman was observed acting irrationally at a local business where she demanded to speak with the president of the company claiming that she had new ideas for product development. The patient reports that she has not slept for days and that her mood is "fabulous." Urine human chorionic gonadotropin is positive. Illicit substances were not detected.

22. Which of the following is most likely to be present on Mental Status Examination (MSE)?

    (A) racing thoughts
    (B) depressed mood
    (C) auditory hallucinations
    (D) daytime sleepiness
    (E) weight loss

23. Which of the following medical disorders can present with similar symptoms?

    (A) hyperglycemia
    (B) thyroid disorder
    (C) rheumatoid arthritis
    (D) diabetes mellitus
    (E) cirrhosis

Questions 24 and 25

A 24-year-old man with a history of seizure disorder and polysubstance abuse has been incarcerated for assaultive behavior. The patient is evaluated by a neurologist, who prescribes phenytoin (Dilantin).

24. Which of the following conditions is associated with this medication?

    (A) leukocytosis
    (B) hypertension
    (C) gingival hyperplasia
    (D) hepatic failure
    (E) Ebstein anomaly

25. The patient returns 1 month later for a follow-up examination and reports that he experienced a

generalized seizure. Laboratory investigation reveals that the phenytoin level is 6.5 mg/dL (normal, 10–20 mg/dL). Which of the following is the most appropriate intervention at this time?

    (A) Increase the phenytoin dose to achieve a therapeutic level.
    (B) Discontinue phenytoin and begin divalproex sodium.
    (C) Add a benzodiazepine as an adjunct medication.
    (D) Ask the patient about compliance with medications.
    (E) Add phenobarbital.

26. A 24-year-old woman with a history of schizophrenia tells you that she would like to become pregnant. What is the chance for familial transmission of schizophrenia?

    (A) 0.1%
    (B) 1%
    (C) 2%
    (D) 5%
    (E) 10%

27. A 70-year-old man with a history of major depression is brought to the emergency department by his family, who is concerned because he was found wandering in the streets near his home. During the MSE, attention is best assessed by asking the patient to do which of the following?

    (A) perform serial-sevens subtraction
    (B) recite his Social Security number
    (C) spell a five-letter word forward and backward
    (D) perform digit recall
    (E) repeat the examiner's first name

28. An 18-year-old patient experiences a sudden onset of euphoria, grandiose delusions, a decreased need for sleep, and paranoia. Which of the following conditions is most associated with these symptoms?

(A) schizophrenia, paranoid type
(B) cannabis intoxication
(C) MDD with psychotic features
(D) schizoaffective disorder
(E) cocaine intoxication

29. A Malayan man experiences a dissociative episode characterized by an outburst of homicidal behavior toward his friend, whom he believed was insulting his appearance. Which of the following conditions is most associated with this presentation?

(A) substance intoxication
(B) dissociative identity disorder
(C) Ganser syndrome
(D) factitious disorder
(E) culture-bound syndrome

Questions 30 and 31

A 26-year-old woman is diagnosed with schizophrenia. The psychiatrist decides to treat her symptoms with a high-potency antipsychotic medication. The patient experiences abnormal involuntary movements associated with the use of the antipsychotic drug she has been prescribed.

30. Realizing that side effects may affect further medication compliance, the psychiatrist should prescribe which of the following?

(A) clozapine
(B) risperidone (Risperdal)
(C) benztropine (Cogentin)
(D) methylphenidate (Ritalin)
(E) a cholinergic agonist

31. Despite the intervention, the patient abruptly stops taking her antipsychotic medication. The psychiatrist decides to change the patient's medication. Which of the following may be considered?

(A) haloperidol
(B) clozapine
(C) loxapine (Loxitane)
(D) pimozide (Orap)
(E) perphenazine (Trilafon)

Questions 32 and 33

A 30-year-old woman with a history of unstable interpersonal relationships, suicidal gestures, and marked impulsivity is referred to you for dialectical behavioral therapy (DBT).

32. Which of the following disorders is this patient likely to be suffering from?

(A) avoidant personality disorder
(B) bipolar disorder
(C) passive-aggressive personality disorder
(D) borderline personality disorder
(E) schizoid personality disorder

33. The foundations of DBT include which of the following?
(A) The patient is doing the best that she can.
(B) The patient may fail in therapy.
(C) At times the patient does not want to improve.
(D) The patient should not learn new behaviors.
(E) The patient is responsible for causing all of her own problems.

34. A 21-year-old man presents with a 4-week history of paranoid delusions and auditory hallucinations that comment on his appearance. After thorough evaluation, you diagnose him with schizophrenia, paranoid type, and prescribe haloperidol 5 mg bid. One week later, the patient returns for a follow-up examination and reports that, although his symptoms have improved, he now experiences muscle stiffness in his arms and neck. You prescribe benztropine 1 mg bid and schedule a follow-up appointment in 2 weeks. One week later, the patient's mother calls you and reports that her son is more agitated and confused. Physical examination reveals tachycardia, dilated pupils, and flushed skin.

The next appropriate measure would be which of the following?

(A) discontinue benztropine and prescribe amantadine (Symmetrel)
(B) increase haloperidol to 5 mg tid
(C) increase benztropine to 2 mg bid
(D) discontinue haloperidol and prescribe risperidone
(E) prescribe lorazepam 1 mg bid

35. A 28-year-old male medical student is found to have an enlarged testicle during a routine physical examination. The student reports that it has been gradually enlarging for several months. The physician asks why he did not report these findings earlier. "I'm sure it's nothing," the student replies. This response is an example of which of the following?

(A) a mature defense
(B) a neurotic defense
(C) a narcissistic defense
(D) an immature defense
(E) confidence

36. A 45-year-old Asian-American woman is brought to the emergency department by her husband, who reports that for the past 3 days his wife has not been sleeping well, has been experiencing bad dreams, and appears "in a daze" with a sense of feeling "numb." The patient endorses feeling anxious but does not know why. She has been unable to perform her usual activities of daily living. One week ago, the patient was discharged from the hospital after experiencing an anaphylactic reaction to IV contrast dye while undergoing an imaging procedure for sinusitis. Although she cannot recall specifics, her husband verifies the history, adding that the doctors "thought she was

going to die." Upon returning to the hospital, she experiences intense fear about revisiting the same hospital from which she was recently discharged. The most appropriate diagnosis to consider is which of the following?

(A) PTSD
(B) acute stress reaction
(C) generalized anxiety disorder (GAD)
(D) adjustment disorder
(E) depressive disorder

37. A 40-year-old woman without a past psychiatric history is admitted to the hospital for treatment of depression. During morning rounds, the patient appears unresponsive and does not respond to verbal stimuli. There are no signs of trauma or overdose. A review of her chart reveals that the patient was well the night before and went to sleep without incident. You determine that the patient's unresponsiveness is psychogenic. Which of the following findings is most likely to be apparent on examination?

(A) an abnormal electroencephalogram (EEG)
(B) nonsaccadic eye movements
(C) elevated temperature
(D) decreased respirations
(E) cold-caloric-induced nystagmus

38. A 24-year-old woman experiences fatigue, weight gain, and hyperphagia during the winter months. She reports a sad mood and "can't wait" until her vacation to Florida. The most likely diagnosis is which of the following?

(A) dysthymia
(B) sundowning syndrome
(C) anxiety disorder
(D) stress disorder
(E) seasonal affective disorder

39. A 27-year-old woman is brought to the emergency department by her parents, who report that their daughter is unable to recall her name. The emergency department physician reports that a complete neurologic workup is within normal limits. Collateral information reveals that the patient had episodes in which she would take unplanned trips, sometimes for days, without notice, and would return unable to recall the episode. A review of her medical chart notes a past history of possible sexual abuse as a child. Urine toxicology is negative and she does not take any medications. Which of the following is the most likely diagnosis?

(A) partial complex seizure disorder
(B) delirium
(C) dissociative fugue
(D) PTSD
(E) depressive disorder

40. A 26-year-old female graduate student reports to you a 4-week history of a depressed mood that has caused her significant difficulty in attending her classes. The patient reports difficulty falling asleep at night, weight loss, and passive suicidal ideation. A careful review of her history reveals that for the past 2 years she also experienced brief and distinct periods of an elevated and expansive mood, a decreased need for sleep, and an increase in goal-directed activities. Which of the following is the most appropriate diagnosis to consider?

(A) MDD
(B) bipolar I disorder, current episode manic
(C) bipolar II disorder, current episode depressed
(D) cyclothymic disorder
(E) dysthymic disorder

41. You are asked to evaluate a 30-year-old male prisoner who reports a depressed mood and suicidal ideation. During your examination, you note that the prisoner responds to your questions with approximate answers. Which of the following is the most appropriate diagnosis to consider?

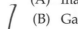

(A) malingering
(B) Ganser syndrome
(C) Capgras syndrome
(D) Munchausen syndrome
(E) fugue state

42. A 75-year-old man is admitted to the hospital following a serious suicide attempt. The patient exhibits clinical features of depression and has a past history of suicide attempts. The medical chart reveals that he is prescribed levodopa/ carbidopa, digoxin, aspirin, and a medication for cardiac arrhythmia. The most appropriate treatment at this time is which of the following?

(A) prescribe risperidone
(B) administer supportive psychotherapy
(C) prescribe nortriptyline (Pamelor)
(D) prescribe diazepam (Valium)
(E) administer electroconvulsive therapy (ECT)

43. A 38-year-old woman presents to your office with a 2-week history of symptoms of depression characterized by hypersomnolence and reaction sensitivity. She reports to you that she recently enrolled in graduate school and is having trouble with many of her classes. Which of the following diagnoses should be considered?

(A) adjustment disorder
(B) major depression with atypical features
(C) dysthymic disorder
(D) major depression with melancholic features
(E) sleep disorder

44. A 33-year-old man changes his first name to honor a musician whom he idolizes. He recently bought the same guitar as the musician and formed a rock band to play his music. During practice, the man dresses like his idol. This behavior is an example of which of the following?

(A) identification
(B) regression
(C) fixation

(D) projection

(E) idealization

45. A 60-year-old man with schizophrenia sits motionless in his chair. The patient is mute and reacts very little to his environment. His eyes appear fixated on a distant object. At times, he assumes bizarre postures and imitates the movements of others. What is the best description of his behavior?

(A) partial complex seizure

(B) absence seizure

(C) catatonia

(D) cataplexy

(E) catalepsy

46. During an examination to evaluate muscle rigidity, a male patient is somewhat resistant to movement of his arms but maintains the arm in the position in which you place it. This is an example of which of the following?

(A) catalepsy

(B) cataplexy

(C) rigidity

(D) dystonia

(E) malingering

Questions 47 and 48

A 42-year-old healthy man is taking a medication to help him sleep at night. Unexpectedly, he experiences painful, persistent penile erection.

47. Which of the following medications is most likely to cause this condition?

(A) fluoxetine (Prozac)

(B) sertraline

(C) paroxetine (Paxil)

(D) trazodone (Desyrel)

(E) nortriptyline

48. Which of the following statements regarding this condition is correct?

(A) It is self-limiting.

(B) It is dose dependent.

(C) It may require surgery.

(D) It occurs after long-term therapy.

(E) It is related to dopamine blockade.

Questions 49 and 50

A 60-year-old man reports a history of excessive worry about his daughter since she moved away to college 1 year ago. His wife of 40 years verifies his complaint, adding that "he worries about everything." Recently, his wife made plans to travel abroad to visit friends. The patient is unable to accompany his wife because of respiratory problems caused by years of heavy smoking and is anxious about her leaving. He reports difficulty falling asleep, excessive daytime fatigue, and difficulty concentrating at work.

49. Which of the following should be considered to treat his symptoms?

(A) buspirone (BuSpar)

(B) fluoxetine

(C) alprazolam (Xanax)

(D) diazepam

(E) lorazepam

50. Two weeks later, the patient reports that the medication you prescribed has helped everything but his difficulty falling asleep. He reports that during the past week he has slept only 4 hours per night. After careful consideration, you decide to prescribe a 1-week supply of medication to help him sleep. Which of the following medications is most appropriate to consider?

(A) clorazepate (Tranxene)

(B) zolpidem (Ambien)

(C) oxazepam (Serax)

(D) diphenhydramine (Benadryl)

(E) temazepam (Restoril)

Questions 51 and 52

A 25-year-old woman is scheduled for a gynecologic procedure. Upon discharge from the hospital, she is likely to receive pain medication. For 1 year, you have been prescribing a monoamine oxidase inhibitor (MAOI) to treat a single episode of depression with excellent results.

51. Which of the following medications may cause a fatal drug interaction in this patient?

    (A) codeine
    (B) acetaminophen
    (C) oxycodone
    (D) meperidine (Demerol)
    (E) ibuprofen

52. The patient tolerates the procedure well and 2 months later reports to you that she is pregnant. Which of the following interventions is most appropriate?

    (A) MAOIs are safe in pregnancy and should be continued.
    (B) Antidepressant therapy should be discontinued.
    (C) Discontinue the MAOI and initiate treatment with fluoxetine.
    (D) Discontinue the MAOI during the first trimester only.
    (E) Discontinue the MAOI and begin maintenance ECT.

Questions 53 and 54

A 62-year-old homeless man presents to the emergency department with impaired gait and nystagmus. His vital signs are stable and an ophthalmologic examination is within normal limits. The patient is unable to recall the date and has difficulty sustaining attention without evidence of amnesia.

53. Which of the following is the most appropriate initial intervention?

    (A) Perform a breath analysis.
    (B) Obtain a head computed tomographic scan.
    (C) Perform a lumbar puncture.

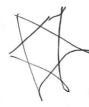

Breath test only for cops you should give IM thiamine

(D) Administer parenteral thiamine.
(E) administer IV dextrose.

54. Which of the following language deficits is characteristic of Broca aphasia but not of Wernicke aphasia?

    (A) nonfluency
    (B) impaired repetition
    (C) impaired writing
    (D) impaired naming
    (E) impaired reading comprehension

55. A 34-year-old executive reports drinking up to six cups of caffeinated coffee per day. He boards a plane scheduled for an 18-hour flight on which only decaffeinated beverages are served. Which of the following symptoms is the executive most likely to experience?

    (A) depressed mood
    (B) muscle cramping
    (C) headache
    (D) irritability
    (E) nausea

Questions 56 and 57

A 25-year-old man with a history of medication-responsive schizophrenia presents to the emergency department with severe muscle stiffness and an elevated temperature. The patient appears confused, is diaphoretic, and vital signs are unstable. A urine toxicology screen is provisionally negative.

56. Which of the following is the most essential intervention?

    (A) Administer IV dantrolene sodium.
    (B) Apply cooling blankets.
    (C) Administer naloxone (Narcan).
    (D) Administer bromocriptine.
    (E) Discontinue medications.

57. Which of the following laboratory abnormalities is most likely to be present?

    (A) anemia
    (B) leukopenia

(C)   elevated creatine phosphokinase (CPK)

(D)   decreased transaminases

(E)   elevated blood urea nitrogen (BUN)

58.   An 18-year-old man presents to the emergency department after being involved in a motor vehicle accident. The medical chart reports a history of substance use. Which of the following tests can confirm your diagnosis of substance abuse?

(A)   serum liver function studies

(B)   breath analysis

(C)   urine toxicology screen

(D)   naloxone injection

(E)   elevated heart rate

59.   A 72-year-old man without a prior psychiatric history presents to the outpatient clinic with a recent history of cognitive deficits. The patient has had a stable level of consciousness and denies any current or past substance abuse. The patient has not been prescribed any new medications. The medical chart reveals a history of megaloblastic anemia and a subtotal gastrectomy for severe peptic ulcer disease. Which of the following initial interventions is most appropriate?

(A)   Order a magnetic resonance imaging scan of the brain to confirm dementia, Alzheimer type.

(B)   Order a reversible workup for dementia.

(C)   Discuss long-term extended-care facility admission.

(D)   Obtain a forensic examination to evaluate competency.

(E)   Obtain a neurologic consult.

60.   A 37-year-old woman presents to the emergency department complaining of severe diarrhea and a coarse tremor. The medical chart notes a history of bipolar I disorder. The most appropriate intervention aimed at establishing a diagnosis is which of the following?

(A)   Obtain a serum medication level.

(B)   Prescribe antidiarrheal medication.

(C)   Obtain a urine toxicology screen.

(D)   Obtain a urine pregnancy test.

(E)   Obtain renal function studies.

61.   A young healthy man is diagnosed with bipolar I disorder and is prescribed lithium carbonate to treat his symptoms of mania. Which of the following laboratory tests should be obtained before initiating treatment with lithium?

(A)   EEG

(B)   creatinine clearance

(C)   liver function studies

(D)   24-hour urine volume

(E)   thyroid-stimulating hormone

62.   A 27-year-old woman has been prescribed fluoxetine for depression for the past year. She comes to you complaining of medication side effects and wishes to discontinue her antidepressant. As her physician, you discuss with her the appropriate risks and benefits, and you discontinue her treatment. Two weeks later, she returns complaining of depressive symptoms characterized by sleep and appetite changes, poor concentration, and a depressed mood for most of the day. You decide that she is experiencing a recurrent major depressive episode and decide to prescribe her a different class of medication to treat her symptoms. After discussing the appropriate precautions with her, you prescribe an MAOI. Within 1 week, she begins experiencing irritability, abdominal pain and diarrhea, and autonomic instability characterized by hypertension and tachycardia. Her temperature is 103.5°F. The patient also reports experiencing myoclonic-like jerking of her muscles and vivid visual hallucinations of colorful flowers spinning toward the sky. She states that she has followed your directions carefully while taking this medication. Which of the following can account for this presentation?

(A)   neuroleptic malignant syndrome (NMS)

(B)   tyramine-induced hypertensive crisis

(C)   malignant hyperthermia

(D)   serotonin syndrome

(E)   hallucinogen abuse

Questions 63 and 64

A 17-year-old girl is referred to the school nurse for frequent episodes of vomiting in the bathroom during lunch breaks. Her friends report that, despite a preoccupation with her body image, she eats "twice as much as anybody else." The parents are called to the school and recall that a recent bill from their charge account at the local pharmacy indicated a large number of laxative purchases. The girl reports that her mood is fine, and her records at school indicate that she is an above-average student.

63. Medical complications of this disorder are most often due to which of the following?

   (A) chronic vomiting
   (B) weight loss
   (C) ritualistic fasting
   (D) suicide gestures
   (E) substance abuse

64. Which of the following medications is the most appropriate initial treatment for her symptoms?

   (A) antiemetics
   (B) antidepressants
   (C) antianxiety agents
   (D) appetite stimulants
   (E) hypnotic medications

Questions 65 and 66

A 16-year-old female high school student is referred by her parents for an evaluation. One year prior to the evaluation, the girl began restricting her food intake and started a rigorous exercise program to improve her appearance. Aspiring to be a model, the girl lost 25 lb but remained preoccupied with her appearance despite weighing only 85 lb. Her friends reported that she constantly referred to herself as being "fat" and did not seem interested in dating. The girl continued to lose weight and was reluctant to discuss her condition.

65. The girl is most likely to experience which of the following?

   (A) normal breast development
   (B) three consecutive missed periods
   (C) the loss of feelings of hunger

   (D) body weight 85% of expected normal
   (E) sexual promiscuity

66. The mortality rate associated with this disorder may be as high as which of the following?

   (A) 5%
   (B) 10%
   (C) 20%
   (D) 25%
   (E) 30%

Questions 67 and 68

A 50-year-old woman reports a depressed mood, poor appetite, and weight loss 1 month following the death of her husband. After his death, she began to feel that she would be "better off dead." At times, she believes that she can hear his voice calling to her. She denies any feelings of worthlessness but feels guilty about not being able to do the right things for him before he died. When talking with others, she believes that her feelings are normal.

67. Which of the following describes this condition?

   (A) uncomplicated bereavement
   (B) complicated bereavement
   (C) major depressive episode
   (D) adjustment disorder with depressed mood
   (E) dysthymic disorder

68. Which of the following is the most appropriate course of action?

   (A) no treatment
   (B) prescribing antidepressant medication
   (C) prescribing sedative-hypnotic medication
   (D) admission to a hospital
   (E) evaluating for a sleep disorder

69. A 25-year-old man reports a 5-year history of excessive hand washing and a preoccupation with feeling clean. The thought of contracting an infectious disease persists throughout the day even though he makes attempts to ignore it. His condition has progressively worsened and has caused significant impairment while at work and

at home. Which of the following medications is the best initial choice to treat his symptoms?

(A) antipsychotics

 (B) antianxiety agents

(C) antidepressants

(D) antiepileptic agents

(E) lithium

Questions 70 and 71

A 52-year-old obese man experiences excessive daytime sleepiness and a depressed mood. His wife reports that he snores loudly and is restless while sleeping. There is no evidence of substance abuse, and the patient does not have a prior psychiatric history.

70. Which of the following is the most likely cause of his symptoms?

 (A) depression

(B) abnormal circadian rhythm

(C) periodic limb movements of sleep

(D) airway obstruction

(E) nocturnal myoclonus

71. Which of the following is the treatment of choice for his symptoms?

(A) breathing air under positive pressure

(B) nasal surgery

(C) benzodiazepine medication

(D) antidepressant medication

(E) uvulopalatoplasty

Questions 72 and 73

A patient with chronic paranoid schizophrenia who has been stable for years on a low-potency antipsychotic agent begins experiencing parkinsonian-like side effects. His physician prescribes a drug to alleviate some of these side effects. One week later, the patient is seen in the emergency department with dilated pupils, dry mouth, warm skin, and tachycardia. He is experiencing visual hallucinations.

72. The most appropriate intervention is which of the following?

(A) Administer IV atropine.

(B) Administer an anticholinesterase medication.

(C) Administer IV dantrolene sodium.

(D) Administer haloperidol.

(E) Administer a benzodiazepine.

73. After the appropriate intervention, the patient experiences nausea and vomiting and has a seizure. Which of the following medications should be administered next?

(A) atropine

 (B) lorazepam

(C) physostigmine

(D) epinephrine

(E) prochlorperazine (Compazine)

74. A 40-year-old woman suffers from depression and obsessive ritualistic behavior. The physician decides to prescribe an SSRI. Which of the following medications might the physician consider?

 (A) buspirone

(B) phenelzine (Nardil)

(C) clomipramine (Anafranil)

(D) doxepin (Sinequan)

(E) fluvoxamine (Luvox)

Questions 75 and 76

A 56-year-old man with a long history of alcohol abuse and liver disease is ordered by the court to enroll in an inpatient detoxification program for alcohol dependence. He begins to experience clinical signs and symptoms of withdrawal.

75. Which of the following medications is the most appropriate to prescribe during his treatment?

(A) chlordiazepoxide (Librium)

 (B) phenobarbital

(C) disulfiram (Antabuse)

(D) lorazepam

(E) alprazolam

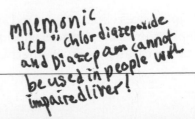
mnemonic
"LCD" chlordiazepoxide and Diazepam cannot be used in people with impaired liver!

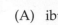

76. Soon after his admission, the man begins to report hallucinations and becomes agitated. Which of the following medications should be prescribed to treat these symptoms?

    (A) sertraline
    (B) clonazepam (Klonopin)
    (C) haloperidol
    (D) lithium
    (E) fluoxetine

77. A 48-year-old woman successfully completes an inpatient program for alcohol detoxification for which she was prescribed chlordiazepoxide. Upon discharge, the patient is prescribed a medication that disrupts alcohol metabolism. Soon after discharge, the patient attends an office party where she reports having a few drinks. She has been compliant with her prescribed medication and does not have any active medical problems. Which of the following symptoms is the patient likely to experience?

    (A) high blood pressure
    (B) euphoria
    (C) blurred vision
    (D) vomiting
    (E) urinary retention

78. A 22-year-old man with a history of bipolar disorder is prescribed lithium carbonate to treat his symptoms. During a weekend rugby tournament, he hurts his knee and an orthopedic physician prescribes a medication to reduce his symptoms of pain and swelling. Although the patient reports relief from this medication, he begins to experience abdominal pain, diarrhea, and drowsiness. Which of the following medications may contribute to the production of these symptoms?

    (A) ibuprofen
    (B) acetaminophen
    (C) aspirin
    (D) codeine
    (E) meperidine

79. A patient experiences clinical signs and symptoms of depression. The physician decides to prescribe a medication whose mechanism

includes significant blockade of serotonin reuptake. Which of the following antidepressants should be considered?

    (A) maprotiline (Ludiomil)
    (B) amitriptyline (Elavil)
    (C) bupropion (Wellbutrin)
    (D) desipramine (Norpramin)
    (E) clonazepam

80. A patient who is human immunodeficiency virus (HIV)-positive reports a depressed mood, low energy, and hopelessness. Which of the following medications can the physician prescribe to achieve rapid relief of some of his symptoms?

    (A) methylphenidate
    (B) fluoxetine
    (C) bupropion
    (D) buspirone
    (E) nefazodone (Serzone)

Questions 81 and 82

A college-aged man reports that he and his friends have been experimenting with the new drug craze on campus called "huffing." His roommate reports that he has been accumulating typewriter correction fluid, nail polish remover, and model airplane glue.

81. Which of the following is experienced by a person after huffing?

    (A) staring into space
    (B) tolerance
    (C) depressed reflexes
    (D) increased appetite
    (E) diminished response to pain

82. Which of the following is the current treatment for this type of drug abuse?

    (A) antidepressant agents
    (B) dialectic behavioral therapy
    (C) abstinence
    (D) exposure and response prevention
    (E) antipsychotic agents

83. A 30-year-old man with schizophrenia exhibits symptoms that have not been stable over time.

[handwritten margin note: Does well in his most interesting class since able to stay focused during interesting class]

He complains of hair loss that began after he started taking one of his medications. Which of the predominant symptoms would support the diagnosis of the paranoid subtype?

(A) immobility

(B) inappropriate affect

(C) disorganized speech and behavior

(D) posturing

(E) prominent hallucinations or delusions

84. You are treating a 32-year-old woman for bipolar I disorder with a combination of medications. She complains of hair loss. This side effect is a reversible side effect of which of the following medications?

(A) divalproex sodium

(B) ziprasidone (Geodon)

(C) carbamazepine

(D) clozapine

(E) olanzapine (Zyprexa)

85. A young man experiences erectile dysfunction and is told that the medication he is prescribed is likely to be the cause. Which of the following medications is associated with erectile dysfunction?

(A) amantadine

(B) methylphenidate

(C) SSRIs

(D) antihistamines

(E) cholinergic agents

Questions 86 and 87

A 21-year-old male college student without prior medical or psychiatric history is evaluated for poor work performance. The student reports to the dean that he finds it hard to follow through with assignments and is easily distracted by environmental stimuli. The dean comments to the student about how frequently he interrupts others during conversations and observes that it seems that the student is not paying attention to what he is saying. Overall, his grades are poor except in the class he considers "the most interesting class I have ever had." He often forgets required materials for classes and his assignments are frequently late. The student's parents report that he was incompletely

evaluated for similar difficulties while in public school. The student seemed to improve when the family moved out of the area and he attended private school.

86. Which of the following is the most likely diagnosis?

(A) attention deficit hyperactivity disorder (ADHD)

(B) bipolar I disorder

(C) bipolar II disorder

(D) conduct disorder

(E) learning disability

87. The patient is prescribed methylphenidate for symptoms of inattention and hyperactivity. After an adequate trial and dose, the patient does not fully benefit from the medication. Which of the following actions is the most appropriate?

(A) Add a low-dose amphetamine.

(B) Add an anxiolytic medication.

(C) Add an antidepressant.

(D) Discontinue methylphenidate and prescribe a mixed amphetamine compound.

(E) Discontinue methylphenidate and prescribe an antidepressant.

88. A 19-year-old man is brought to the emergency department by the police for an evaluation. The written police report states that the patient has been calling 911 for the past 4 weeks reporting that he is being spied on by aliens from a distant planet. The patient reports that he is receiving messages from the aliens through his radio and that he hears voices in his head commenting on his appearance. He has not been sleeping well at night because he has been "guarding his bedroom." You note that his affect is flat, and he appears tired during your examination. A urine toxicology screen is negative. Which of the following is the most likely diagnosis?

(A) schizophrenia

(B) bipolar I disorder with psychotic features

(C) schizoaffective disorder

(D) brief psychotic disorder

(E) MDD with psychotic features

[handwritten note at bottom: schizophrenia 6 months of decline of functioning and 1 month of psychotic sx → del/hall;]

89. An 18-year-old woman with recently diagnosed schizophrenia is acutely psychotic and in labor with her first child. The obstetric service requests a psychiatric consultation for a safe medication to control the patient's psychosis while she is in labor. Which of the following would be relatively safe?

    (A) haloperidol
    (B) chlorpromazine (Thorazine)
    (C) thioridazine (Mellaril)
    (D) droperidol (Inapsine)
    (E) trihexyphenidyl (Artane)

psychosis while in labor → haloperidol;

DIRECTIONS (Questions 90 through 100): Each set of items in this section consists of a list of lettered headings followed by several numbered words or phrases. For each numbered word or phrase, select the ONE lettered option that is most closely associated with it. Each lettered option may be selected once, more than once, or not at all.

Questions 90 through 92

Match the appropriate test to assess for intelligence in each age group.

    (A) Wechsler Preschool and Primary Scale of Intelligence (WPPSI)
    (B) Wechsler Adult Intelligence Scale—Revised (WAIS-R)
    (C) Wechsler Memory Scale (WMS)
    (D) Wechsler Intelligence Scale for Children (WISC)

90. A 4-year-old girl whose parents wish to have her evaluated for entrance into an "elite" kindergarten.

91. A 65-year-old female physician who is now concerned about memory difficulties.

92. An 8-year-old boy whom the school system wants evaluated for possible special needs in the classroom.

Questions 93 through 95

Match the clinical presentation with the appropriate neuropsychological test.

    (A) Minnesota Multiphasic Personality Inventory-2 (MMPI-2)
    (B) WISC
    (C) Rey-Osterrieth Test
    (D) Beck Depression Inventory
    (E) Blessed Rating Scale
    (F) WAIS-R
    (G) Boston Diagnostic Aphasia Examination
    (H) Rorschach Test
    (I) Mini-Mental Status Examination (MMSE)
    (J) Bender-Gestalt Test
    (K) Wisconsin Card Sorting Test (WCST)
    (L) Wada Test

93. A 35-year-old woman with a protein S deficiency shows evidence of left side hemineglect.

94. A 7-year-old boy with difficulty in school needs further evaluation of academic potential.

95. You would like to address the deficits of a 69-year-old man with nonfluent speech and formulate a specific treatment plan.

Questions 96 through 100

Select the drug most likely to cause the associated symptoms.

    (A) lysergic acid diethylamine (LSD)
    (B) phencyclidine (PCP)
    (C) cocaine
    (D) marijuana
    (E) opiates
    (F) nicotine

96. An 18-year-old high school student with conjunctival redness, increased appetite, dry mouth, tachycardia, and a sensation of slowed time.

97. A 31-year-old man with miosis, bradycardia, hypotension, hypothermia, and constipation.

98. An assaultive 26-year-old man with vertical nystagmus, echolalia, paranoid ideation, and hallucinations.

99. A 16-year-old girl with abdominal cramps, confusion, palpitations, and muscle twitching. *11*

Nicotine → "muscle twitching

100. A 21-year-old man with tachycardia, dilated pupils, hallucinations, and complaints of chest pain.

Answers and Explanations

1. **(D)** Antipsychotics are indicated for acute treatment of agitation and violence sometimes seen in manic patients. Haloperidol works quickly doses (20–30 minutes). Doses of 2–5 mg by mouth (PO) or intramuscularly (IM) are usual initial. It may be given IV as well, especially in the intensive care unit (ICU). Hydroxyzine is an antihistamine; it is not effective in mania. Lithium, divalproex sodium, and carbamazepine have all been shown to control mood fluctuations in manic patients. However, these agents take days to work and are not effective in the acute management of this patient.

2. **(A)** Lithium is not associated with significant blood dyscrasias, although it can cause a modest benign increase in the white blood cell (WBC) count. Carbamazepine is commonly associated with reduced WBC count, but the incidence of agranulocytosis is approximately 1 in 10,000. Agranulocytosis is a rare complication with divalproex sodium, a bit more common is benign thrombocytopenia. Antipsychotic medication is occasionally associated with a decrease in leukopoiesis, but the WBC count usually returns to normal with continued treatment. Agranulocytosis can also occur in the setting of antipsychotic medication use in approximately 1 in 10,000 cases (clozapine has a higher incidence). Lorazepam is not associated with WBC abnormalities.

3. **(D)** This patient is most likely suffering from somatization disorder, which often coexists with other psychiatric illnesses such as anxiety, depressive, and personality disorders. The suspected presence of a somatization disorder should prompt a search for other treatable illnesses. In managing patients with somatization disorder, it is important to accept that symptoms are not consciously produced and to let patients know that you realize their symptoms are a source of great consternation. Regardless of history, any patient presenting to a physician with physical complaints deserves a reasonable physical investigation; patients with somatization disorder are as likely, if not more likely, to develop identifiable medical conditions. However, rather than repeat tests, it may be necessary to contact previous treaters. Sending this patient away for a year would not be helpful; rather regular, frequent checkups and fostering a therapeutic alliance and support are in order.

4. **(C)** Women are as much as 20 times more likely to receive the diagnosis of somatization disorder than are men. Rarely will any therapy or intervention "cure" the patient of somatization disorder; at best, patients learn to minimize the impact somatization has on their lives. Somatization disorder is common in lower socioeconomic groups. Conversion symptoms are common in somatization disorder and are included in the diagnostic criteria. Patients with this disorder benefit from regular, scheduled visits that allow them to forge a trusting therapeutic alliance.

5. **(C)** This patient is most likely suffering from schizotypal personal disorder. This personality disorder with its attendant social isolation and subtle distortions of reality may indeed resemble schizophrenia in remission; the diagnosis can be sorted out by a thorough history. Frank hallucinations of any type are uncommon; only

subtle distortion of environmental cues is seen. Although men may be slightly more at risk for being diagnosed with schizotypal personality disorder, the disparity is not stark. As with any personality disorder, schizotypal personality disorder represents a lifelong maladaptive approach to life and does not suddenly express itself well into adulthood.

6. **(D)** In schizotypal personality disorder, the subtle disconnection from reality, which may be exacerbated in times of stress as in this case, can be treated with low doses of neuroleptics. These patients lack the capability, stable sense of self, and trust to be able to engage in, or benefit from, psychoanalysis. Antidepressant medication of any type, including tricyclics and SSRIs, are helpful in the schizotypal patient who displays significant affective (mood) symptoms, which is not seen in this case. There is no evidence of anxiety that would make benzodiazepines useful.

7. **(D)** This patient is most likely suffering from schizophrenia. Symptoms of schizophrenia are commonly divided into positive and negative symptoms. Flat affect, a negative symptom, represents an absence, in this case, of a normally reactive and variable affect. Auditory hallucinations, delusions (including paranoid delusions), and loose associations are all positive symptoms.

8. **(C)** The exacerbation seen is most likely precipitated by medication noncompliance. Stress from work or a viral illness may indeed contribute to a relapse, but they are less strongly predictive of a reemergence of psychotic symptoms than medication noncompliance. Nicotine has been shown to lower neuroleptic levels, which has been offered as a reason cigarette smoking is rampant among patients with schizophrenia. However, this patient's smoking decreased, which if anything would be expected to increase neuroleptic levels.

9. **(B)** Classically, patients with hepatitis secondary to alcohol abuse or dependence have elevated liver enzymes (such as gamma-glutamyl transpeptidase, aspartate transaminase, or alanine transaminase). However, in advanced alcoholism, the liver may be "burnt out" and liver function tests may reveal low or normal levels of these enzymes. As a result of liver damage, prothrombin time is typically increased. Hypomagnesemia, not hypermagnesemia, is more likely to be found in alcoholism, usually as a result of dietary deficiency. In the patient having a withdrawal seizure, the problem is absence, not presence, of alcohol. His blood alcohol is expected to be zero. The alcoholic is more likely to have thrombocytopenia than thrombocytosis.

10. **(B)** As a result of vitamin deficiencies and the direct insult alcohol exacts on the nerve function, peripheral neuropathy can be seen in 10% of heavy drinkers. Another important nervous system effect of alcohol and its metabolites is cerebellar degeneration, which can be suggested by an unsteady gait and nystagmus. Alcoholic fatty liver—a swollen liver resulting from the deposition of fats and proteins in the hepatocytes—reverses with abstinence from alcohol. Although there is some evidence that a glass of wine each day may impart some protective cardiac effects, heavy drinking is certainly destructive to the cardiovascular system. It raises the blood pressure and levels of triglycerides, thereby increasing the risk of myocardial infarction. Heavy drinking also lowers WBC count and interferes with many specific aspects of the immune system; for example, it compromises T-cell function.

11. **(B)** The patient does not have a history of mental illness, which gives you information about past behaviors, especially suicidality. She is unable to contract for safety, and attempts to contact collaterals have been unsuccessful. Collateral information is essential to validate the present history as well as to provide data about baseline mental status. In the absence of collateral input, from either family or healthcare professionals, and the important fact that she remains suicidal, the patient should not be discharged from the emergency department. The patient does not exhibit psychotic behavior and is not a management problem. The administration of an antipsychotic medication can cause side effects and may affect

future compliance with psychotropic medications. A thorough history, physical, and MSE, in conjunction with sound judgment based on the available facts, supplants judgment based on a telephone presentation or decisions by managed care organizations.

12. **(D)** TCAs inhibit reuptake of norepinephrine and serotonin to varying degrees. Structurally, they can be divided into tertiary amines (amitriptyline, clomipramine, doxepin, imipramine, and trimipramine) and secondary amines (desipramine, nortriptyline, and protriptyline). Tertiary amines tend to inhibit reuptake of serotonin to a greater degree than norepinephrine, and secondary amines primarily inhibit reuptake of norepinephrine. Bupropion is an antidepressant that inhibits both norepinephrine and dopamine reuptake.

13. **(C)** This scenario represents a case of Munchausen syndrome by proxy, in which one person feigns illness in another to vicariously gain medical attention. Commonly, the victim is a child and the perpetrator is the child's mother. Apparent bleeding, seizures, and central nervous system (CNS) depression are typical presentations. The disorder is underdiagnosed and typically takes more than a year to diagnose due both to the elusive and crafty planning of the perpetrator and the unwillingness of health-care providers to accuse the ostensibly caring parent. *Conversion disorder* is characterized by the presence of one or more neurologic symptoms that are left unexplained by a known medical or neurologic disorder. It is associated with such comorbid psychiatric disorders as MDD, anxiety disorder, or schizophrenia, and adolescents and young adults suffer from this disorder most commonly. Paralysis, blindness, and mutism are the most common conversion disorder symptoms. The diagnosis requires the association of psychological factors to the initiation and exacerbation of conversion symptoms. In this case, there are no data to support this diagnosis.

14. **(C)** The mental status of the mother has been described as depressed, anxious, and suicidal. Borderline and histrionic personality disorders are the most common Axis II diagnoses associated with Munchausen syndrome by proxy and most sufferers demonstrate a dissociation of affect. Schizophrenia has been reported in only a few cases. Of the choices listed, depression is the most likely; bipolar disorder and PTSD have not been clearly described in the literature. Epilepsy is not associated with the disorder to any significant extent.

15. **(B)** *Panic disorder* is characterized by the sudden unexpected occurrence of panic attacks and periods of intense anxiety or fear accompanied by somatic symptoms, commonly causing the misdiagnosis of a medical illness such as myocardial infarction. The frequency of panic attacks varies widely from many per day to a few per year. Panic disorder is often associated with *agoraphobia*, the fear of being alone in public places. The lifetime prevalence is up to 3%. Concerns of death from cardiac or respiratory disorders occur frequently. *Delirium* is characterized by the sudden onset of a disturbance of consciousness with cognitive changes caused by a general medical condition. *Acute stress disorder* is diagnosed in individuals who have experienced a traumatic event and subsequently develop symptoms within 4 weeks of the event that remit after 1 month. The traumatic event must be reexperienced by the patient, and this causes the patient to avoid stimuli that arouse recollections of the trauma. Other criteria necessary for the diagnosis are the presence of dissociative symptoms and marked anxiety or increased arousal not better accounted for by other medical or psychiatric illnesses.

16. **(A)** Tricyclic and tetracyclic medications, MAOIs, SSRIs, and the benzodiazepines are effective in the treatment of panic disorder. Beta-adrenergic drugs like propranolol are not effective for the treatment of panic disorder. Haloperidol, an antipsychotic agent; lithium, a mood stabilizer; and clonidine, an alpha-2-adrenergic agonist, are ineffective. Of the choices listed, sertraline, an SSRI, is most effective.

17. **(A)** Hypertensive crisis is a potentially life-threatening complication that occurs when patients taking an MAOI eat tyramine-containing

foods such as wine, beer, pickled foods, and aged cheese. Clinical features include hypertension, severe occipital headache, stiff neck, nausea, vomiting, and sweating. IV phentolamine, an alpha-adrenergic receptor-blocking drug, is given to control hypertension. It has been shown to be more effective than beta-blockers or calcium channel blockers. Admission to an ICU and supportive measures are indicated. Although muscle rigidity can occur, the use of dantrolene, a muscle relaxant, is not indicated.

18. **(E)** Clozapine is an effective antipsychotic medication that has been associated with fewer extrapyramidal side effects than the conventional antipsychotics (which primarily act by blocking dopamine type 2 receptors). About 5% of patients taking more than 600 mg/day of clozapine experience clozapine-associated seizures. Tachycardia, hypotension, sedation, fatigue, and weight gain have all been associated with clozapine treatment. Clozapine, unlike the conventional antipsychotic agents, does not affect prolactin secretion and thus does not cause galactorrhea.

19. **(A)** Agranulocytosis is a potentially life-threatening side effect of clozapine treatment. It is defined as a decrease in the number of WBCs, with a specific decrease in the number of neutrophil granulocytes. It occurs in 1–2% of all patients treated with clozapine. The other choices are bone marrow disorders that are not associated with clozapine.

20. **(E)** *Schizotypal personality disorder* is characterized by a pervasive pattern of social and interpersonal deficits. Individuals demonstrate a reduced capacity to establish any close relationships, and eccentric behavior is present. The presence of odd beliefs or magical thinking separates schizotypal personality disorder from schizoid personality disorder. Paranoid ideation is common in both schizotypal and paranoid personality disorders but not in the others. *Schizoid personality disorder* represents a pervasive pattern of detachment from social relationships and a restricted range of expressed emotions. *Avoidant personality disorder* represents

a pervasive pattern of behavior characterized by social inhibition, feelings of inadequacy, and hypersensitivity to negative evaluation. *Narcissistic personality disorder* represents a pervasive pattern of grandiosity, lack of empathy, and a need for admiration.

21. **(B)** *Borderline personality disorder* is a pervasive pattern of instability of interpersonal relationships, self-image, affect, and marked impulsivity. *Antisocial personality disorder* describes individuals with long histories of disregard for the rights of others and often dishonesty used in attempts to gain something for themselves. Patients with *histrionic personality disorder*, like those with borderline personality disorder, may display excessive emotionality and attention-seeking behavior, but their core symptoms center around superficial seductiveness and theatricality. Those with *dependent personality disorder* require an excessive amount of advice, reassurance, and approval from others. *Schizoid personality disorder* represents a pervasive pattern of detachment from social relationships and a restricted range of expressed emotions.

22. **(A)** This patient is most likely suffering from bipolar I disorder. Racing thoughts, pressured speech, expansive mood, a decreased need for sleep, and an increase in goal-directed activity are all common manifestations of mania. The patient is usually energized during the day even after only a few hours of sleep. Weight loss and depressed mood are characteristic of a depressive disorder. Auditory hallucinations may be present in severe cases of mania but are usually a symptom of a psychotic disorder such as schizophrenia.

23. **(B)** Many disorders can mimic symptoms of mania. A complete history, physical examination, and routine laboratory tests can sufficiently rule out most medical causes of mania. They include endocrine disorders such as thyrotoxicosis and Cushing disease, hypoglycemia, electrolyte disorders, substance abuse and withdrawal, medications such as steroids and anticholinergic agents, nutritional deficiencies, and CNS insults.

24. **(C)** Gingival hyperplasia is associated with administration of phenytoin. Other, dose-related symptoms include nystagmus, dizziness, slurred speech, ataxia, mental confusion, and decreased coordination. Hepatic failure is associated with divalproex sodium, and Ebstein anomaly is associated with lithium therapy.

25. **(D)** Before any pharmacologic changes are considered, the physician must assess compliance with medications. The subtherapeutic phenytoin level may be due to patient noncompliance, especially if side effects are being experienced.

26. **(E)** The risk of schizophrenia among first-degree relatives of patients with the disease may be as high as 10%, compared with a 1% risk in the general population.

27. **(D)** *Attention* is the ability to focus one's perception on an outside or inside stimulus. A simple test of attention is digit recall. Most people can recall a 7-digit number forward and 5–7 digits in reverse. *Concentration* refers to sustained attention to an internal thought process. The serial-sevens examination, in which the examiner asks the patient to subtract 7 from 100 and continue the subtraction process for as many calculations as possible, is a good test of concentration. Another test of concentration is to have the patient spell a five-letter word forward and backward. Asking the patient to recall the examiner's name is an example of recent memory, and asking him to recall his Social Security number is a test of remote memory.

28. **(E)** Cocaine intoxication can appear like a manic episode associated with bipolar I disorder with an increase in energy, euphoria, grandiosity, and impaired judgment. The acute onset of symptoms makes the diagnosis of major depression unlikely. A diagnosis of schizophrenia requires the presence of symptoms during a significant portion of the previous month, which is not evident. In this case, the patient experiences a sudden onset of euphoria that is not characteristic of schizophrenia. Negative symptoms (e.g., flattened affect, avolition, alogia) are more common in schizophrenia. The diagnosis of schizoaffective disorder requires that during the period of illness there are symptoms that suggest a diagnosis of both schizophrenia and a mood disorder (major depressive episode, manic episode, or a mixed episode). Cannabis intoxication can present with euphoria, paranoia, and impaired judgment in association with physical symptoms of conjunctival injection, increased appetite, dry mouth, and tachycardia. A decreased need for sleep does not suggest cannabis intoxication.

29. **(E)** *Culture-bound syndromes* denote recurrent, locality specific patterns of behavior. The syndrome of *amok* is a culture-bound syndrome of Malayan origin that refers to a violent or furious outburst with homicidal intent. Four defining characteristics are prodromal brooding, a homicidal outburst, persistence in reckless killing without an apparent motive, and a claim of amnesia. The attack typically results in multiple casualties and is most common in young men whose self-esteem has been injured. *Ganser syndrome* is characterized by a patient who responds to questions by giving approximate or outright ridiculous answers. Additional features include altered consciousness, hallucinations, conversion phenomenon, and amnesia for the episode. *Dissociative identity disorder* is a chronic state in which two or more separate ongoing identities or personalities alternate in consciousness. It usually occurs in patients who experienced severe and repeated abuse as young children.

30. **(C)** Neuroleptic-induced extrapyramidal side effects due to the blockade of dopamine are common in the treatment of psychosis. The higher-potency neuroleptic drugs are more likely to cause extrapyramidal side effects than the lower-potency neuroleptics. Extrapyramidal side effects are diminished by agents such as benztropine, antihistamines, benzodiazepines, and dopamine agonists. There are four types of extrapyramidal side effects: acute dystonic reactions, akathisia (restlessness), pseudoparkinsonism, and tardive dyskinesia or tardive dystonia. In this case, the treatment of the involuntary movements involves evaluation of dose and type of neuroleptic. Reducing the dose, substituting with a higher-potency agent, or adding an antiparkinsonian drug are all feasible therapeutic interventions.

31. **(B)** Atypical antipsychotic agents are thought to act on various subpopulations of dopamine neurons as well as on various dopamine receptor subtypes and other neurotransmitter systems. They are considered atypical agents because they are associated with a lower risk of extrapyramidal symptoms. Clozapine, introduced to the United States in 1989, is the first antipsychotic to be labeled atypical. The other choices are all considered typical antipsychotics.

32. **(D)** Borderline personality disorder is a pattern of instability in interpersonal relationships, self-image, affect, and marked impulsivity. DBT, a manualized treatment for chronically parasuicidal patients that incorporates elements of cognitive, behavioral, and supportive therapies, is a form of cognitive-behavioral treatment for borderline personality disorder. Avoidant personality disorder represents a pervasive pattern of behavior characterized by social inhibition, feelings of inadequacy, and hypersensitivity to negative evaluation. Schizoid personality disorder represents a pervasive pattern of detachment from social relationships and a restricted range of expressed emotions. Bipolar disorder is an affective illness characterized by alternating periods of mania and major depression. Passive-aggressive personality disorder describes a pervasive pattern of negativistic attitudes and passive resistance to demands for adequate performance.

33. **(A)** General principles of DBT include believing that the patient wants to improve and is doing the best she or he can. The patient is encouraged to take responsibility and solve her or his own problems. Patients may not have caused all of their problems, but they are encouraged to solve them anyway. Patients learn new behaviors in a relative context and believe that they cannot fail in therapy.

34. **(A)** The patient is experiencing anticholinergic toxicity as evidenced by dilated pupils, dry or flushed skin, agitation, confusion, and tachycardia. Additional manifestations include disorientation and urinary retention. More severe toxicity may result in hyperthermia or coma. In this case, the patient reported benefit from haloperidol but experienced extrapyramidal side effects, common to the high-potency antipsychotic medications. Benztropine, an anticholinergic medication, is prescribed to alleviate extrapyramidal side effects, but in this patient it caused anticholinergic side effects. Amantadine is an antiviral medication that is used to help alleviate extrapyramidal side effects and should be instituted to replace benztropine.

35. **(C)** *Denial*, a narcissistic defense, is a common unconscious emotional defense mechanism used to avoid becoming aware of a painful aspect of reality. Denial can be used in both normal and pathologic states. As a defense mechanism it serves to keep internal or external reality out of the conscious to avert stress and anxiety. Regression, an immature defense, is an emotional and physical retreat from adult standards of behavior toward an infantile level of passivity and dependence. At times, regression represents a retreat from the arduous task of recovery. *Rationalization* is a neurotic defense mechanism in which unacceptable behavior, feelings, or thoughts are logically justified by elaborate and reassuring answers. *Suppression*, a mature defense, is a conscious act of controlling and inhibiting unacceptable impulses, emotions, or ideas.

36. **(B)** The essential feature of acute stress disorder is the development of anxiety and dissociative symptoms within 1 month of exposure to an extremely traumatic stressor. Diagnosis should be considered if the symptoms persist at least 2 days and cause significant distress or impairment. While experiencing the stressor, the individual must experience three of these five symptoms: a subjective sense of numbing, detachment, or absence of emotional responsiveness; a reduction in awareness of surroundings; derealization; depersonalization; or dissociative amnesia. In addition, the person must reexperience the event in some way (e.g., bad dreams), must experience anxiety or increased arousal, and must experience a marked avoidance of the stimuli that arouse recollections of the traumatic event. The diagnosis of PTSD requires more than 1 month of symptoms. Adjustment disorder can be considered for

those individuals who do not meet criteria for acute stress disorder but develop similar symptoms in excess of what is to be expected given the nature of the stressor. GAD is characterized by excessive anxiety and worry that occur for at least 6 months. MDD can exist in the context of an acute stress reaction. However, in this case, the symptoms are not suggestive of a depressive illness.

37. **(E)** Psychogenic unresponsiveness can be delineated from coma by obtaining an EEG, which is normal in a psychogenic state. On physical examination, deep tendon reflexes may be suppressed. In patients who are awake, cold water introduced into the ear produces nystagmus with the fast component away from the ear. In coma, the eyes either do not react or they may slowly and smoothly deviate toward the ear in which the cold water was introduced. Voluntary eye movements called saccades are rapid and smooth. Saccadic eye movements are elicited in patients by asking them to stare at an object at one side of the visual field and then ask them to shift their gaze to the opposite visual field. Typically, eye movements in coma or persistent vegetative states are spontaneous and random.

38. **(E)** Seasonal affective disorder describes a seasonal pattern of symptoms associated with major depressive episodes in MDD, bipolar I disorder, and bipolar II disorder. The essential feature is the onset of depressive symptoms at characteristic times of the year. More common in women, most episodes begin in the fall or winter and remit in the spring. Major depressive episodes that occur in a seasonal pattern are typically characterized by anergy, hypersomnia, overeating, weight gain, and carbohydrate craving. Age is a strong predictor, with young persons at higher risk.

39. **(C)** The essential features of dissociative fugue are sudden and unexpected travel away from home or one's usual place of daily activities with a subsequent inability to recall the episode accompanied by confusion about personal identity or the assumption of a new identity. The disorder is more common in women and is often associated with a childhood history of sexual

abuse. Partial complex seizures tend to be brief and do not last as long as the clinical picture presents. Delirium is characterized by a disturbance of consciousness and a change in cognition that develops over a short period of time.

40. **(C)** This patient does not meet full criteria for major depression (e.g., 4/5 *Diagnostic and Statistical Manual of Mental Disorders, Fourth Edition, Text Revision* [DSM-IV-TR] criteria), so she cannot be diagnosed with bipolar II disorder, which is characterized by the occurrence of one or more major depressive episodes accompanied by at least one episode of hypomania (a distinct period of a persistently elevated, expansive, or irritable mood that lasts at least 4 days). Bipolar II disorder differs from bipolar I disorder in that, although the manic and hypomanic episodes of these two disorders have identical list criteria, bipolar II disorder is not severe enough to cause marked impairment in social or occupational functioning or to cause hospitalization. Dysthymic disorder is also ruled out by the presence of manic symptoms making cyclothymic disorder the best choice.

41. **(B)** The hallmark of Ganser syndrome is that the patient responds to questions by giving approximate or ridiculous answers. Often confused with malingering, Ganser syndrome is primarily described in the prison population. It involves the production of answers to questions that are relative but not quite correct (e.g., $4 \times 5 = 19$). It is classified in the DSM-IV-TR as a dissociative disorder not otherwise specified. Munchausen syndrome is a factitious disorder with physical symptoms. Capgras syndrome describes a content-specific delusion in which the patient believes that a significant other, usually a family member, has been replaced by an identical imposter.

42. **(E)** ECT provides safe and effective treatment of MDD in the elderly, especially in a patient with a high risk of suicide or medical contraindications (e.g., heart disease) to the use of psychotropic medications. Nortriptyline, a TCA, is lethal in overdose and should not be prescribed in an acutely suicidal patient. Cardiac arrhythmia is also a contraindication to TCA use.

43. **(B)** The specifiers of melancholic features and atypical features can be applied to a current or recent major depressive episode that occurs in the course of MDD and to a major depressive episode in bipolar I or bipolar II disorder. The atypical features specifier can also be applied to dysthymic disorder. The essential features of the atypical specifier are mood reactivity and two of the following four features: increased appetite or weight gain, hypersomnia, leaden paralysis, and rejection sensitivity. The essential feature of a major depressive episode with melancholic features is a loss of interest or pleasure in all or almost all activities or a lack of reactivity to usually pleasurable stimuli.

44. **(A)** *Identification* is an unconscious defense mechanism in which the person incorporates the characteristics and qualities of another person or object into his or her own ego system. The defense serves to strengthen the ego. *Regression*, an immature defense, is an emotional and physical retreat from adult standards of behavior toward an infantile level of passivity and dependence. *Projection* is the false attribution of one's own unacceptable feelings to another. *Fixation* refers to an overactive attachment to a person or object; *idealization* is the attribution of near-perfect, unrealistic attributes to that person or object.

45. **(C)** The essential feature of the catatonia observed in patients with schizophrenia is a marked psychomotor disturbance involving motor immobility, excessive motor activity, mutism, negativism, peculiar voluntary movements, echolalia (parrot-like senseless repetition of words or phrases), or echopraxia (imitation of movements of another person). Catalepsy is just one potential symptom of catatonia, and is not a complete answer. Cataplexy is a sudden and brief loss of muscle tone involving either a few muscle groups or most of the antigravity muscles of the body. The fact that the patient occasionally mimics the movements of others makes seizure activity unlikely.

46. **(A)** *Catalepsy* is a general term for the assumption of an immobile position that is constantly maintained, especially after an examination.

Cataplexy is a sudden and brief loss of muscle tone involving either a few muscle groups or most of the antigravity muscles of the body. *Dystonia* is a stiffening of muscle groups sometimes seen after administration of typical neuroleptics. The patient does not seem to have a secondary gain for his symptoms making malingering unlikely.

47. **(D)** Priapism can occur with a number of antidepressant or antipsychotic agents but occurs most often with the use of trazodone (1 in 1000 to 1 in 10,000 incidence). The three SSRIs (fluoxetine, sertraline, and paroxetine) listed can cause impotence, but are unlikely to cause priapism. Nortriptyline is a TCA not associated with priapism.

48. **(C)** The condition usually occurs within the first 4 weeks of treatment but can happen as late as 18 months into treatment. The condition is independent of dose. Priapism is a medical emergency and may require surgery. The condition may respond to intracavernosal injection of an alpha-adrenergic agonist to promote detumescence and constriction of veins.

49. **(A)** The patient is most likely suffering from GAD. Treatment of GAD includes antidepressants, benzodiazepines, buspirone, and cognitive-behavioral therapies. However, benzodiazepines should be avoided in patients with respiratory compromise, because these medications can exacerbate breathing-related disorders. Alprazolam, diazepam, and lorazepam are all benzodiazepines. Buspirone, a nonbenzodiazepine anxiolytic, is a logical alternative and has been demonstrated to be effective in the treatment of GAD. Beta-blocking agents such as propranolol are effective but should not be first-line therapy in patients with chronic obstructive pulmonary disease or other respiratory disorders.

50. **(B)** The long-term use of benzodiazepines (temazepam, oxazepam, and clorazepate) for sleep is controversial especially in patients with substance abuse or breathing-related disorders. Zolpidem is not a member of the benzodiazepine class but does produce its effects

at the gamma-aminobutyric acid (GABA)-benzodiazepine receptor and as a result has a much lower risk of dependence. Zaleplon (Sonata) is a newer nonbenzodiazepine hypnotic that interacts with the GABA-benzodiazepine receptor complex. It has an ultrashort half-life of 1 hour. A nonbenzodiazepine medication is a logical alternative in cases in which respiratory function is compromised. Diphenhydramine should be avoided in the elderly because of its anticholinergic effects.

51. **(D)** Hypertensive crisis is a life-threatening emergency that may result from the combination of meperidine and an MAOI. The combined use of these medications is absolutely contraindicated. The treatment of hypertensive crisis is with IV alpha-adrenergic blocking agents and ICU admission and support. All of the other medications are safe in combination with MAOIs.

52. **(C)** The use of any medications in pregnancy requires examining the risks and benefits of treatment. The use of MAOIs is contraindicated in pregnancy partly because they can exacerbate pregnancy-induced hypertension. Although ECT is safe in pregnancy, maintenance ECT is indicated after an initial course is completed. The safety of newer antidepressants such as paroxetine in pregnancy has not yet been completely established, but studies of fluoxetine suggest that it is relatively safe. Specific recommendations regarding the course of treatment for a single episode of MDD do not exist. Many physicians find that the treatment of a single episode requires 9–12 months of pharmacotherapy. The return of symptoms suggests a recurrent MDD that requires longer-term pharmacotherapy. Of course, patient preference plays a role as well.

53. **(D)** The patient presents with clinical symptoms of Wernicke encephalopathy, a medical emergency, characterized by ophthalmoplegia, ataxia, and delirium and caused by thiamine deficiency. If the thiamine deficiency is not corrected, Wernicke-Korsakoff syndrome emerges characterized by amnesia, ataxia, and nystagmus. The syndrome results from chronic thiamine deficiency with resultant pathology in the mammillary bodies and the thalamus. A history of alcohol abuse is common but other causes of thiamine deficiency such as starvation, prolonged vomiting, and gastric carcinoma can cause this syndrome. The use of IV dextrose prior to the administration of thiamine may aggravate Wernicke encephalopathy. The other interventions may be appropriate if thiamine does not resolve the symptoms.

54. **(A)** *Aphasia* is characterized by the loss of language abilities produced by brain dysfunction. Cardiovascular disorders, brain tumors, infection, trauma, and degenerative diseases are the most common causes. *Broca aphasia* is characterized by short, nonfluent output with intact comprehension. Reading comprehension is preserved. *Wernicke aphasia* presents as fluent speech output with poor reading comprehension. Repetition, naming, writing, and reading aloud are impaired in both disorders. Wernicke aphasia results from lesions of the posterior superior left temporal gyrus (Wernicke area). Broca aphasia results from a lesion of the middle third of the left inferior frontal gyrus (Broca area).

55. **(C)** Caffeine withdrawal occurs after the abrupt cessation or a marked reduction in the use of caffeinated products. Studies estimate that up to 75% of caffeine users will experience symptoms of withdrawal at some point. Caffeine withdrawal symptoms have their onset 12–24 hours after the last dose, and symptoms peak in 24–48 hours. Symptoms typically remit in 1 week. Although all the possible choices are associated with caffeine withdrawal, up to 50% of sufferers experience headache, the most common symptom.

56. **(E)** This patient is most likely suffering from NMS. Death, reported in up to 30% of cases, usually results from the failure to recognize the syndrome or from delayed treatment. Discontinuation of the offending agent and supportive treatment in an ICU setting is imperative. Cooling measures reduce hyperthermia. IV dantrolene sodium and oral bromocriptine have been used but their benefits are unclear. The exact frequency remains unknown with some studies

suggesting up to 1.9% of all patients treated with antipsychotics experience this syndrome. NMS may be more frequent in men and younger patients. Naloxone does not have a place in the treatment of NMS.

57. **(C)** An elevated serum CPK demonstrates muscle injury. Leukocytosis is also seen. Elevated BUN may be seen in dehydration resulting from NMS but is not as common as CPK elevation.

58. **(D)** Physical dependence emphasizes the presence of tolerance or withdrawal. Naloxone injection can precipitate opiate withdrawal in dependent persons. Positive urine toxicology or breath analysis can identify only substance abuse not dependence. Elevated liver function studies can be present in individuals who abuse alcohol but can also be present in other non-substance-related disorders. Elevated heart rate can be present in many withdrawal syndromes or medical disorders and is not specific for any substance.

59. **(B)** Dementia is an organic and global decline of functioning without impaired consciousness. (This differentiates it from delirium characterized by a waxing and waning consciousness.) The most common type of dementia (50–60%) is the Alzheimer type. Vascular dementia is the second most common type of dementia, occurring in 10–20% of cases. Other degenerative processes that cause dementia are Parkinson disease, Huntington disease, and Pick disease. Infectious, metabolic, endocrine, neoplastic, and toxic processes can also cause dementia. In this case, the history of cognitive decline without impaired consciousness suggests a diagnosis of dementia. The history reveals a megaloblastic anemia, the cause of which may be a vitamin B_{12} deficiency possibly secondary to a subtotal gastrectomy. Folate deficiency can also cause megaloblastic anemia. Vitamin deficiencies such as B_{12} and folate can cause clinical signs of dementia but represent one of a few possible reversible causes of this process. A complete reversible workup for dementia should also include thyroid function studies and a rapid plasma reagin to test for syphilis. Alzheimer disease is confirmed only by autopsy.

60. **(A)** Lithium, commonly used to treat bipolar disorder, can be dangerous in intoxication, which is a neurotoxic event and can lead to death or permanent damage to the nervous system particularly the cerebellum. Cardiovascular and renal manifestations may also be present. Lithium has a low therapeutic index with a therapeutic range of 0.5–1.5 mEq/L. Plasma concentrations above the therapeutic range, especially greater than 2.0 mEq/L, precipitate severe CNS and renal impairment. Early clinical signs of intoxication include dysarthria, coarse tremor, and ataxia. Impaired consciousness, fasciculations or myoclonus, seizures, and coma are ominous manifestations. The goal of treatment is removal of lithium from the body. Gastric lavage, rehydration, and hemodialysis are possible interventions. Given the danger of lithium intoxication, a serum drug level should be obtained before any of the other interventions.

61. **(E)** Baseline medical tests should be obtained and documented before starting many psychotropic medications including the mood stabilizers lithium, carbamazepine, and divalproex sodium. Assessment of thyroid function, complete blood count, electrolytes, ECG, and renal function studies (BUN, creatinine, urinalysis) are important before the initiation of lithium. Older patients require additional tests, including EEG, thyrotropin-releasing hormone test, 24-hour urine volume determination, and creatinine clearance. Lithium-induced polyuria results from the inhibition of the effect of antidiuretic hormone. Reversible T-wave changes on the ECG are common.

62. **(D)** The serotonin syndrome occurs when an SSRI is combined with another drug that can potentiate serotonin, such as the monoamine oxidase-inhibiting drugs, pentazocine, L-tryptophan, lithium, and carbamazepine. Symptoms of the syndrome include abdominal pain, diarrhea, diaphoresis, hyperpyrexia, tachycardia, hypertension, myoclonus, irritability, agitation, seizures, and delirium. Coma, cardiovascular collapse, and death have been reported. In this case, the serotonergic effects of fluoxetine are potentiated by the

MAOI. Fluoxetine has a prolonged half-life with active metabolites that require up to 6 weeks' clearance time. Treatment with the MAOI was initiated before adequate washout of the fluoxetine and resulted in the serotonin syndrome. Management involves discontinuation of the offending agent and supportive care. There is no evidence that the patient is continuing to take her MAOI and eat a tyramine-heavy diet, that she has been abusing hallucinogens, or that she is taking antipsychotics that might induce any of the remaining choices.

63. **(A)** *Bulimia nervosa*, more common than anorexia nervosa, consists of repeated episodes of binge eating of large amounts of food associated with the feeling of being out of control. The patient usually purges by self-induced vomiting or repeated laxative or diuretic use and engages in excessive amounts of exercise to prevent weight gain. Unlike individuals with anorexia nervosa, individuals with bulimia nervosa usually maintain a normal body weight. Medical complications of bulimia nervosa are usually secondary to either chronic vomiting or laxative abuse. Fluid and electrolyte imbalances (alkalosis, hypokalemia, hypochloremia, dehydration); dental caries and enamel loss; gastrointestinal disturbances such as esophagitis, Mallory-Weiss tears, and constipation; and sore throat are also common.

64. **(B)** Antidepressant medications reduce binge eating and purging independent of the presence of a mood disorder. Imipramine, desipramine, MAOIs, and fluoxetine have been effective in controlled studies. The other choices treat symptoms of the illness without treating the underlying disorder.

65. **(B)** Anorexia nervosa is clinically characterized by a deliberate self-imposed starvation in the pursuit of being thin, driven by a fear of being fat. The patient refuses to maintain accepted normal body weight appropriate for age and height. Failure to achieve 85% of expected body weight, the intense fear of being fat, a disturbed perception of the body weight or shape (or denial of the seriousness of the current low body weight), and amenorrhea in postmenarchal females are diagnostic criteria. Underdeveloped breasts, abnormal insulin secretion, endocrine disorders, and poor sexual development with a marked decreased interest in sexual activity are also associated with this disorder. For anorexia nervosa to be diagnosed, a postmenarchal female must have missed at least three consecutive periods. Patients do not lose their feelings of hunger despite their refusal to eat properly.

66. **(C)** The mortality rate for anorexia nervosa ranges from 5% to 20%.

67. **(A)** *Bereavement* refers to the reaction to the death of a loved one. Some individuals develop symptoms of a major depressive episode. For example, 50% of all widows and widowers meet criteria for major depression within the first year. The bereaved usually refers to feeling depressed as being normal. If the symptoms of a major depressive episode begin within 2 months of the loss and do not persist beyond the 2-month period, they are considered the result of bereavement unless associated with marked impairment of any of the following: thoughts of death other than feelings that they would be better off dead or should have died with the deceased person, expressing guilt other than about the actions taken or not taken by the survivor at the time of the death, a morbid preoccupation with worthlessness, marked psychomotor retardation, or hallucinations other than that he or she hears the voice of (or sees the image of) the deceased individual. Complicated bereavement is chronic and unremitting distress. Chronic grief may occur if the relationship between the bereaved and the deceased was close or ambivalent, if they were dependent on one another, or if few other support systems are available. Bereavement reactions are very intense after sudden or unexpected deaths. Prolonged denial, anger, or guilt complicates the course of bereavement. Adjustment disorder requires the development of symptoms within 3 months of an identifiable stressor, with marked distress in excess of what would be expected from experiencing the stressor: In this case, the symptoms are considered acceptable reactions to the death of a spouse.

Dysthymic disorder requires 2 years of symptoms marked by a depressed mood.

68. **(A)** Most bereaved do fine without treatment. Support and reassurance usually come from family, friends, or clergy. When the bereaved feel unable to move beyond the grief, psychotherapeutic measures are appropriate. The treatment of anxiety or insomnia with medications remains controversial and no controlled studies have established clear efficacy. However, medications may be warranted if cognitive or other higher functions of daily living are substantially affected.

69. **(C)** The treatment of patients with obsessive-compulsive disorder (OCD) requires integrating multiple treatment modalities including medications, psychotherapy, and collateral support systems. The best-studied medication to treat obsessions is clomipramine, a TCA. SSRIs have also been effective in treating symptoms of OCD, but at doses higher than those used to treat depression. MAOIs are helpful for those who suffer from comorbid anxiety. Lithium has not been proven to be helpful in the treatment of OCD. Antipsychotic agents are used in conjunction with antidepressants but are not usually indicated as individual agents. Anxiolytic agents are of little use in treating obsessions. Antiepileptics are not indicated for the treatment of OCD.

70. **(D)** *Sleep apnea* is defined as the cessation of respirations lasting at least 10 seconds. The presence of more than five episodes of apnea per hour of sleep is diagnostic. Sleep apnea is classified as obstructive, central, or a mixed picture of both types. Classified as a breathing-related sleep disorder, sleep apnea leads to excessive sleepiness or insomnia. Characterized by upper airway obstruction, obstructive sleep apnea is associated with snoring, morning headache, excessive movements at night, and mental dullness. The typical patient is a middle-aged obese man.

71. **(A)** Nasal continuous positive airway pressure (CPAP) is the treatment of choice for obstructive sleep apnea. No medications are consistently effective in normalizing sleep in these patients. The use of nasal CPAP appears to prevent long-term morbidity and mortality and provides restorative sleep. Surgical procedures are reserved for CPAP treatment failures.

72. **(B)** Anticholinergic toxicity can be caused by many psychotropic medications. The low-potency agents chlorpromazine and thioridazine and the TCAs amitriptyline and imipramine are particularly anticholinergic. The syndrome often results when an anticholinergic medication is coadministered with an antipsychotic medication to prevent or treat extrapyramidal side effects such as parkinsonism and dystonia. Clinical features include decreased secretions, agitation, dry skin, flushing of the skin, hyperthermia, tachycardia, dilated pupils, urinary retention, constipation, and hypotension. Seizures, hallucinations, and coma may result from severe intoxication. Drugs that inhibit the enzyme that breaks down acetylcholine (anticholinesterase medications such as physostigmine) reverse the syndrome and are usually administered IV with appropriate monitoring. Atropine would further increase the heart rate; haloperidol would likely worsen anticholinergic symptoms and benzodiazepines are reserved for use in agitation and anxiety.

73. **(A)** Anticholinesterase toxicity, manifesting as nausea, vomiting, bradycardia, and seizures, result from excessive action of acetylcholine at specific receptors. Atropine, an antimuscarinic agent, can reverse the symptoms. Physostigmine would worsen the toxicity. Although prochlorperazine would combat vomiting, it would not treat the underlying condition and might worsen the anticholinergic toxicity. Similarly, epinephrine would treat the bradycardia without treating the underlying condition.

74. **(E)** SSRI medications are used to treat a variety of medical and psychiatric disorders. Fluvoxamine is an SSRI particularly indicated for both depression and OCD. Doxepin and clomipramine are TCAs and phenelzine is an MAOI. Buspirone is a nonbenzodiazepine medication used to treat anxiety disorders.

75. **(D)** Because they act at the same GABA receptors as alcohol, the benzodiazepines are the preferred medications used in detoxification from alcohol. For uncomplicated detoxification, the long-acting benzodiazepines such as chlordiazepoxide and diazepam are appropriate because they are essentially self-tapering. The shorter-acting benzodiazepines such as lorazepam or oxazepam are used in patients with impaired liver function, because they are not oxidized to long-acting metabolites and do not accumulate. Patients with unstable medical problems, cognitive impairment, or old age are also candidates for the shorter-acting medications. Phenobarbital was formerly used for detoxification and has been replaced by benzodiazepines. Disulfiram, which interferes with the metabolism of alcohol, is reserved for long-term behavioral therapy of alcohol dependence.

76. **(B)** The patient is experiencing hallucinations due to alcohol withdrawal. Benzodiazepines will treat the underlying withdrawal as well as the hallucinations. An antipsychotic is unnecessary and may also reduce the seizure threshold. The patient shows no evidence of a mood disorder that would be best treated with sertraline or fluoxtine (SSRIs), or lithium, a mood stabilizer.

77. **(D)** Ethanol is metabolized in the liver to acetaldehyde, which is enzymatically converted to acetate by the enzyme aldehyde dehydrogenase. Disulfiram is a medication that irreversibly inhibits the action of alcohol dehydrogenase. Acetaldehyde accumulates and accounts for the aversive effects associated with the disulfiram-ethanol reaction. Flushing, sweating, dyspnea, hyperventilation, tachycardia, hypotension, nausea, and vomiting are common symptoms. Extreme reactions can result in respiratory depression, cardiovascular collapse, myocardial infarction, seizures, and death. Blurred vision and urinary retention are anticholinergic effects associated with antipsychotic, antidepressant, and antiparkinsonian medications. Hypertension is associated with but not characteristic of the disulfiram-ethanol reaction. Disulfiram is not recommended for patients with moderate to severe liver disease, renal failure,

severe cardiac disease, pregnancy, or peripheral neuropathy. In this case, the patient was prescribed chlordiazepoxide and presumably had preserved liver function.

78. **(A)** Many nonsteroidal anti-inflammatory drugs can decrease the clearance of lithium and produce significant increases in serum levels. Ibuprofen, indomethacin, ketoprofen, diclofenac, phenylbutazone, naproxen, and piroxicam have all been reported to produce such potential dangerous interactions. The symptoms of abdominal pain, diarrhea, and drowsiness indicate mild to moderate (1.5–2.0 mEq/L) lithium toxicity. Acetaminophen, aspirin, and the opiates do not interfere with lithium clearance. Meperidine, however, can cause dangerous interactions with MAOIs.

79. **(B)** Clinically effective antidepressant medications potentiate the actions of serotonin, norepinephrine, and dopamine in the brain. The antidepressant action of amitriptyline, a TCA, is to significantly block the reuptake of serotonin and to a lesser degree norepinephrine. Bupropion is a weak inhibitor of dopamine reuptake with modest effects on norepinephrine. It does not have any effect on serotonin. Lorazepam is an anxiolytic medication whose actions are mediated by GABA receptors. Maprotiline is a TCA with modest effects on norepinephrine and no effect on serotonin. Desipramine, a TCA, has potent effects on norepinephrine reuptake and has weak effects on the serotonergic system.

80. **(A)** Medically ill patients with depressive disorders may respond to psychostimulants, an excellent choice if the patient is unable to tolerate TCAs. The rapid onset of action and rapid clearance are beneficial. Nefazodone, fluoxetine, and bupropion are effective antidepressants but may take 4–6 weeks to accomplish beneficial results. Buspirone is a nonbenzodiazepine anxiolytic medication not indicated in the treatment of depression.

81. **(C)** Inhalant abuse is commonly a social activity undertaken in groups. Volatile or toxic solvents such as toluene (found in glues and adhesives), trichloroethane (found in correction fluid), or hydrocarbons (gasoline) are placed in a bag and the fumes are inhaled. The practice is known as *huffing*, *sniffing*, or *bagging*. Effects are almost immediate because the substances are rapidly absorbed. Signs and symptoms of intoxication include visual disturbances, dyscoordination (a drunken appearance), depressed reflexes, euphoria, and nystagmus. An increased appetite suggests marijuana use, and staring into space and euphoria are associated with PCP use.

82. **(C)** Abstinence is the only treatment for inhalant abuse. Antipsychotic agents are of no use and may aggravate organic presentations of inhalant abuse. Agitation can be managed by benzodiazepine medications such as lorazepam.

Inhalant tx is abstinence

83. **(E)** The five subtypes of schizophrenia (paranoid, catatonic, residual, disorganized, and undifferentiated) are based on the presence or absence of predominant symptoms. The paranoid type is marked by prominent hallucinations or delusions; the disorganized type is marked by disorganized speech and behavior and inappropriate affect; and the catatonic type is marked by waxy flexibility or motoric immobility, excess motor activity, negativism, bizarre posturing, and echolalia or echopraxia. The residual type is marked by the absence of predominant hallucinations or delusions, disorganized speech, or catatonic behavior. The undifferentiated type is reserved for patients who meet criteria for schizophrenia but do not meet criteria for the other four types.

Paranoid Schiz → hall and del people after them

84. **(A)** Divalproex sodium, indicated for the treatment of simple or complex absence seizures or as an adjunct medication in the treatment of partial seizures, can cause sometimes significant hair loss that is usually reversible. Common side effects associated with divalproex sodium are nausea, vomiting, and indigestion. Sedation and mildly elevated serum transaminase levels are also seen. Hepatic failure resulting in fatalities has occurred, usually during the first 6 months of treatment. Divalproex sodium is also used in the treatment of migraine headache and as a mood stabilizer. Hair loss is not associated with

valproate causes hair loss that's reversible;

carbamazepine, clozapine, olanzapine, or ziprasidone, although these too have side effects.

85. **(C)** Sexual dysfunction has become an increasingly common side effect associated with many antidepressant medications. It may be underreported for many reasons. Decreased libido, erectile dysfunction, ejaculatory dysfunction, and anorgasmia have been reported. None of the other choices are associated with sexual dysfunction to the same degree as the SSRIs, and some of the choices may be used to reverse the dysfunction. Various pharmacologic strategies aimed at treating these side effects include the alpha-2-antagonist yohimbine; the dopamine agonists methylphenidate and amantadine; bupropion; cyproheptadine (an antihistamine with serotonin antagonist properties); and bethanacol, a cholinergic agonist.

86. **(A)** ADHD is a disorder of unclear etiology. As many as 9% of children suffer from this disorder, and up to 60% of those diagnosed carry the diagnosis into adulthood. The disorder is characterized by symptoms of inattention, hyperactivity, and impulsivity that are inappropriate for age. Although the DSM-IV-TR criteria suggest that symptoms must have been present before the age of 7 years, many cases are not diagnosed until adolescence or adulthood. In these cases, a retrospective history from both the patient and the family often support the presence of early life symptoms. Although some symptoms are reminiscent of the manic component of bipolar disorder, these disorders represent two separate entities. A careful history by astute physicians will secure the proper diagnosis. Depressive, anxiety, and substance-abuse disorders are common comorbid conditions that often make the diagnosis of ADHD more difficult. The absence of prominent mood symptoms and the relative degree of impairment help distinguish ADHD from other disorders.

private school gave more attention so it improve with ADHD.

87. **(D)** The approach to the treatment of the core symptoms of ADHD has been the initiation of a trial of a psychostimulant medication. Often, if one stimulant fails to treat symptoms, another stimulant is prescribed. Many patients benefit

Always D/C methylphenadate then add a combination mixed amphetamine compound.

[Margin handwritten note, left side:] → 1 month of hallucinations and Delusions and 6 months of decline in function) Schizophrenia is characterized by

from one stimulant and not another. The appropriate choice in this case would be to try a second type of stimulant before alternative strategies are implemented.

88. **(A)** The median age of onset for the first psychotic episode of schizophrenia is in the early to mid-twenties for men and the late twenties for women. The onset can be abrupt or insidious. Estimates of prevalence have ranged from 0.2% to 2.0%. Schizophrenia is characterized by a 1-month period of two of the following symptoms: delusions, hallucinations, disorganized speech, disorganized behavior, and negative symptoms such as affect flattening, alogia, or avolition. Continuous signs of the disturbance should be present for 6 months, with a decline in functioning in at least two areas (work, school, interpersonal, or self-care). A prodrome often precedes the acute phase of the disorder. Distinguishing schizophrenia from mood disorders with psychotic symptoms (e.g., bipolar I disorder with psychotic features) and schizoaffective disorder can often be difficult in that a mood disturbance is common during the prodromal and active phases of schizophrenia. If psychotic symptoms occur exclusively without the presence of mood symptoms, then schizophrenia is more likely. Schizoaffective disorder describes the presence of a major depressive episode, a manic episode, or a mixed episode concurrent with symptoms that are characteristic of schizophrenia: delusions, hallucinations, disorganized speech or behavior, or negative symptoms. A brief psychotic disorder is defined by the presence of delusions, hallucinations, disorganized speech or behavior, or catatonic behavior lasting for at least 1 day but less than 1 month.

89. **(A)** In the context of labor, high-potency typical antipsychotics are considered relatively safe to use to control psychosis. For a mother suffering psychosis during delivery, the benefit of using high-potency antipsychotics outweighs the risk because strictly speaking during delivery, it is unclear if there is any risk in using these medications. Thorazine and droperidol could lower blood pressure significantly. A related issue is postpartum psychosis characterized

by an agitated, highly changeable psychosis that usually develops between the third and fourteenth day postpartum and can lead to the fatal complication of infanticide. The incidence of postpartum psychosis in primiparous women is about 1 in 500. For those affected after the first pregnancy, subsequent pregnancies carry a risk of about 1 in 3.

90–92. [90 (A), 91(C), 92 (D)] Wechsler developed a variety of scales each to be used depending on the age of the examinee. WPPSI is designed for children ages 4–6.5, the WISC is for children ages 5–15, and the WAIS-R is for people age 15 and older. The WMS was designed to evaluate a variety of memory deficits in adults.

[Handwritten above 93:] Protein S Def - Stroke - Rey Osterrieth test

93. **(C)** The Rey-Osterrieth figure is sensitive to deficits in copying and lack of attention to detail in people with right-sided parietal lobe lesions. It appears that this young woman may have had a stroke in this area resulting from her protein S deficiency, hypercoagulable state.

94. **(B)** The appropriate test to evaluate intelligent quotient (IQ) is the WISC.

95. **(G)** The Boston Diagnostic Aphasia Examination is a series of tests given by an experienced clinician to evaluate and make treatment recommendations for individuals with aphasia. The MMPI-2 **(A)** is an objective test interpreted by skilled evaluators used in personality assessment. It is the most widely used and highly standardized test of personality structure. The Beck Depression Inventory **(D)** is a 21-item test, with three responses per item, that is an easily used screening tool to evaluate for depression. The Blessed Rating Scale **(E)** is a tool that asks friends or families of the patient to assess the ability of the patient to function in his usual environment. The WAIS-R **(F)** is used to provide an assessment of IQ of people older than 15. The Rorschach Test **(H)** is a projective test used to assess personality structure. The MMSE **(I)** is a quick, easily administered test that allows for immediate assessment of dementia. Scores of less than 24 are suggestive of a dementing process. The Bender-Gestalt Test **(J)** involves copying figures, which helps to determine if

[Handwritten at bottom of page:] psychosis while in Labor haloperidol;

organic brain disease is present. The Wisconsin Card Sorting Test **(K)** assesses executive functions of the brain such as mental flexibility and the ability to abstract and reason. These capacities are believed to be located in the frontal lobes. Damage to the frontal lobes can lead to abnormalities on this test. Wada Test **(L)** is used to evaluate hemispheric language dominance prior to surgical amelioration of seizure focus. Whereas most right-handed individuals show left hemispheric dominance for language, left-handed individuals may either be right or left dominant. The test consists of injecting sodium amytal into the carotid artery and observing the transient effects on speech. Injection into the left carotid artery will anesthetize the left side of the brain; those with left hemispheric language dominance will show interrupted speech.

96. **(D)** Cannabis (marijuana) is the most commonly abused illicit drug in the United States. The onset of action after smoking is immediate, and symptoms include conjunctival injection, mild sedation, dose-dependent hypothermia, dry mouth, increased appetite, tachycardia, and euphoria. A sensation of slowed time and paranoid ideation can also occur.

97. **(E)** The onset of action for opiates can be almost immediate when smoked, about 5 minutes when injected and longer if taken orally. Symptoms include miosis, bradycardia, hypotension, hypo-thermia, and euphoria. Intoxication can lead to fatal respiratory depression.

98. **(B)** PCP is an hallucinogen that produces a dissociative anesthesia. It can cause unpredictable behavior, assaultiveness, and belligerence. Agitation, nystagmus (vertical or horizontal), tachycardia, a numbed response to pain, muscle rigidity, hyperacusis, hypertension, echolalia, and anticholinergic effects are associated symptoms.

99. **(F)** Nicotine found in tobacco smoke produces symptoms of excitement. Intoxication may produce symptoms of confusion, muscle twitching, weakness, abdominal cramps, depression, palpitations, coma, and respiratory failure. Use of hallucinogens (e.g., LSD, MDMA [3,4-methylenedioxy-N-methylamphetamine, or "Ecstasy"]) causes symptoms that usually begin 1 hour after ingestion and generally last 8–12 hours. Most hallucinogenic drugs have stimulant-type effects and produce elevated vital signs and increased activity. Hallucinations and a heightened sense of perception of objects and colors are typical.

100. **(C)** As a sympathomimetic agent, cocaine increases the heart rate and dilates the pupils. It can also cause constriction of the coronary arteries. The hallmark of cocaine intoxication is hallucinations.

CHAPTER 9

Practice Test 2
Questions

DIRECTIONS (Questions 1 through 4): Each set of items in this section consists of a list of lettered headings followed by several numbered words or phrases. For each numbered word or phrase, select the ONE lettered option that is most closely associated with it. Each lettered option may be selected once, more than once, or not at all.

(A) citalopram
(B) fluoxetine
(C) mirtazapine
(D) nefazodone
(E) paroxetine
(F) sertraline
(G) venlafaxine

1. Has a warning causing hepatotoxicity

2. May increase blood pressure in higher doses

3. Has the most specific serotonin reuptake

4. Has a half-life of approximately 7 days

DIRECTIONS (Questions 5 through 94): Each of the numbered items in this section is followed by answer choices. Select the ONE lettered answer or completion that is BEST in each case.

5. An 18-year-old woman recently diagnosed with a first episode of schizophrenia agrees to take a neuroleptic medication to help decrease her hallucinations, but she is adamantly opposed to taking any medication that may cause her to gain excessive weight. Which of the following atypical neuroleptic medications is not associated with significant weight gain?

(A) quetiapine (Seroquel)
(B) olanzapine (Zyprexa)
(C) risperidone (Risperdal)
(D) ziprasidone (Geodon)
(E) clozapine (Clozaril)

6. A 72-year-old woman complains to her physician that she has been seeing "little people" walking around her house over the past few days; moreover, she saw one while waiting in the doctor's office. Examination proves her to be alert and oriented. What term best describes this phenomenon?

(A) illusion
(B) hallucination
(C) flashback
(D) formication
(E) hallucinosis

7. A 25-year-old patient presents to her primary care doctor complaining of a sudden onset of intense fear and a feeling that she was going to die while stuck in traffic earlier in the week. She was short of breath, diaphoretic, and tremulous, and she could feel her heart pounding. Her initial impulse was to drive to an emergency department, but her distress subsided on its own in about 20 minutes. An appropriate course of action for the primary care doctor is which of the following?

(A) Prescribe a short-acting benzodiazepine for the next such episode.

(B) Refer the patient to a psychiatrist.

(C) Reassure the patient that her symptoms are most likely benign and not a cause for concern.

(D) Prescribe a selective serotonin reuptake inhibitor (SSRI) and ask to see the patient back in 1 week.

(E) Conduct a thorough medical screening for heart and lung disease.

[handwritten left margin: primary care doctor should do a thorough medical screen of heart and lungs; But psychiatrist should do choice "C"]

8. You are seeing a 45-year-old man with an unknown psychiatric history. On Mental Status Examination (MSE), he speaks coherently and articulately, but makes no sense because many of the words he uses are of his own invention. This patient demonstrates which of the following?

(A) word salad

(B) negative symptoms

(C) dysarthria

(D) neologisms

(E) clang associations

9. A 34-year-old woman is diagnosed with dysthymic disorder. Which of the following statements regarding this patient is likely true?

(A) She has had a feeling of depression, for most of the day, for at least the past 6 months.

(B) At some point in her illness, she may have experienced mood-congruent delusions.

(C) Her presenting complaint was suicidality.

(D) She has a comorbid diagnosis of alcohol dependence.

(E) Her presenting complaint was of poor appetite, insomnia, fatigue, poor concentration, and a feeling of hopelessness.

10. A man brings his wife to the doctor because she believes that her husband is actually an imposter who looks exactly like her husband. The term for this delusion is which of the following?

(A) koro

(B) amok

(C) Capgras syndrome

(D) pseudocyesis

(E) couvade syndrome

11. A 49-year-old woman with diabetes presents to her primary care physician. She says that as a result of divorcing her husband 1 month ago, she has been sleepless, agitated, and depressed. In her twenties, she drank alcohol abusively but she has not had any alcoholic drinks in many years. In terms of the classification of psychiatric disease within the *Diagnostic and Statistical Manual of Mental Disorders, Fourth Edition, Text Revision* (DSM-IV-TR) multiaxis system, which of the following statements is true?

(A) Her Axis II diagnosis is adjustment disorder.

(B) Alcohol abuse, in remission, should be placed on Axis I.

(C) Diabetes should be included on Axis IV.

(D) Recent divorce should be included on Axis V.

(E) Her Global Assessment of Functioning (GAF) should be included on Axis III.

Questions 12 and 13

You are asked to evaluate a 12-year-old boy who has a history of Tourette disorder and complex vocal and motor tics. On evaluation, you note the patient intermittently making obscene gestures and repeating your phrases.

12. In your report, you should describe the motor tics as which of the following?

    (A) blepharospasm
    (B) bruxism
    (C) copropraxia
    (D) echopraxia ✓
    (E) torticollis

13. When noting the vocal tics that were observed, which of the following is the term best used?

    (A) coprolalia
    (B) echolalia
    (C) palilalia
    (D) parapraxis ✓
    (E) dysarthria

Questions 14 and 15

A wealthy middle-aged woman presents to you after being arrested for shoplifting. The patient says she has been stealing for years, although she would have no difficulty affording the objects stolen. She states that she steals "on the spur of the moment" and that these impulses seem foreign and distressing.

14. What is this form of impulse control disorder is called?

    (A) pyromania
    (B) trichotillomania
    (C) intermittent explosive disorder ✓
    (D) kleptomania
    (E) pathologic gambling

15. The fact that these impulses are distressing to her indicate that they are which of the following?

    (A) ego-syntonic
    (B) ego-dystonic ✓
    (C) mood congruent
    (D) mood incongruent
    (E) delusional

16. A 49-year-old man comes to you complaining of headaches, memory loss, disorientation, and occasional paralysis that affects his arms and lasts several hours. During the MSE, you notice that the patient is giving approximate answers to many questions (e.g., there are six toes on the foot and 2 + 2 = 5). You also notice that the patient is talking past the point. Feeling that this is a dissociative-type disorder, which of the following could you label it?

    (A) amok
    (B) Ganser syndrome
    (C) piblokto
    (D) malingering
    (E) fugue state

Questions 17 and 18

A 19-year-old woman presents with complaints of fear, apprehension, and trembling without predisposing situations noted. On examination, you note brown skin, smoky brown rings on the outer cornea, and occasional rapid, seemingly purposeless movements. After completing your workup, your diagnosis is Wilson disease.

17. In preparing your report, the ocular findings are best termed which of the following?

    (A) Kayser-Fleischer rings
    (B) arcus senilis
    (C) xanthelasma ✓
    (D) Brushfield spots
    (E) subconjunctival hemorrhage

18. Which of the following is the best term for rapid, jerky movements that worsen with voluntary movement?

    (A) chorciform
    (B) athetoid
    (C) hemiballismus ✓
    (D) myoclonus
    (E) myotonia

Questions 19 and 20

A 21-year-old woman is brought to the psychiatric emergency department after calling the police to turn herself in. She claims that she was responsible for the loss of her neighbor's pregnancy. She believes her negative thoughts toward the woman caused her miscarriage. On further questioning, she tells you that she felt threatened by her neighbor because she believed her thoughts could be heard through the walls. She feels that this is an invasion of her privacy.

19. The delusion that the patient's thoughts toward the neighbor were the responsible factors for the lost pregnancy is best termed which of the following?

    (A) magical thinking
    (B) ideas of reference
    (C) displacement
    (D) projection
    (E) reaction formation

20. Which of the following is the best term for the patient's fear that her thoughts could be overheard?

    (A) thought broadcasting
    (B) thought insertion
    (C) thought control
    (D) transference
    (E) echolalia

Questions 21 and 22

A 25-year-old man who is hospitalized for bipolar disorder tells you that he has his doctorates in six fields and currently is the richest person in the world. He states that he speaks 28 languages, one of which is an angelic language. He tells you that he is concerned, however, because a well-known supermodel is infatuated with him and she will not leave him alone. He wishes to leave the hospital to spend some time with her.

21. Which of the following is the best term for the patient's belief that a famous supermodel is in love with him?

    (A) erotomania
    (B) satyriasis

    (C) nymphomania
    (D) thought broadcasting
    (E) alexia

22. The patient's incorrect perception of his wealth and education is most likely a form of which of the following?

    (A) micropsia
    (B) macropsia
    (C) palinopsia
    (D) delusion of grandeur
    (E) delusion of infidelity

Questions 23 and 24

A devout husband finds that his wife is having an affair with his best friend. One week later, he finds that he cannot walk. A thorough neurologic workup fails to reveal a cause to his sudden paraplegia. His neurologic examination is not consistent with upper or lower motor neuron findings. Despite this dramatic disability, he seems quite unaffected by it emotionally.

23. Which of the following is the best label for the sudden neurologic symptom without evidence of etiology?

    (A) projection
    (B) conversion
    (C) sublimation
    (D) dissociation
    (E) rationalization

24. This patient's disregard for the severity of his symptoms is called which of the following?

    (A) déjà entendu
    (B) jamais vu
    (C) déjà vu
    (D) la belle indifférence
    (E) folie à deux

25. A 67-year-old woman with pulmonary carcinoma and secondary brain metastases recently drafted a will in the presence of her family attorney. She has a history of major depressive disorder (MDD) that is now in remission. She decides that her children who are well-established in their careers do not need any

inheritance and that her estate would best serve charity. To secure the validity of the will, the patient asks her psychiatrist to submit a letter to her attorney regarding her competency. Which of the following is most important in determining a person's testamentary capacity?

(A) knowledge of natural heirs to the estate
(B) the presence of a conservator of person
(C) history of mental illness
(D) actus reus
(E) presence of a judge to witness the signing of the will

26. Which of the following is an exception to informed consent?

(A) nonemergent situations
(B) patient waiver of informed consent
(C) inability to read or write
(D) presence of a language barrier
(E) a living will

27. A deputy sheriff serves you a subpoena for the records of one of your patients who is the defendant in a civil liability lawsuit. Which of the following is the most appropriate course of action?

(A) Release the patient's records to the plaintiff because the subpoena overrides patient consent.
(B) Hand over only the information that is relevant to the case.
(C) Contact the patient and ask if she or he would like the information released.
(D) Release the patient's records directly to the court.
(E) Refuse to tell the sheriff if you are the patient's physician to maintain confidentiality.

28. A 23-year-old graduate student you have been seeing in long-term psychotherapy has stopped paying his bills despite being reimbursed by

his insurance company. Which of the following is the next appropriate course of action?

(A) Notify a collection agency to obtain reimbursement.
(B) Contact the patient's insurance company and demand that they issue you another payment.
(C) Inquire with family members whether the patient has financial problems.
(D) Directly address this issue with the patient at the next scheduled appointment.
(E) Send the patient a letter of termination and instruct him to no longer call your office.

Questions 29 and 30

You are asked to perform a "competency to stand trial" evaluation of an 18-year-old man who was arrested for violently assaulting his girlfriend. The patient has no past psychiatric history, and friends report that he has never demonstrated any violent tendencies. The patient reports that his relationship with his girlfriend "went downhill" shortly after they graduated from high school and his girlfriend stopped calling him. On MSE, his affect is constricted and his mood is reported as "crazy." Thought processes are goal-directed, and he denies any hallucinations or delusions. The patient is unable to correctly perform simple calculations. Each time he is asked to multiply, subtract, or add a pair of numbers, his answers are wrong by one or two digits. For example, he responds "22" when asked to multiply 7 by 3.

29. Intentionally feigning symptoms to avoid prosecution is consistent with which of the following disorders?

(A) factitious disorder
(B) malingering
(C) factitious disorder
(D) conversion disorder
(E) Munchausen by proxy

30. Which of the following statements best distinguishes malingering from conversion disorder?

(A) Malingerers seek primary gain incentives, whereas individuals with conversion disorder seek secondary gain incentives.

(B) Malingerers are usually friendly and cooperative, whereas individuals with conversion disorder are uncooperative.

(C) Malingering and conversion disorder can be distinguished based on the absence of an underlying neurologic problem.

(D) Malingering represents an unconscious process, whereas conversion disorder results from conscious feigning of symptoms.

(E) Malingerers avoid evaluation and treatment, whereas patients with conversion disorder are usually eager for evaluation and treatment.

31. A 7-year-old girl is brought to the emergency department for evaluation of a sore throat and fever. Her parents took her to the pediatrician's office about 1 week ago and he recommended fluids and bed rest. Within the last 2 days, the patient developed dysphagia and severe abdominal pain. History from the parents indicates the patient has been anxious and impulsive over the last month. There has also been a marked decline in school performance, and she has not been interested in playing with her friends. Physical examination is remarkable for significant erythema over the posterior pharynx with gray exudate. There are abrasions in the region of the patient's labia. Complete blood count shows a white blood cell (WBC) count of 14,000/μL with a left shift. Which of the following is the next appropriate step?

(A) Detain the parents while you notify the police.

(B) Arrange for a family meeting to determine a safe disposition.

(C) Refer the patient to the family's pediatrician.

(D) Notify the probate court to have the patient legally removed from the alleged perpetrator.

(E) Contact the state's Child Protective Services while keeping the patient safe.

Questions 32 and 33

A 48-year-old male is brought into the emergency room (ER) via an ambulance. He smells of alcohol, is covered in vomit, and not responsive to questions. He is unsteady and uncooperative with the physical examination, but he is noted to have disconjugate eye movements.

32. Which of the following would be the most appropriate next step in the management of this patient?

(A) Administer thiamine intramuscularly (IM) before IV fluids and glucose.

(B) Administer thiamine intravenously (IV) before IV fluids and glucose.

(C) Administer thiamine IV after IV fluids and glucose.

(D) Administer naloxone IV before IV fluids and glucose.

(E) Administer naloxone IV after IV fluids and glucose.

33. The above patient is stabilized and admitted to the ICU. After 3 days, he begins to become confused again, with visual hallucinations, tremors, diaphoresis, and elevated blood pressure and pulse. Which of the following is the most appropriate treatment for this patient?

(A) Administer a barbiturate.
(B) Administer a benzodiazepine.
(C) Administer additional thiamine.
(D) Administer an antipsychotic.
(E) Administer hydralazine.

34. A young White male, age unknown, is brought into the emergency room unresponsive to questioning. His vitals demonstrate a normal temperature, a low pulse and blood pressure, and decreased respirations. He appears pale with

pupils that are constricted and minimally responsive. Administration of which of the following would be most likely to improve his condition?

- (A) antabuse
- (B) benzodiazepines
- (C) flumazenil
- (D) naloxone
- (E) thiamine

35. A 77-year-old woman without prior psychiatric history is brought into her family physician's office with her husband. He is concerned that she is "depressed" and needs treatment. He describes her withdrawing emotionally over the past year or two, with a gradual decline in her ability to care for herself. They have been unable to take part in their usual social activities, and the patient "just wanders around the house during the day." He has also noticed that she is forgetful, often misplacing items, and mixing up names of acquaintances. When asked, the patient denies any difficulties, stating she feels "fine," and that her husband worries too much. She adamantly refutes problems with her memory, instead blaming him for "moving things around in our house." She has no significant medical problems. Upon MSE, she is pleasant and cooperative with questions, although defensive at times. Her affect is neutral but full. There is no suicidal or homicidal ideation, and she denies any psychotic symptoms. Her Mini-Mental State Examination is 20/30. Her physical is essentially unremarkable. Which of the following is the most appropriate primary treatment for this patient?

- (A) citalopram
- (B) galantamine
- (C) ginkgo biloba
- (D) memantine
- (E) ziprasidone

Questions 36 and 37

You are asked to see a 37-year-old woman with end-stage ovarian cancer because she has told her oncologist that she wants to die. When you approach the patient's bed, you see a cachectic but smiling woman surrounded by her husband and two young daughters. She has a history of depression but is not under any treatment for it now. "I am ready to go, Doctor," she says to you. Her oncologist has told you that he would like to try a new chemotherapy for which the patient is a good candidate but the patient has refused.

36. Which of the following statements is most accurate regarding suicide statistics?

- (A) Suicide is the second leading cause of death among individuals aged 15–24.
- (B) Suicide is common in children under the age of 13.
- (C) Women are more likely to commit suicide than men.
- (D) Men are more likely to attempt suicide than women.
- (E) Risk of suicide decreases with increasing age.

37. According to the American Medical Association's (AMA) Code of Medical Ethics, physician-assisted suicide is which of the following?

- (A) justifiable if a patient's suffering becomes intolerable despite adequate pain control
- (B) unethical
- (C) defined as euthanasia
- (D) a matter on which the AMA has no official position
- (E) not an ethical issue and must be left to state legislatures

38. A 16-year-old girl is brought to your office by her parents to get a pregnancy test. She consents for the evaluation but requests that you keep the results confidential. Beta-human chorionic gonadotropin is positive. The patient's parents demand to know the results. Which of the following should you do?

(A) Notify the parents of the results because they pay her medical bills.

(B) Encourage the patient to discuss the results with her parents.

(C) Report the results to Child Protective Services.

(D) Invoke testimonial privilege.

(E) Disclose the results in a meeting with the patient and her parents.

Questions 39 and 40

After you ask her how many siblings she has, a patient launches into a long discussion first on her sister Sally, then one of Sally's old boyfriends, Mark, who is now an accountant, she says, which in turn leads her to a monologue on accountants and bankers, whom she says are all "in cahoots with the IRS and CIA—you can't trust 'em!" You note that she never comes back to answering the question fully until you prompt her to. She further tells you that she believes "the government has experimentally planted alien eggs in my ovaries, you know. I know they've told you. They think I don't know."

39. Which of the following is an example of the above patient's thought processes when asked about her siblings?

(A) trichotillomania
(B) flight of ideas
(C) tangentiality
(D) circumstantiality
(E) isolation of affect

40. Delusions as in the above patient's case are an example of

(A) a perceptual disturbance
(B) a disturbance in thought content
(C) disorganized thought processes

(D) a cognitive deficit
(E) impaired judgment

Questions 41 and 42

41. A 35-year-old woman presents to your office with a referral from a psychologist for psychiatric treatment. She has been suffering "the blues" for several months including crying spells and insomnia. She is convinced that her fiancé is about to break up with her because she has been eating more than usual. Sometimes, however, she feels "just fine." The treatment of choice for this patient is which of the following?

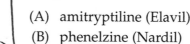

(A) amitryptiline (Elavil)
(B) phenelzine (Nardil)
(C) fluoxetine (Prozac)
(D) divalproex sodium (Depakote)
(E) fluoxetine and ziprasidone (Geodon)

42. The patient responds well to treatment and after several months returns to your office for a follow-up visit. She tells you she has just been married and would like to become pregnant. She and her husband have been having unprotected sex for a month. You proceed to do which of the following?

(A) Tell her to stop her medication immediately.
(B) Ask how important pregnancy is to her.
(C) Refer her for electroconvulsive therapy (ECT).
(D) Discuss the risks and benefits of continuing her treatment during pregnancy.
(E) Add another antidepressant to prevent postpartum depression.

43. A 45-year-old man is brought to the psychiatric emergency room by police after being found screaming and cutting down a tree in the town square. He tells you that the ghost of his wife, who died 3 months ago, is living in the tree. The man has no previous psychiatric history, but reports being "very depressed" since the death of his wife and having considered suicide. He is disheveled and appears to have ignored his personal hygiene for some

time. His vital signs are normal. Which of the following do you decide to do?

(A) Prescribe an antipsychotic.
(B) Prescribe an antidepressant.
(C) Prescribe an antipsychotic and an anti-depressant.
(D) Obtain a urine toxicology screen.
(E) Ask him the **CAGE** questions to rule out alcoholism.

Questions 44 and 45

44. You are seeing a 56-year-old man with a history of alcoholism. He complains about not being able to sleep and requests a sleeping aid. He has no other signs of depression and reports that "everything is going well." You decide to give him which of the following?

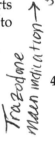

(A) trazodone (Desyrel)
(B) alprazolam (Xanax)
(C) diazepam (Valium)
(D) zolpidem (Ambien)
(E) zalpelon (Sonata)

45. The side effect of this medication that you warn him about is which of the following?

(A) impotence
(B) retrograde ejaculation
(C) priapism
(D) incontinence
(E) anorgasmia

Questions 46 and 47

46. You are seeing a 9-year-old boy with a history of depression and suicidal ideation. He has been taking fluoxetine (Prozac) for 6 months and has had a good response. His mother asks to see

you after his appointment and tells you that she is concerned about news reports saying that SSRIs increase the risk of suicide in children. She asks you to consider stopping the medication. Which of the following is the best course of action?

(A) Stop the fluoxetine immediately as the patient is a minor and it is his mother's wish.
(B) Switch to paroxetine (Paxil) because it does not increase suicide risk.
(C) Ask the mother, "What's really bothering you about your son being on antide-pressants?"
(D) Switch to amitryptiline (Elavil).
(E) Discuss the risks and benefits of fluoxe-tine and other SSRIs in the pediatric population.

47. A month later, the boy and his mother return to your office. She informs you that after her son's last appointment, she has been giving him St. John's wort because she believes he needs a "natural remedy." Which of the following should you do?

(A) Tell the mother to stop the St. John's wort immediately.
(B) Tell the mother there is no evidence that St. John's wort is an effective treatment for depression.
(C) Tell the mother to watch out for side effects including photosensitivity and dizziness.
(D) Refer the case to social services for child abuse.
(E) Increase the dose of his antidepressant as St. John's wort will lower blood con-centrations of the antidepressant.

Question 48

A 60-year-old patient has suffered from bipolar illness for decades, developing along the way severe reactions to each of the mood stabilizers you have tried him on. He is currently in the midst of a severe manic episode. His family is "at wit's end," according to a daughter. You suggest ECT to which the patient agrees. His daughter, however, says she has heard of "depressed and psychotic people who had it done to them, with little or no benefit. And it seems so barbaric."

48. You respond by saying your advice is to still consider ECT. Which of the following describes the factor you base this on?

   (A) Bipolar illness, especially in a manic episode, has an extremely high rate of response to ECT, perhaps higher than either of the other two disorders the daughter mentioned.
   (B) ECT is proven to be safer in bipolar illness than in any other of the disorders for which ECT is used.
   (C) ECT is proven to have more lasting results in bipolar disorder than in the other two.
   (D) Bipolar illness is shown to respond best in late life to ECT.
   (E) ECT is shown to have more lasting effects than medications.

49. Treating bipolar illness is believed to do which of the following?

   (A) have no change on the likelihood of further episodes
   (B) have no effect on future episodes
   (C) decrease the likelihood of further episodes as well as the severity of them
   (D) increase the patient's response to medications or ECT in the future
   (E) decrease the patient's response to medications or ECT in the future

Questions 50 and 51

A 60-year-old widow is brought to your clinic by her daughter, who reports that her mother said to her this afternoon that she "wanted to end it all." She reports thoughts of overdosing on her pills, which she has stockpiled. This woman has no prior history of suicide attempts but has had thoughts of suicide on multiple prior occasions over the course of her near-lifelong history of depression. She lost her husband to a sudden heart attack 1 year ago, but her daughter says that she still has many very supportive friends whom she spends significant amounts of time with. She still carries on her avid hobby of gardening, although "at a slower pace" because of her worsening arthritis. She expresses worries over a recent "big drop" in the value of retirement stocks she has.

50. Which of the following is the most significant factor mitigating her risk for suicide?

   (A) her social supports
   (B) her gardening hobby
   (C) her race
   (D) her slower movements secondary to arthritis
   (E) the fact that she has not attempted suicide before, despite her long history of depression

51. Important medical causes of depression to rule out in this and any depressed patient include which of the following?

   (A) vitamin B_{12} and tryptophan deficiency
   (B) thyroid illness and malignancy
   (C) adrenal illness and basement membrane disorders
   (D) vascular disease and phospholipid metabolism disorders
   (E) infectious illness and lipid disorders

Questions 52 and 53

A 20-year-old college sophomore is brought to the emergency department after being found passed out in her bathroom. She had been vomiting, which she admits now was self-induced. History is significant for a breakup 4 months ago with her boyfriend of 2 years. Her weight is in the 82nd percentile for her height. She is amenorrheic. There is no history of binge eating.

52. Which of the following do you most expect her examination to show?

    (A) dental decay
    (B) pitting fingernails
    (C) pectus excavatum
    (D) palpable spleen
    (E) café au lait spots

53. Additional social history would be most likely to reveal that she is which of the following?

    (A) a gymnast
    (B) a victim of rape
    (C) an identical twin
    (D) a genius
    (E) carefree

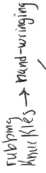

personality D/O → Borderline PD

54. A 14-month-old girl presents with her parents who report that she has become less responsive to them and less interactive with her 6-year-old brother. In addition, her gait has become clumsy, and most recently, she has been noted to habitually rub her knuckles together. The parents also bring the chart from their daughter's pediatrician with a note indicating that although her head circumference was normally sized at birth, it has now fallen into the 10th percentile for her age. The girl most closely fulfills criteria for which of the following?

    (A) autistic disorder
    (B) childhood disintegrative disorder
    (C) Rett syndrome
    (D) Asperger syndrome
    (E) childhood-onset schizophrenia

rubbing knuckles → hand-wringing

55. A 24-year-old man with a history of schizophrenia presents to the emergency department. He had previously taken haloperidol (Haldol), but now refuses to take it. Because the patient did not take the haloperidol, you decide to try fluphenazine (Prolixin), which seems to mitigate his symptoms. One week later, he leaves the hospital. He continues the medications you prescribed and on a follow-up visit you notice he moves slowly and has a festinating gait. The receptor most likely to account for the above side effect is which of the following?

    (A) nigrostriatal D$_2$ receptors
    (B) mesolimbic D$_2$ receptors
    (C) basal ganglia acetylcholine receptors
    (D) D$_4$ receptors
    (E) 5-hydroxytryptamine-2 (5-HT$_2$)

56. A 16-year-old boy began having repetitive eye blinking at the age of 6. By age 12, he began blurting stereotyped phrases such as "Balls!" and "Shitty!" as well as making kissing noises. Concomitant with this, he had increasing difficulty with paying attention in school and occasionally displayed wild, disinhibited behavior. Which of the following is the treatment of choice for the primary condition evident in this case?

    (A) pimozide (Orap)
    (B) methylphenidate (Ritalin)
    (C) fluoxetine (Prozac)
    (D) topiramate (Topamax)
    (E) clonidine (Catapres)

57. A 12-year-old boy has recently been arrested for setting fire to a neighbor's barn. He has been in trouble before for playing with fireworks in the neighborhood, and when he was 10 years old he was suspended for lighting matches at his school. Which is the most frequently diagnosed DSM-IV-TR diagnosis associated with fire setting in children?

    (A) a pervasive developmental disorder
    (B) mental retardation
    (C) conduct disorder
    (D) a tic disorder
    (E) destructive personality disorder of childhood

Questions 58 and 59

A 9-year-old boy with a history of normal developmental milestones has been wetting his bed for the last 6 months. His parents report that the bed-wetting initially occurred sporadically, but for the last 2 months it has been happening about every other night.

58. Which of the following is the most accurate description of this boy's problem?

    (A) primary diurnal enuresis
    (B) primary nocturnal enuresis
    (C) secondary diurnal enuresis
    (D) secondary nocturnal enuresis
    (E) primary diurnal encopresis

59. Once medical causes have been ruled out, which of the following is the pharmacologic treatment of choice for this condition?

    (A) clonidine
    (B) haloperidol (Haldol)
    (C) carbamazepine (Tegretol)
    (D) diphenhydramine (Benadryl)
    (E) imipramine (Tofranil)

Questions 60 and 61

An 11-year-old boy was adopted at age 6 months. His biological mother suffered from severe alcohol dependence. He has been in a special education school due to his global learning difficulties and his intelligence quotient (IQ) has recently been measured at 60.

60. According to his IQ measurement, the patient would be diagnosed as having which of the following?

    (A) borderline intellectual functioning
    (B) mild mental retardation
    (C) moderate mental retardation
    (D) severe mental retardation
    (E) mental retardation, severity unspecified

61. Given the history of prenatal alcohol exposure in this patient, which of the following might you expect?

    (A) microcephaly
    (B) cleft palate
    (C) chromosome 13 translocation
    (D) congenital blindness
    (E) prominent jaw

62. A 5-year-old girl has come under the care of state Child Protection Services. Her mother was known to be using crack cocaine and IV heroin, and supporting her habit with prostitution. The girl's temporary foster parents reported to state workers that she was indiscriminately social with adults and unusually clingy. In her social interactions with other 5-year-old children at her preschool, she was described as being inappropriately aggressive with them. This case most closely illustrates a diagnosis of which of the following?

    (A) mixed receptive-expressive language disorder
    (B) reactive attachment disorder of infancy and early childhood
    (C) childhood disintegrative disorder
    (D) attention deficit hyperactivity disorder (ADHD)
    (E) conduct disorder

Questions 63 and 64

A 12-year-old girl has recently come under psychiatric care for her depression and treatment of alcohol abuse. During the course of her evaluation, she revealed that she had a 3-year-long sexual relationship with her stepfather beginning when she was 8 years old.

63. Which of the following generalizations related to this case is most accurate?

(A) Sexual activity between daughter and father (or stepfather) is the most common form of incest.

(B) The patient is at decreased risk of future sexual abuse or rape due to her heightened defense mechanisms around sexual issues.

(C) The patient has increased risk of developing borderline personality disorder.

(D) The patient has increased risk of developing schizophrenia after adolescence.

(E) The patient's history of alcohol abuse makes her a less reliable historian and her story about the sexual abuse less likely to be true.

64. The patient's stepfather has a decreased likelihood, compared to the general population, of having which of the following?

(A) other paraphilias

(B) alcohol dependence

(C) a history of violence

(D) a sexually gratifying relationship with spouse

(E) a personal history of childhood sexual abuse

65. A 27-year-old law student presents to you as a referral for treatment of depression diagnosed by his primary care physician. On MSE, you find that the patient's speech is pressured and that he quickly jumps from one topic to another. He says that his mood has improved greatly since he last saw his primary care doctor: "In fact, I'm on top of the world." The patient relates that now he does not get much sleep. He reports 3–4 hours a night for the last week, "not that I need that much sleep anyway." The most appropriate single pharmacotherapy strategy for this patient would be which of the following?

(A) lorazepam (Ativan)

(B) imipramine

(C) fluoxetine

(D) divalproex sodium (Depakote)

(E) citalopram (Celexa)

Questions 66 and 67

A 36-year-old woman presents with depressed mood, a sense of hopelessness, and thoughts of suicide for the last month. She also reports increased appetite. She also has been sleeping up to 16 hours a day. On MSE, her mood is sad most of the time, but she laughs in response to humorous statements. The patient did say that last week her mood brightened a bit when she won $150 from playing the lottery.

66. Additional history that would suggest a diagnosis of an atypical major depression versus a melancholic depression would be which of the following?

(A) severe concentration difficulty and cognitive impairment

(B) a normal dexamethasone suppression test

(C) rejection hypersensitivity

(D) the presence of psychotic symptoms

(E) a history of manic symptoms after anti-depressant treatment

67. Which of the following is a psychiatric drug class specifically associated with good treatment response for atypical major depression as in this case?

(A) anticonvulsants

(B) monoamine oxidase inhibitors (MAOIs)

(C) SSRIs

(D) tricyclic antidepressants (TCAs)

(E) typical neuroleptics

Questions 68 and 69

You have been treating a 34-year-old man for depression with an SSRI for the last 2 months. He had been on fluoxetine 20 mg/day for the first month, and then you raised the dose to 40 mg by mouth (PO) qd for the last month. His depressive symptoms have remained refractory despite the increase in dosage. You have decided to change the medication to phenelzine (Nardil), an MAOI, in hopes of eliciting a better antidepressant response.

68. In making the transition from the SSRI to the MAOI, which of the following is the best strategy?

    (A) Begin tapering down the dose of the SSRI and start tapering up on the dose of the MAOI simultaneously.
    (B) Stop the SSRI abruptly and immediately begin tapering up on the MAOI.
    (C) Taper off SSRI and then 5 weeks after the last dose begin tapering up on the MAOI.
    (D) Stop the SSRI abruptly and begin with the MAOI at an equipotent dose the next day.
    (E) Start the MAOI until therapeutic levels have been reached, then taper off the SSRI.

69. With regard to taking the MAOI, which of the following is very important that the patient be aware of?

    (A) may experience stiffness and tremor
    (B) should take the medications with bland food
    (C) should avoid foods rich in tryptophan
    (D) should avoid foods rich in tyramine
    (E) may feel overly sedated

70. A 42-year-old accountant presents for long-term psychotherapy treatment. In the first session, you find that he has been divorced three times. The poor quality of his romantic and other relationships are the focus of his concerns. Over the course of months, you find out that he is a perfectionist and inflexible within relationships. He typically idealizes his partner, then devalues her, before ending the relationship suddenly. At times, he loses "a sense of self" in relationships, not knowing who he is or what he wants. During this time he relies on others to advise him on what he should do. However, if he takes this advice and his plans fail, he uses this to devalue his advising friend. The patient makes it very clear that he sought your treatment as a psychotherapist "because I'll only accept the best in the city." The patient also reports to you that he has some unique abilities of perception that allow him to detect what or who will provide the best possible outcome for him. For example, he picked you as a therapist not only because of your reputation, but also because of your office phone number, which has digits in ascending value order. Which of the following is the most appropriate Axis II DSM-IV-TR diagnosis for this patient?

    (A) borderline personality disorder
    (B) narcissistic personality disorder
    (C) obsessive personality disorder
    (D) personality disorder not otherwise specified
    (E) schizotypal personality disorder

71. A 43-year-old woman is hospitalized during a psychotic episode in which she had the delusion that she was being shot with invisible laser beams from satellites in Earth orbit. According to her family, she had stopped taking her regimen of haloperidol and lithium 4 weeks prior to her admission to the hospital, and she had been telling her family about her concerns regarding the laser beams for the last 2 weeks. Her MSE on presentation to the hospital revealed primarily thought disorder and delusional symptoms without a prominent mood component. The patient's past psychiatric history is significant for three prior hospitalizations over the last 20 years. At the time of her first admission, she presented with a 3-week history of manic symptoms and psychosis. During her second hospitalization, she was suicidal and noted to be depressed with psychotic symptoms. During her third admission, she was again depressed with prominently disorganized

behavior. Which of the following is the most appropriate diagnosis for this patient?

(A) bipolar disorder
(B) MDD
(C) psychotic disorder not otherwise specified
(D) schizoaffective disorder
(E) schizophrenia

Questions 72 and 73

The medical team on an inpatient service calls you to help them with a 72-year-old female patient. They report that at night she becomes confused, thinking that she is in a hotel. She makes demands of the nursing staff that they feel are unreasonable, and she has become disruptive of their other work. She has the most trouble from 10 PM until about 2 AM, when she usually falls asleep. In the morning, she is much better oriented and cooperative. A review of her medications reveals that she is taking cimetidine 400 mg PO bid, furosemide 40 mg PO qd, atenolol 50 mg PO qd, digoxin 0.125 mg PO qd, and diphenhydramine 50 mg PO qhs and 25 mg PO qhs (second dose 3 hours post first dose for insomnia).

72. Which of the following medications most likely to cause this patient's nighttime confusion?

(A) atenolol
(B) cimetidine
(C) digoxin
(D) diphenhydramine
(E) furosemide

73. The neurotransmitter system most directly implicated in the etiology of this medication-induced confusion is which of the following?

(A) acetylcholine
(B) dopamine
(C) gamma-aminobutyric acid (GABA)
(D) serotonin
(E) norepinephrine

74. A clinical research psychiatrist at university A has been running a double-blind placebo-controlled trial of a new antidepressant. The psychiatrist concludes after a statistical analysis of the data that there is no better effect of the drug compared to placebo. The psychiatrist's colleagues at five separate institutions (universities B, C, D, E, and F) have run identical studies and determine that there is a treatment effect of the drug compared to placebo. Given this information, one may conclude that the research trial at university A resulted in which of the following?

(A) high variance
(B) low predictive value
(C) standard error
(D) type I error
(E) type II error

Questions 75 and 76

A 56-year-old man with a long history of paranoid schizophrenia has been taking his chlorpromazine regularly for 27 years. About 5 years ago, he developed writhing movements of his wrists and fingers that disappear when he goes to sleep.

75. Which of the following extrapyramidal syndromes is most consistent with this case?

(A) akathisia
(B) dystonia
(C) neuroleptic malignant syndrome (NMS)
(D) parkinsonism
(E) tardive dyskinesia

76. The anatomic structure in the brain most likely implicated in the etiology of this movement disorder is which of the following?

(A) basal ganglia
(B) cerebellum
(C) frontal cortex
(D) midbrain
(E) motor cortex

77. You are seeing a 55-year-old Vietnam veteran at a Veteran's Administration hospital. He has been hospitalized numerous times previously for drug abuse and psychotic symptoms. During this admission, he complains of not being able to sleep for more than an hour at a time because he feels he is under attack, and fears that someone is going to jump out of the bushes at his apartment complex and "ambush" him. He knows intellectually that this will not happen, but he cannot stop the thoughts. A poor prognostic indicator for a diagnosis of posttraumatic stress disorder (PTSD) is which of the following?

    (A) existence of premorbid personality disorder
    (B) exposure to trauma in middle adulthood
    (C) rapid onset of symptoms
    (D) short duration of symptoms
    (E) strong social supports

78. A 29-year-old man presents to your outpatient psychiatric clinic complaining of anxiety and depression. His social history reveals that he is a junior faculty member of a local university, working about 90 hours per week. He reports stress arising from his marital relationship that is exacerbated by his occupational demands. You identify a central conflict in this patient of issues of intimacy versus isolation borrowing from the theoretical work of which of the following?

    (A) Carl Jung
    (B) Karen Horney
    (C) Erik Erikson
    (D) Jean Piaget
    (E) Sigmund Freud

Questions 79 and 80

A 46-year-old man with a history of complex partial epilepsy is referred to your psychiatric clinic by his neurologist for onset of delusional thinking.

79. You may inform the patient's family that the prevalence of psychotic episodes in patients with complex partial epilepsy is closest to which of the following percetages?

    (A) 1%
    (B) 5%
    (C) 10%
    (D) 20%
    (E) 50%

80. An investigation into the history of this patient's personality traits may reveal classic signs of complex partial epilepsy-associated personality including increased or decreased sexuality, hypergraphia, heightened experience of emotions, and which of the following?

    (A) depression
    (B) hyperreligiosity
    (C) urinary incontinence
    (D) obsessive-compulsive behaviors
    (E) sleep disorders

81. After being called to the emergency department to evaluate a young woman who overdosed on barbiturates, you find her in bed with her eyes closed. She opens her eyes briefly in response to pain and demonstrates flexion from pain but makes no sounds. Which of the following numbers represents her Glasgow Coma Scale score?

    (A) 7
    (B) 6
    (C) 5
    (D) 4
    (E) 3

82. A 46-year-old man with a history of schizophrenia had been maintained on thioridazine (Mellaril) 700 mg qd since he was diagnosed at the age of 20. Over the last 8 months, he has been complaining of hearing derogatory voices, and his dose has been increased to 800 mg qd. He has no signs of tardive dyskinesia. What is the most harmful side effect associated with 1000 mg or more of thioridazine?

(A) constipation

(B) dry eyes

(C) urinary retention

(D) pigmentary retinopathy

(E) nephrogenic diabetes insipidus

83. A 24-year-old man is admitted to the psychiatric ward with new-onset command suicidal auditory hallucinations. He is given haloperidol 10 mg IM. Fifteen hours later, he develops torticollis. What is the best treatment for this occurrence?

(A) acetaminophen

(B) labetalol (Normodyne)

(C) benztropine

(D) a lower-potency neuroleptic

(E) penicillamine

Torticollis → Neck spasmas dystonia

84. A 28-year-old woman with a history of bipolar disorder is admitted to the medical service because of weakness, mental status changes, and a serum sodium of 154 mmol/L. Over the last 2 weeks, she has had polyuria, excessive thirst, and polydipsia. What drug is most likely associated with this medical condition?

(A) lithium carbonate

(B) haloperidol

(C) diazepam (Valium)

(D) valproic acid

(E) buspirone (BuSpar)

Questions 85 and 86

A 47-year-old man who is addicted to heroin has been admitted to the inpatient psychiatric ward for detoxification.

85. What is the most effective treatment of autonomic dysregulation during detoxification?

(A) haloperidol

(B) thioridazine

(C) amantadine (Symmetrel)

(D) clonidine

(E) pimozide

86. If the patient did not want detoxification but did want to stop using heroin, which of the following medications would be most appropriate for maintenance?

(A) lorazepam

(B) alprazolam (Xanax)

(C) methadone

(D) sertraline (Zoloft)

(E) lithium

Questions 87 and 88

A 75-year-old man with Alzheimer disease presents to your clinic complaining of depression. He has a past medical history including diabetes mellitus, two myocardial infarctions, atrial fibrillation, and one coronary artery bypass graft.

87. Assuming this patient is suffering from depression, which antidepressant class would you most want to avoid?

(A) SSRIs

(B) TCAs

(C) butyrophenones

(D) dibenzodiazepines

(E) benzodiazepines

88. Blockade of which neurotransmitter system would most likely result in a cognitive decline in this patient?

(A) histamine

(B) serotonin

(C) dopamine

(D) acetylcholine

(E) norepinephrine

89. A 35-year-old woman presents to the emergency department after taking an overdose of lithium. Which of the following signs is most associated with lithium toxicity?

(A) acute dystonia

(B) abdominal pain

(C) paresthesias

(D) paranoid delusions

(E) leg pain

Questions 90 and 91

A 67-year-old woman presents to your office with a long history of depression. She has tried a number of different antidepressant medications in the past but has not had a remission with any of them. Currently, she is on lithium, venlafaxine (Effexor), nortriptyline (Pamelor), lorazepam, risperidone, and benztropine. She is starting to believe that her next-door neighbors are out to harm her. You want to offer her ECT.

90. Which of her medications would be the best to continue given the ECT?

    (A) lithium
    (B) venlafaxine
    (C) haloperidol
    (D) lorazepam
    (E) clozapine

91. Which of the following is a relative contraindication to ECT?

    (A) a space-occupying lesion of the brain
    (B) a history of seizures
    (C) diabetes mellitus
    (D) a small-bowel obstruction
    (E) catatonia

Questions 92 and 93

A 26-year-old man presents to the psychiatric emergency department with paranoia, visual hallucinations, feelings of unreality, depersonalization, and extreme agitation. A urine toxicology screen is positive for phencyclidine (PCP).

92. What is the best treatment for extreme agitation in this patient?

    (A) a phenothiazine antipsychotic
    (B) a butyrophenone antipsychotic
    (C) trihexphenidyl (Artane)
    (D) trazodone (Desyrel)
    (E) fluoxetine

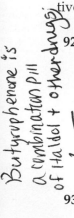

Butyrophenone is a combination pill of Haldol + other drugs

93. If this patient were not extremely agitated, what would be the best treatment?

    (A) vitamin B$_{12}$
    (B) IV haloperidol
    (C) supportive care
    (D) vitamin E
    (E) cheese

94. A 45-year-old woman is admitted to the psychiatric inpatient ward. She is severely depressed, believes that her neighbors are conspiring to murder her, and occasionally can hear a man's voice that says she should die. After talking with the neighbors, you find out that they are the ones who brought the patient to the hospital. They have been good friends for 20 years and have noticed the patient has not been leaving the house much, has taken to looking out of her windows with suspicious glances, and has not cleaned her house in the last 2 months. Which of the following medication combinations would be proper treatment for this patient?

    (A) sertraline and lithium
    (B) paroxetine (Paxil) and thyroid augmentation
    (C) fluoxetine and risperidone
    (D) sertraline and lorazepam
    (E) lorazepam and clozapine

DIRECTIONS (Questions 95 through 100): Each set of items in this section consists of a list of lettered headings followed by several numbered words or phrases. For each numbered word or phrase, select the ONE lettered option that is most closely associated with it. Each lettered option may be selected once, more than once, or not at all.

Questions 95 through 98

Match the clinical vignette with the most likely substance-induced disorder.

    (A) cannabis intoxication
    (B) cocaine intoxication
    (C) cocaine withdrawal
    (D) alcohol intoxication
    (E) alcohol withdrawal
    (F) heroin intoxication

(G) heroin withdrawal

(H) 3,4-methylenedioxymethamphetamine (MDMA) (Ecstasy) intoxication

(I) PCP intoxication

(J) methamphetamine intoxication

(K) inhalant intoxication

(L) nicotine intoxication

(M) nitrous oxide intoxication

(N) psilocybin withdrawal

95. A 23-year-old man is brought to the emergency department by the police. He shows agitation, vertical nystagmus, and analgesia.

96. A 62-year-old homeless man admitted to a psychiatric unit begins having visual hallucinations, tremor, and seizures.

97. A 43 year-old woman presents to the psychiatric emergency department complaining of depression and suicidality. She is observed to be fatigued, irritable, and with a dysphoric effect.

98. A 30-year-old musician presents in the outpatient clinic. He complains of fever, diarrhea, and myoclonus of extremities for the last 24 hours.

Questions 99 and 100

Choose the medication most likely associated with side effects in the following scenarios.

(A) benztropine

(B) clozapine

(C) desipramine (Norpramin)

(D) fluoxetine

(E) haloperidol

(F) lorazepam

(G) lithium

(H) nefazodone (Serzone)

(I) olanzapine

(J) phenelzine

(K) valproic acid

(L) venlafaxine

99. A 34-year-old man with schizophrenia presents with fever and chills. He is found to be bacteremic and has a WBC count of 900/μL.

100. A 41-year-old woman on medications for her affective disorder presents with fatigue, weight gain, cold intolerance, constipation, and decreased concentration.

[handwritten annotations: "Depressed and suicidal Tina → inpatient psychiatry)"; "severe signs of alcohol withdrawal talked about with Georgia."]

Answers and Explanations

1. **(D)** Nefazodone is an antidepressant, which has the advantage of not causing sexual dysfunction like most antidepressants. Unfortunately, it has a black-box warning for hepatitis and liver failure, which is not predictable, so it requires regular monitoring of liver function tests and therefore is not used as frequently.

2. **(G)** Venlafaxine is an antidepressant that inhibits the reuptake of serotonin as well as, in higher doses, norepinephrine. It therefore can cause increased blood pressure in doses above 300 mg daily.

3. **(A)** Although all of the listed antidepressants likely increase serotonin as a therapeutic mechanism, they all affect other neurotransmitters to a certain extent. Citalopram tends to more specifically affect the serotonin system.

4. **(B)** Fluoxetine stands out as having a significantly longer half-life than the other listed antidepressants. This translates into fewer "withdrawal" symptoms if suddenly stopped. It also may be an advantage in cases of occasional poor compliance. The long half-life does not appear to affect the time to significant clinical improvement, which remains several weeks for antidepressants.

5. **(D)** Quetiapine, olanzapine, clozapine, and risperidone have all been shown to cause weight gain as a side effect. The only atypical antipsychotic to date that has not been shown to cause significant weight gain is ziprasidone.

6. **(E)** Although this woman is having hallucinations—perceptions created without any corresponding sensory stimuli—her experience is best characterized as hallucinosis. *Hallucinosis* is a hallucination occurring in a patient who is completely alert and oriented, and most commonly occurs in alcohol withdrawal or chronic alcohol abuse. An *illusion* is a misinterpretation of something that is already there (e.g., a floor lamp being seen as a standing person). A *flashback* is a sensory reexperience of a past, emotionally intense event (e.g., a war veteran's having a flashback of the sights and sounds of a battle). *Formication* is the tactile experience of bugs crawling over, or within, one's body.

7. **(E)** This patient has described a panic attack. Panic attacks are characterized by a sudden onset of intense fear, dread, or anxiety, and accompanied by a variety of physical symptoms. Although virtually any organ system can seem to be the source of distress in panic disorder, common symptoms include diaphoresis, palpitations, shortness of breath, tremulousness, flushing, chest pain, and dizziness. Regardless of the clinical setting or psychiatric history, patients presenting with symptoms suggestive of panic disorder must be thoroughly worked up to rule out physiologic pathology as the source of the symptoms. Untreated, panic disorder tends to run a chronic course and can cause severe disability.

8. **(D)** *Neologistic speech*, a positive symptom of schizophrenia, consists of words made up by the patient, having meaning only to him. *Word salad* is an illogical, incoherent collection of words or phrases. *Clang associations* are words or phrases strung together because of the

sounds they make, not because of the meaning they convey. *Dysarthria* is a problem with pronunciation and articulation of words; it does not imply an inherent inability to understand and use language; for example, a dysarthric person could conceivably write a coherent and meaningful sentence.

9. **(E)** *Dysthymia* is a low-grade, chronic, intermittent depression. The symptoms must be present in adults for at least 2 years. Like depression, other than a subjective feeling of depressed mood, or the blues, the key features of dysthymia are alterations in appetite and sleep, feelings of hopelessness, difficulty concentrating, and low energy or fatigue. Although dysthymia and MDD share a number of features, it is generally the severity and duration of symptoms that distinguish the two disorders. In the presence of alcohol dependence, it would be difficult to convince any clinician that the mood disturbance is not due to the effects of the drug, and would exclude a diagnosis of dysthymia.

10. **(C)** Patients with Capgras syndrome suffer from the delusion that someone familiar is an identical-appearing replacement. *Koro* is a traumatic fear that the penis is shrinking into the body cavity. *Amok* is a violent fit followed by amnesia. *Pseudocyesis* is the physiologic signs and symptoms of pregnancy developing in the absence of pregnancy. *Couvade syndrome* occurs when the husband of a pregnant woman goes into a sort of labor. Koro, amok, and couvade syndrome are culture bound, that is, they describe unusual, recurrent patterns of behavior that resist placement in any Western diagnostic category (the DSM).

11. **(B)** The multiaxis system of diagnosis in criteria uses the signs and symptoms of psychiatric illness to assign diagnosis and to provide a snapshot picture of a particular patient. It was originally intended to lend objectivity to psychiatric diagnoses, principally in the service of research; today, it is widely used clinically. Axis I includes psychiatric illnesses that appear in a defined period or periods and result in some diminished function as compared to previous functioning. Common Axis I diagnoses are

schizophrenia, generalized anxiety disorder, and drug-related illnesses, such as alcohol abuse. Axis II represents long-standing pervasive problems in mental life such as personality disorders and mental retardation. Axis III is for all medical conditions, which may or may not relate directly to the psychiatric diagnosis. Axis IV is for psychosocial stressors. Axis V, the GAF, is a numerical value, from 1 (lowest) to 100 (highest), characterizing the overall level of impairment resulting from the conditions described on Axis I through Axis IV. The multiaxis representation of this patient would appear as:

- *Axis I:* Adjustment disorder, alcohol abuse, in remission
- *Axis II:* Deferred
- *Axis III:* Diabetes
- *Axis IV:* Psychosocial stressor (recent divorce)
- *Axis V:* GAF: 70

12. **(C)** Both *copropraxia* and *echopraxia* are terms used in relation to movements and are specifically used in reference to obscene gestures and repeating another's movements, respectively. *Bruxism* is the grinding of the teeth. *Blepharospasm* is the spasm of the periorbital muscles causing sustained or exaggerated blinking. *Torticollis* is a spasm of the neck muscles such as the sternocleidomastoid on one or both sides. This usually brings the neck to one side or another but can also pull forward or backward.

13. **(B)** *Coprolalia* and *echolalia* are terms used in relation to language or speech and are specifically used in reference to obscene speech and repeating another's words, respectively. *Palilalia* is also a repetition of words but is the repetition of one's own words as the person appears to get stuck on the same word or phrase. *Parapraxis* is a slip of the tongue, and dysarthria refers to a problem of word articulation, usually secondary to cerebellar or motor control abnormalities.

14. **(D)** All of the terms listed are impulse control disorders of various forms. The content of each is listed below:

- *Pyromania:* Fire setting that is deliberate, more than once
- *Trichotillomania:* Hair pulling with appreciable hair loss
- *Kleptomania:* Stealing objects not out of need or monetary value
- *Pathologic gambling:* Maladaptive gambling behavior
- *Intermittent explosive disorder:* Aggressive impulses resulting in assault or the destruction of property

15. **(B)** *Ego-syntonic* and *ego-dystonic* refer to whether thoughts or behaviors are distressing or not distressing to the patient. In this case, the impulses are distressing and would therefore be classified as ego-dystonic. *Mood congruency* usually refers to delusions or hallucinations in mood disorders and whether they are themes consistent with the mood. *Delusions* are fixed, false beliefs that are not shared by others.

16. **(B)** *Ganser syndrome* is a dissociative disorder described by Ganser in three prisoners. It is characterized by approximate answers and talking past the point and is associated with amnesia, disorientation, fugue, and conversion symptoms. Amok and *piblokto* are dissociative trance disorders that are described as disturbances in consciousness and are indigenous to particular cultures. Malingering is difficult to distinguish in these situations, but in this case a secondary gain is not identifiable. *Logorrhea* is excessive speech.

17. **(A)** *Kayser-Fleischer rings* are golden brown or gray-green rings of pigment at the corneal limbus that can be present in a disorder of copper metabolism such as Wilson disease. *Arcus senilis* is a light gray ring beginning superiorly and extending to the limbus. It can resemble a corneal arcus, which is associated with hypercholesterolemia, but in an elderly patient it is often a normal finding. Also associated with hypercholesterolemia is *xanthelasma*, raised yellow areas around the eyelids. *Brushfield spots* are lighter-colored areas in the outer third of the iris that can be associated with Down syndrome, but can also be a normal

variant. *Subconjunctival hemorrhage* is the finding of blood in the areas of the eye surrounding the iris.

18. **(C)** *Hemiballismus* is an uncontrolled swinging of an extremity. It is usually sudden, and once initiated it cannot be controlled. *Choreiform movements* are involuntary, irregular, and jerky but lack the ballistic-like nature of hemiballismus. *Athetoid movements*, or athetosis, are slow, snake-like movements of the fingers and hands. *Myoclonus* is a sudden muscle spasm, and *myotonia* is prolonged muscle contraction.

19. **(A)** Magical thinking and ideas of reference are two types of delusions that can be found in psychotic disorders. *Magical thinking* is the belief that one's thoughts can control outside events. *Ideas of reference* is the belief that other people or the media are referring to or talking about the person experiencing this delusion. Reaction formation, displacement, and projection are all types of defense mechanisms. *Reaction formation* is the formation of thoughts that are opposite to anxiety-provoking feelings. *Displacement* is the transferring of a feeling toward an object that is less threatening, such as the family pet or one's spouse or children. *Projection* is the false attribution of one's own unacceptable feelings to another.

20. **(A)** *Thought broadcasting* is the delusion that one's thoughts can be heard by others. It is often seen in schizophrenia. *Thought insertion* and *thought control* also can be seen in schizophrenia and are delusions that others can insert thoughts into a patient's mind or that another can control the patient's thoughts or behaviors, respectively. *Transference*, in strict terms, is the reexperiencing of past experiences with the analyst in the setting of psychoanalytic psychotherapy. In general, this term has come to mean the transferring of emotions and feelings that one has from one's past to the physician or care provider. Echolalia is the repetition of another's words or phrases.

21. **(A)** *Erotomania* is the term used to describe a delusion in which individuals falsely believe that another person is in love with them.

Nymphomania is insatiable sexual desire in a woman, and *satyriasis* is its male counterpart. Thought broadcasting is the delusion that one's thoughts can be heard by others. *Alexia* is an inability to read.

22. **(D)** This patient demonstrates *delusions of grandeur*, that is, an elevated sense of one's position or wealth. A *delusion of infidelity* is an unfounded belief that one's spouse or significant other is being unfaithful. *Micropsia* and *macropsia* are misperceptions of visual stimuli. Objects appear smaller (micropsia) or larger (macropsia) than they are in reality. Palinopsia is the persistence of the visual image after the stimulus has been removed.

23. **(B)** A *conversion disorder* is often a dramatic set of physical symptoms, usually neurologic, that result from unconscious conflicts. *Sublimation* is a defense mechanism employed to deal with unacceptable feelings or desires that one may possess and to channel these motivations into socially acceptable behaviors. Like sublimation, *rationalization* is a defense against undesired motivations, but in this case these motivations are concealed by elaborate and reassuring explanations that avoid the actual underlying motives. *Dissociation* is a defense mechanism that deals with stressors via a breakdown of the usual integration of memory, behavior, and perception.

24. **(D)** *La belle indifférence* is the indifference shown toward a deficit or loss of function classically seen in a conversion disorder. *Déjà entendu* is the feeling that one is hearing what one has heard before. It is usually associated with anxiety states or fatigue. *Déjà vu* is a similar experience but refers to the sensation that something has been seen before. *Jamais vu* is the opposite of déjà vu in that it refers to something that should be familiar but seems quite unfamiliar. *Folie à deux* is a shared delusion aroused in one person by the influence of another.

25. **(A)** *Testamentary capacity* (the level of competence required to make a valid will) is based on the presence of all of the following: (1) an understanding of the nature of the will;

(2) knowledge of one's assets; (3) knowledge of natural heirs; (4) absence of acute psychosis (i.e., delusions), which might compromise rational decision making; and (5) freedom from undue influence or coercion. The validity of the will may be undermined by demonstrating that the individual failed to meet any of the above criteria. The presence of a conservator of person and history of mental illness are important only insofar as they bear upon any of the noted factors. A history of mental illness is not sufficient to invalidate one's testamentary capacity. *Actus reus* refers to the voluntary act of committing a crime and is an element used in determining criminal responsibility. The presence of a judge at the signing of a will is not required.

26. **(B)** Informed consent is crucial in maintaining patient autonomy in decision making. Elements involved in obtaining informed consent include providing the patient with information regarding the risks and benefits of treatment, alternative treatment options (including no treatment), and establishing the competency of the patient to make a voluntary decision. Exceptions to informed consent include (1) emergency situations in which obtaining informed consent would jeopardize patient safety, (2) patient waiver of informed consent, and (3) situations in which disclosing information would directly harm the patient (also known as *therapeutic privilege*; it is seldom used). The other choices are not valid exceptions to informed consent.

27. **(C)** Confidentiality is an integral part of the physician-patient relationship and is especially important in establishing the trust of a psychotherapeutic relationship. The physician-patient privilege should be breached only in specific instances such as the patient's waiving of the privilege (i.e., patient initiates litigation, consent to release information is obtained, there is a duty to protect, emergency situation, or in cases in which the court orders release). In this case, the information should not be released unless the patient has waived his physician-patient confidentiality privilege. Lying to or misleading the court is unethical and may subject one to prosecution. The remaining choices fail to maintain confidentiality.

28. **(D)** When a patient has stopped paying his or her bill, the physician should directly address the issue with the patient. Failure to pay one's bills may reflect underlying issues for which the patient has entered into psychotherapy or that are related to psychiatric symptoms. Contacting a collection agency before addressing the issue with the patient is inappropriate. If a patient continues to refuse payment after discussing the issue, the patient should be notified in writing of the outstanding balance and a referral to a collection agency might be made. To preserve confidentiality, care should be taken to disclose the minimum information needed for collection (i.e., date of service and charge) without referring to diagnosis or treatment rendered. Asking the insurance company to pay you after a check has been disbursed to the patient is futile because the insurance company's obligation toward the insured has been fulfilled. Disclosing the existence of a professional relationship with the patient to his family is a breach of confidentiality. Terminating the therapeutic relationship before exploring the dynamics behind the patient's payment delinquency might harm any future therapeutic alliance.

29. **(B)** *Malingering* is the intentional production of symptoms for secondary gain (e.g., to avoid work, to evade criminal prosecution, or to gain financial rewards). A diagnosis of malingering should be suspected in medicolegal cases, in individuals with antisocial personality disorder, when symptoms are out of proportion to objective findings, or when a patient in distress does not cooperate with evaluation/treatment. *Factitious disorder* can be differentiated from malingering based on the absence of external incentives. In factitious disorder, symptoms are intentionally feigned to satisfy an intrapsychic incentive to assume the sick role. *Munchausen syndrome* is a factitious disorder characterized by repeated acts of feigning illnesses to gain medical attention. Intrapsychic gain obtained by the act of getting medical attention through feigning medical illness in another individual (usually a child or elderly person) is sometimes referred to as *Munchausen by proxy*. Conversion disorder describes the production of neurologic or other medical symptoms resulting from intrapsychic needs or conflicts. In contrast to factitious disorder and malingering, symptoms associated with conversion disorder are not consciously produced.

30. **(E)** Individuals with malingering tend to be suspicious and uncooperative with diagnostic evaluations. Furthermore, they do not typically follow up with recommended treatment regimens and refuse opportunities to return to social or work activities. Malingerers consciously feign symptoms for financial incentives or to avoid work/social obligations (*secondary gain*). In contrast, conversion disorder is the unconscious or involuntary production of symptoms resulting from intrapsychic needs or conflicts. Individuals with conversion disorder are more likely to be friendly, cooperative, interested in evaluations that may "find the answer," and avidly follow up with prescribed treatments. The other choices are not accurate statements distinguishing between malingering and conversion disorder.

31. **(E)** Sexual abuse is estimated to occur with an incidence of 0.25% of children per year. Known acquaintances (e.g., fathers, stepfathers, and male relatives) are often the perpetrators. In this vignette, the patient likely has acquired *Neisseria gonorrhoeae* from a male perpetrator. Other physical findings may include injuries to the genitalia (i.e., hymen, vagina) or the perineum. Psychiatric manifestations of sexual abuse may include anxiety, agitation, aggressive or impulsive behavior, and exhibitionism. When sexual abuse of a child is suspected, the first step is to ensure the safety of the child and immediately notify the state's Child Protective Services. Reporting is mandatory in cases of physical and sexual child abuse. The other choices fail to protect the child and do not satisfy state-mandated reporting statutes.

32. **(A)** This case represents Wernicke encephalopathy, a condition seen in chronic alcohol dependency. The etiology is acute thiamine deficiency and it presents with the classic triad of confusion, ataxia, and opthalmoplegia. Although it is usually reversible with thiamine replacement,

it is important to administer the thiamine prior to giving fluids and glucose. Administration of glucose and fluids first may provoke a worsening of symptoms resulting in permanent damage.

33. **(B)** The patient is experiencing symptoms consistent with severe alcohol withdrawal, namely delirium tremens (DT), characterized by delirium, confusion, combativeness, and elevated vitals signs. DT carries a significant mortality if not treated. The treatment of choice is IM or IV benzodiazepines. Although barbiturates may also treat withdrawal, they have a narrower therapeutic index, with a higher risk of sedation and respiratory depression. Neither the antipsychotic or thiamine will treat the underlying alcohol withdrawal, and giving hydralazine may be dangerous as it may mask the symptoms.

34. **(D)** The patient is presenting with evidence of overdose with opiates, which is characterized by the triad of somnolence, respiratory depression, and pinpoint pupils. Opiate intoxication can be rapidly reversed with IV administration of an opiate antagonist, such as naloxone. Antabuse blocks acetaldehyde dehydrogenase and is given to alcoholics as an aversive stimulus to avoid alcohol consumption. Benzodiazepines would be used in cases of severe alcohol withdrawal, or DT, which would demonstrate elevated vital signs. Flumazenil is a benzodiazepine antagonist used in the emergency treatment of overdose with benzodiazepines, which does not cause pupilary constriction. Thiamine would be given in cases of Wernicke encephalopathy, caused most commonly by chronic, heavy alcohol consumption. It presents with a triad of confusion, ataxia, and opthalmoplegia.

35. **(B)** This elderly woman is showing signs of dementia, likely Alzheimer disease, the most common cause of dementia. The primary treatment modality is to begin an anticholinesterase inhibitor, such as galantamine. Memantine, an *N*-methyl d-aspartate (NMDA) receptor antagonist, is a newer medication that may be added to the regimen. Antidepressants and antipsychotic medications may be used for associated depression or agitation/psychosis, respectively,

but they are not primary treatments. Ginkgo biloba has not been shown to be effective for the memory deficits in dementia.

36. **(A)** Suicide is the second leading cause of death among individuals aged 15–24; only accidents account for more deaths in this population. Risk factors for completed suicide include (1) age >45, (2) male gender, (3) separated/divorced >married, (4) White race >Black race, and (5) Jews/Protestants >Catholics. The lifetime suicide rate in individuals with a diagnosis of a major psychiatric disorder (i.e., schizophrenia, bipolar I disorder, MDD) is estimated at 10–15%. Suicide in children younger than age 13 is rare. Women attempt suicide up to four times more frequently than men; however, men are three times more likely to succeed at suicide than are women.

37. **(B)** Physician assisted suicide involves the doctor's facilitating a person's death by providing the information or equipment necessary to end his or her life. The AMA's Code of Medical Ethics strongly condemns such action as "fundamentally incompatible with the physician's role as healer." Rather, the ethical obligation of the physician is to adequately respond to a patient's end-of-life issues. The AMA's Code of Medical Ethics emphasizes that participation in physician-assisted suicide would have detrimental implications to both society and the practice of medicine. Euthanasia occurs when a physician carries out the killing of a patient to relieve intolerable and refractory suffering. Euthanasia is not the mere facilitation of the terminal act, but involves the actual administration of the fatal agent. Like physician-assisted suicide, it is condemned by the AMA's Code of Medical Ethics. Recently, a Michigan physician was found guilty of second-degree murder for giving a lethal injection at the request of a patient suffering from Lou Gehrig disease.

38. **(B)** Physician-patient confidentiality in the treatment of minors must be maintained unless otherwise mandated by law (e.g., cases of abortion in some states) or when parental involvement is necessary in making complex and life-threatening medical decisions. In this case,

the physician must respect the patient's confidentiality but should remain cognizant of the implications this will have on the family system. Therefore, it is most appropriate to encourage the minor to discuss the issue with her parents. At this point, there is no indication of child harm or neglect that would mandate reporting to Child Protective Services. Testimonial privilege refers to the privilege invoked to protect physician-patient confidentiality when medical information is subpoenaed without patient consent. The remaining two choices fail to maintain physician-patient confidentiality.

39. **(C)** *Tangentiality* is similar to circumstantiality in its representing speech/thoughts that are logically connected but that drift off the point. Tangentiality differs from circumstantiality in that the speaker never comes back to the point.

40. **(B)** Delusions are disturbances in thought content and are fixed, false beliefs not held by others. They are included in none of the other choices, which are categories of the MSE.

41. **(C)** Because of their side effect profile, the treatment of choice in major depression is the SSRIs such as fluoxetine (Prozac). Although MAOIs such as phenelzine are thought to be somewhat more effective in atypical depression—for example, eating more, rather than decreased appetite—they carry the risk of hypertensive crisis when combined with foods containing tryptophan. Amitryptiline and other tricylic antidepressants include the risk of arrhythmias and can be lethal in overdose, unlike the SSRIs. And while the patient reports periods during which she is "just fine," there is nothing to indicate a cycling pattern that would require a mood stabilizer such as divalproex sodium. Similarly, being convinced that her fiancé is about to leave her is not psychotic, but is instead a mild mood-congruent delusion that does not require an adjunct antipsychotic such as ziprasidone.

42. **(D)** Fluoxetine is a class C drug, meaning that it is potentially harmful to the developing fetus, according to animal studies, although no definitive studies in humans are available. A

discussion of the risks and benefits of treatment is therefore most appropriate. It does not have the withdrawal syndrome known to occur with paroxetine, but still stopping it immediately should be avoided. Asking the patient how important pregnancy is to her would be inappropriate, since it is a personal choice and, according to the information provided in the vignette, it is not something that puts her in danger of any kind. ECT may be an option but not before a discussion of the risks and benefits of her current treatment. Finally, there is no indication that she is at particular risk for postpartum depression and there is no evidence in the literature that adding a second antidepressant in pregnancy will prevent this disorder.

43. **(D)** There are many reasons why this man could be exhibiting psychosis (cutting down a tree that his wife's ghost lives in) and depression. It's more than possible that he is suffering from some kind of severe grief disorder, although 3 months is too short to make this diagnosis. It is also possible that his wife's death unmasked a psychotic depression, or that alcoholism has led to some kind of dementia. Regardless of the eventual diagnosis, it is important to first rule out other irreversible causes of his behavior such as drug abuse. Certainly it is premature to prescribe any medications for him at this time.

44. **(A)** Although there are a number of sleeping aids available, many are benzodiazepines. Because these overlap with alcohol in binding to GABA receptors—hence their use in alcohol withdrawal—these should be avoided in patients with a history of alcoholism. The same is true of zolpidem, which has been shown to have similar abuse potential to diazepam. Zalpelon is relatively contraindicated in those with severe liver dysfunction, which is a potential issue in a patient with a history of alcoholism. Trazodone, which was developed as an antidepressant, has been shown to be an effective sleeping aid and is therefore useful in this population.

45. **(C)** Trazodone carries a 1 in 1000 to 1 in 10,000 risk of priapism. The other sexual side effects among the choices are known to occur with

the SSRIs, but not particularly with trazodone. Incontinence is not a significant side effect of any antidepressant.

46. **(E)** All of the SSRIs have been in the news recently, mostly because of controversy over data on increased suicidal gestures among children taking these medications. Paroxetine has been the focus of many of the reports. However, fluoxetine is the only medication indicated for treatment of childhood depression, which makes switching to paroxetine or amitryptiline incorrect in this setting. Fluoxetine does not have the withdrawal syndrome known to occur with paroxetine, but still stopping it immediately should be avoided. Asking the child's mother what is "really bothering her" is unlikely to be productive, as it is somewhat accusatory and a leading question.

47. **(C)** Although many people think of "natural remedies" such as St. John's wort as safe, these supplements can have risks of significant side effects. In particular, St. John's wort side effects include increased photosensitivity, stomach upset, rashes, fatigue, restlessness, headache, dry mouth, dizziness, and confusion. These side effects are more likely when St. John's wort is combined with SSRIs. St. John's wort has been shown to have some benefits in mild depressions and is thought to act like an MAOI. The precise pharmacokinetics of St. John's wort are unknown, but if anything, doses of SSRIs should be decreased while patients are taking the supplement because of possible potentiation of side effects. As with any antidepressant, it is not a good idea to stop it abruptly. There is no reason to think that child abuse is involved, as the child's mother is not putting her son in danger.

48. **(A)** Bipolar manic episodes have perhaps the highest rate of response to ECT. The safety of ECT depends on underlying medical conditions, not on the disorder being treated. Its effects are not longer lasting than those of medications.

49. **(C)** This question refers to *kindling*, the hypothesis that each decompensation in a mental illness leads to increased risk to have another, and

likely more severe episode. Conversely, treatment of the decompensations is theorized to be protective against the above. There is no known effect on the response to ECT or medications in the future.

50. **(E)** Lack of suicide attempt history is her most significant protective factor; a lesser protective factor is social support. Other factors do not play much of a role.

51. **(B)** There are many potential medical causes of depression; the only choice here that lists two well-described such causes is B. Vitamin B_{12} deficiency and adrenal disease as well as vascular disease have also been shown to also be potential causes.

52. **(A)** This patient is most likely suffering from anorexia. Excessive dental decay is common in patients with anorexia or bulimia who purge by self-induced vomiting. Although the other choices may be present in severe starvation, excessive dental decay is most common and appears earliest.

53. **(A)** Occupations such as modeling, ballet, and gymnastics, which encourage thinness, have disproportionately high rates of anorexia. Patients with certain personality disorders, including borderline personality disorder, have a higher likelihood of being victims of abuse or trauma. Education and "type A" personalities are not correlated with eating disorders, nor is being a twin.

54. **(C)** Rett syndrome has been described only in girls. Diagnostic criteria require symptom onset between ages 5 months and 4 years with apparently normal prior development. Criteria for autism do not require deceleration of head growth. In childhood disintegrative disorder, as in Rett syndrome, development is initially normal. However, in childhood disintegrative disorder, development is normal for at least the first 2 years after birth. In Asperger syndrome, there is no delay in language. Childhood schizophrenia cannot be diagnosed in children meeting criteria for a pervasive developmental disorder who do not have prominent delusions and hallucinations.

55. **(A)** Nigrostriatal D_2 receptors that are blocked by neuroleptic medications cause an imbalance between dopamine and acetylcholine, which accounts for the parkinsonian symptoms. Mesolimbic D_2 receptor blockade is believed to account for the antipsychotic effect of neuroleptics and does not cause extrapyramidal symptoms. Typical neuroleptics block both nigrostriatal and mesolimbic dopamine, whereas atypical neuroleptics preferentially block mesolimbic dopamine, accounting for decreased extrapyramidal symptom liability.

56. **(A)** This patient is most likely suffering from Tourette syndrome. Pimozide, a dopamine blocker, has been shown to most clearly suppress tic activity compared to agents affecting other neurotransmitter systems. Although methylphenidate may help this patient's apparent ADHD symptoms, it may also exacerbate his tic disorder. Fluoxetine, topiramate, and clonidine may be effective for comorbid conditions found with Tourette disorder but have not been found to be specifically helpful for this primary condition.

57. **(C)** Fire setting in a repeated pattern in children often accompanies other behaviors that are defiant of rules and authority, as in conduct disorder. Although fire setting may occur in children diagnosed with pervasive developmental disorder, mental retardation, or tic disorder, it is much more unusual. Destructive personality disorder of childhood is not a DSM-IV-TR diagnosis and here serves as a distracter.

58. **(D)** *Secondary enuresis* means that the child achieved continence for over a year and then lost it, as the case suggests. *Nocturnal* means the incontinence happens at night. *Primary enuresis* means that the patient has never achieved complete continence. *Diurnal enuresis* is daytime incontinence. *Encopresis* is the repeated passage of feces into inappropriate places.

59. **(E)** More than 40 double-blind trials of imipramine have confirmed the drug's efficacy for enuresis. Clonidine is an antihypertensive sometimes used in opiate withdrawal. Haloperidol is a typical antipsychotic. Carbamazepine is an anticonvulsant sometimes used as a mood stabilizer. Diphenhydramine is used for insomnia.

60. **(B)** Borderline intellectual functioning is a term no longer used that referred to IQ in the range of 71–84. In mild mental retardation, IQ ranges from 50 or 55 to approximately 70. In severe mental retardation, IQ ranges from 20 or 25 to 35 or 40. Learning disorder not otherwise specified is diagnosed with global learning impairments, but the disability in specific areas of learning is mild and would not result in such low IQ results as in this case.

61. **(A)** Microcephaly, short palpebral fissures, flat midface, and thin upper lip are all associated with fetal alcohol syndrome (FAS). Cleft palate is not specifically associated with FAS. There are no genetic abnormalities associated with FAS. Congenital blindness is not associated with FAS, although methyl alcohol consumption can cause blindness in adults. Prominent jaw is associated with fragile X syndrome.

62. **(B)** Mixed receptive-expressive language disorder does not imply an abnormality in emotional communication such as in displays of aggression toward other children found in reactive attachment disorder. Patients with childhood disintegrative disorder show histories of decline in language and social communication operating that are more profound than in reactive attachment disorder, and there are no criteria noting an association of symptoms of neglect or abuse. ADHD and conduct disorder are most often diagnosed in school-age children who have histories of reactive attachment disorder.

63. **(C)** The majority of patients diagnosed with borderline personality disorder report histories of sexual abuse. Sexual activity among siblings is the most common form of incest, although parent-to-child incest is the most commonly reported form. A history of sexual abuse is in fact a risk factor for being a future victim of sexual abuse. There is no association of childhood sexual abuse and schizophrenia. Abuse of alcohol or other illicit substances at such a young age as this patient is commonly found in victims of childhood sexual abuse.

64. **(D)** Many incestuous fathers act in the face of disappointing and/or conflicted sexual relationships with their spouses. Incestuous fathers and stepfathers all have increased likelihoods of having alcoholism, impulsive or violent behavior, paraphilias such as exhibitionism and pedophilia, and a personal history of being a victim of sexual abuse.

65. **(D)** This patient has symptoms most consistent with a bipolar mood disorder and therefore would most benefit from lithium or another mood stabilizer such as valproic acid. Lorazepam may be used to treat psychomotor agitation and insomnia of mania but does not generally treat the underlying disorder and has a dependency liability in the long term. Imipramine and fluoxetine, as TCAs and SSRIs, respectively, can exacerbate mania. Chlorpromazine, a typical antipsychotic, may help the patient with his mild thought disorder and his psychomotor agitation but may not treat the underlying mood disorder if given alone.

66. **(C)** Atypical depression is characterized by mood reactivity, rejection hypersensitivity, hypersomnolence, increased appetite, and lead pipe psychomotor retardation. Severe concentration impairment is a feature of melancholic depression. Patients with either melancholic or atypical symptoms may have either a normal dexamethasone suppression test or psychotic symptoms. A manic response to antidepressant treatment may be indicative of a bipolar syndrome rather than a unipolar depression.

67. **(B)** Although not commonly used because of the risk of side effects, MAOIs are actually the most effective class of drugs for treating atypical depression. SSRIs and TCAs are also effective. Some anticonvulsants are used for the treatment of bipolar disorder, but not unipolar depression. Neuroleptics are used to treat psychotic disorders.

68. **(C)** When changing from an SSRI to an MAOI, one must allow a washout period of about five half-lives for the SSRI to be more than 90% eliminated; in the case of fluoxetine, this is 5 weeks. This precaution avoids serotonin syndrome, which can occur when significant blood levels of both drugs are present. Serotonin syndrome, which can be fatal, is marked by symptoms of tremor, diaphoresis, rigidity, myoclonus, autonomic dysregulation, hyperthermia, rhabdomyolysis, renal failure, and coma.

69. **(D)** MAOIs prevent the peripheral breakdown of tyramine, which may be ingested with certain foods such as beer, red wine, aged cheeses, liver, smoked fish, dry sausage, and fava beans. If too much tyramine builds up in the blood, it may activate peripheral sympathetic nerve receptors and cause a hypertensive crisis. Stiffness and tremor are usually associated with typical neuroleptics and are rare with MAOIs. Bland food is a nonspecific request. Eating food rich in tryptophan, a serotonin precursor, is not a problem. MAOIs are not usually particularly oversedating compared to tricyclic or other atypical antidepressants.

70. **(D)** This case deliberately brings together many character traits drawn from "pure" diagnoses of character disorders, including borderline, narcissistic, dependent, obsessive-compulsive, and schizotypal personalities. In clinical practice, a large proportion of patients diagnosable in Axis II do not in fact have any clear-cut character syndrome. Such mixed cases are referred to as *personality disorder not otherwise specified.* Patients with pure borderline personality disorder are known for their intense personal relationships, self-destructive behaviors, anger management issues, and poor senses of self-image. Narcissistic personality disorder is marked by a grandiose sense of self-worth, entitlement, lack of real empathy, and tendency to use others for one's own ends. Patients with obsessive-compulsive personality disorder are perfectionists, inflexible, and overly demanding of themselves and others. Schizotypal patients are known for their quirkiness and seemingly magical thinking styles.

71. **(D)** Remembering the DSM-IV-TR criteria for schizoaffective disorder can be daunting. Generally speaking, patients who at one time

appear to have schizophrenia (i.e., diagnostic criteria for it are met) and at other times appear to have a prominent mood disorder (based on an episode that fulfills either major depression or bipolar disorder with or without psychosis) may be diagnosed with schizoaffective disorder. Technically, the diagnosis requires a period of 2 weeks of psychotic symptoms without affective symptoms. Psychotic disorder not otherwise specified is usually reserved for situations in which the clinician does not have enough historical data to know whether the patient has schizophrenia, a mood disorder with psychotic features, or a medical-related or substance-induced psychosis.

72. **(D)** The elderly are particularly vulnerable to medications known to have psychoactive properties or side effects. This is in part due to the decreased ability of geriatric patients to rapidly metabolize medications and thus the tendency of the drugs to build up to higher steady-state levels than for younger persons. Additionally, elderly persons are generally more vulnerable to the effects of medications that act on the central nervous system (CNS) due to decreased reserve of neurons using particular neurotransmitter systems that may be affected by the drugs. For example, elderly people may be more susceptible to the dopamine-blocking effects of haloperidol that cause parkinsonism because they have a decreased number of dopaminergic neurons that arise from the substantia nigra. The patient in this case is on a number of medications that may have CNS side effects at high doses, especially in the elderly. However, the highly anticholinergic properties of diphenhydramine put this patient at particular risk of memory impairment and confusion. Cimetidine and furosemide are conceivable culprits for her confusion due to their minor anticholinergic activity, but are much less likely. Beta-blockers like atenolol have been associated with depression presumably associated with blockade of central adrenergic receptors. Additionally, in some vulnerable patients, they may reduce cardiac output enough to cause a functional hypoperfusion of the brain causing confusion and dizziness. Digoxin may actually decrease sodium ion conduction in

CNS neurons enough to produce delirium in some patients.

73. **(A)** Delirium related to blockade of acetylcholinergic receptors is the most common cause of medication-induced delirium in the elderly. Acetylcholine is uniquely involved with memory processes in the brain and its involvement in the pathophysiology of Alzheimer disease has been heavily researched. Drugs that alter dopamine neurotransmission are most associated with movement disorder and psychosis-related side effects. Drugs affecting GABA receptors may cause sedation and ataxia as well as memory disturbances. Fortunately, the diversity of drugs that affect these receptors is much narrower than the broad classes of drugs that block acetylcholine receptors. Drugs affecting serotonin may affect sleep, appetite, and mood, but few nonpsychiatric drugs affect this system. Drugs affecting central norepinephrine transmission may rarely be associated with depression.

74. **(E)** Studies that find no statistical difference between groups when there actually is a difference result in a type II error. In this case, the positive findings at the other universities make the finding at university A less likely to be correct. University A may have needed a larger number of subjects in the study to find the treatment effect. Type I errors occur more often than type II errors and cause the researcher to conclude that there is a difference between groups when in fact there is none. *Standard error* is the degree to which the means of several different samples would vary if they were taken repeatedly from the same population. The *variance* is the sum of the differences of each data point from the mean. *Positive predictive value* is the proportion of abnormal test results that are true positive, while *negative predictive value* is the proportion of normal test results that are true negative.

75. **(E)** This patient has signs most consistent with *tardive dyskinesia*, an extrapyramidal syndrome that usually affects perioral or limb musculature and causes choreiform movements. Its onset is usually several years after being on the medication and it is more likely to

affect older patients. *Akathisia* is best described as psychomotor restlessness that may have an onset of hours to days after beginning the neuroleptic. *Dystonia* is an acute reaction to neuroleptics in which particular muscle groups (neck or ocular muscles commonly) contract involuntarily. It can be painful and should be treated immediately with anticholinergics. *NMS* is a potentially lethal medical emergency in which patients may have global rigidity, mental status changes, fever, cardiovascular instability, elevated creatine phosphokinases, and risk of rhabdomyolysis. Parkinsonism may look identical to Parkinson disease (tremor, bradykinesia) and may have onset within weeks to months of beginning the medication.

76. **(A)** The basal ganglia, implicated in the yoking of thought to motor action, and in controlling the initiation and quality of motor action, is theorized to be central to the pathophysiology of extrapyramidal syndromes, including dystonia, parkinsonism, akathisia, and tardive dyskinesia. The cerebellum is important in controlling the coordination of motor movements and posture as well as participating in procedural memory. The frontal cortex is generally considered to be important for decision making, impulse control, short-term memory, and affect regulation. The midbrain contains nuclei that help to ensure CNS homeostasis by regulating neurovegetative, autonomic, and arousal functions. The motor cortex serves as the last stage of cerebral processing of motor information before it descends into the spinal cord. An intact motor cortex is required for initiation of movement.

77. **(A)** Premorbid personality disorders and comorbid Axis I disorders have been shown to increase the risk of acquiring PTSD with exposure to a significant, acute psychological trauma. Exposure to psychological trauma in middle adulthood as opposed to childhood or elderly years is considered the period of least vulnerability to PTSD. Rapid onset of symptoms, short duration of symptoms, and strong social supports are good prognostic indicators for PTSD.

78. **(C)** Erik Erikson is perhaps best known for his description of eight stages of human psychological experience spanning the life span, centered on stage-appropriate developmental conflicts: basic trust versus mistrust (birth to 1 year); autonomy versus shame and doubt (1–3 years); initiative versus guilt (3–5 years); industry versus inferiority (6–11 years); identity versus role diffusion (11 years to end of adolescence); intimacy versus isolation (21–40 years); generativity versus stagnation (40–65 years); and integrity versus despair (65 and older). Carl Jung developed concepts of the collective unconscious, archetypes, individuation, introversion, and extroversion. Karen Horney's work is notable for an emphasis on the idea that a person's personality traits are the result of an interaction of the person with the environment, and that "self-realization" is the therapeutic process that removes distorting influences that prevent character growth. Jean Piaget is known for his work using observations of children and adolescents to build a framework describing cognitive stages of development beginning with the sensorimotor stage at birth and ending with the stage of formal operations. Sigmund Freud is the founder of psychoanalysis, notable for such concepts as ego, id, and superego and drive theory.

79. **(D)** About 20% of patients with complex partial epilepsy experience psychotic symptoms at some time.

80. **(B)** Hyperreligious thinking or preoccupation with moral behavior, altered sexual behaviors, hypergraphia or overelaborative communication styles (also referred to as *viscosity*), and heightened experience of emotions form a classic constellation of personality traits associated with complex partial epilepsy. Urinary incontinence is more often associated with normal pressure hydrocephalus or severe dementia. Sleep disorders, depression, and obsessive-compulsive symptoms may be associated with structural brain injury of frontal and subcortical areas but have not been described as being related particularly to complex partial epilepsy.

81. **(B)** The Glasgow Coma Scale measures level of arousal and ranges from a scale of 3 (deep coma) to 14 (fully alert). The categories assessed

are eye opening, best motor response, and best verbal response. Eye opening ranges from a score of 4 (opening spontaneously) to 1 (not opening at all). In this case the eyes open to pain, so a score of 2 is given. Best motor response is as follows: obeys commands, 5; localizes pain, 4; flexion, 3; extension, 2; and no response, 1. In this case, a score of 3 is given for the response. Best verbal response is also based on a scale ranging from 5 to 1. An oriented patient receives a score of 5 and no response receives a score of 1, as in this case. The scores are then added, and in this case are 2 + 3 + 1 = 6.

82. **(D)** At doses of 1000 mg/day or higher, thioridazine has been associated with pigmentary retinopathy, also known as retinitis pigmentosa. Therefore, doses should not exceed 800 mg/day. Pigmentary retinopathy can cause loss of retinal response to contraction of the visual field. An early sign may be nocturnal confusion. Constipation, dry eyes, and urinary retention are side effects from the anticholinergic properties of thioridazine, but typically are not so severe as to compromise health permanently. Nephrogenic diabetes insipidus is not associated with thioridazine.

83. **(C)** Benztropine 1–2 mg IM is useful in the treatment of acute dystonic reactions. Alternatively, diphenhydramine 50 mg IM or IV can be used. If the symptoms do not resolve within 20 minutes, larger doses can be given. Benzodiazepines can also be tried but are not first-line treatment. For acute laryngeal dystonia, 4 mg of benztropine should be given within 10 minutes, then 2 mg of lorazepam IV if needed. None of the other choices are indicated for the treatment of acute dystonia, although switching to a lower-potency neuroleptic might be considered as prophylaxis against further dystonic reactions. Labetalol is an antihypertensive, acetaminophen is an analgesic and antipyretic, and penicillamine is a chelating agent used to treat Wilson disease.

84. **(A)** The disorder described is diabetes insipidus. Lithium inhibits the effect of antidiuretic hormone on the kidney. Although haloperidol (an antipsychotic), diazepam (a benzodiazepine), valproic acid (an antiepileptic used as a mood

stabilizer), and buspirone (an anxiolytic/antidepressant) may be used to treat various manifestations of bipolar disorder, none of them are associated with diabetes insipidus.

85. **(D)** Clonidine, a central alpha-2-autoreceptor agonist, has been proven useful in the treatment of autonomic hyperactivity associated with opioid withdrawal. Haloperidol, pimozide, and thioridazine are antipsychotics. Amantadine is used to treat Parkinson disease and also as an anti-influenza agent.

86. **(C)** Methadone has been proven to greatly reduce the use of heroin when used as a maintenance medication. Patients maintained on doses lower than 40 mg/day of methadone are far more likely to relapse than those on higher doses. Lorazepam and alprazolam are benzodiazepines, sertraline is an SSRI, and lithium is first-line treatment for bipolar disorder.

87. **(B)** TCAs are considered class 1A antiarrhythmics because they possess quinidine-like effects that decrease conduction time through the bundle of His. They have been shown to increase mortality in cardiac patients. TCAs can also increase the heart rate anywhere from 3 to 15 beats/min, and a patient with compromised cardiac function may suffer from increased oxygen demand. Finally, TCAs are associated with significant orthostatic hypotension, which is further exacerbated in patients with cardiac disease. The SSRIs are safely used in patients with cardiac disease, although attention should be paid to cardiac medicines metabolized through the P-450 cytochrome system such as fluoxetine, which could alter medication levels. The butyrophenones and dibenzodiazepines are antipsychotics. Benzodiazepines are not antidepressants.

88. **(D)** Acetylcholine is the neurotransmitter most implicated in cognitive functioning. Anticholinergic effects of medications are frequently implicated in cognitive decline and drug-induced delirium. All of the neurotransmitters listed may be involved in cognition but acetylcholine is by far the most implicated. Dopamine and histamine are targeted by

antipsychotic medications, and serotonin and norepinephrine are thought to be involved in depression.

89. **(B)** Lithium toxicity is characterized early on by dysarthria, ataxia, coarse tremor, and abdominal pain. Later manifestations include seizures, neuromuscular irritability, and impaired consciousness (delirium to coma). Acute dystonias are associated with the use of typical antipsychotics; paranoid delusions are part of the symptom profile of schizophrenia and sometimes of bipolar disorder. Leg pain is not associated with lithium.

90. **(C)** In general, the typical antipsychotics can be continued without significant side effects during ECT, and in fact can lower the seizure threshold, which facilitates ECT. Lithium has been associated with prolonged delirium post-ECT. There are no good data on venlafaxine during ECT. As a benzodiazepine, lorazepam is an antiepileptic and would hinder ECT. Benztropine could cause cognitive difficulties immediately after ECT. Clozapine, an atypical antipsychotic, can cause tardive seizures when administered with ECT.

91. **(A)** There are no absolute contraindications to ECT. A space-occupying lesion is a relative contraindication to ECT. Other relative contraindications include high intracranial pressure, intracerebral bleeding, recent myocardial infarction, retinal detachment, pheochromocytoma, and high anesthesia risk. The other choices are not considered risks.

92. **(B)** For extreme agitation, the butyrophenone antipsychotic haloperidol is useful. Benzodiazepines are also useful for this symptom. Phenothiazine antipsychotics can cause autonomic instability when given to a patient with PCP intoxication. Trihexyphenidyl is used to combat extrapyramidal symptoms associated with antipsychotic use. Trazodone, used commonly for insomnia, and fluoxetine, an SSRI, are antidepressants.

93. **(C)** Supportive care is the best treatment for PCP intoxication that is not complicated by

extreme agitation or violence. Haloperidol, a typical antipsychotic, is useful for extreme agitation. Despite urban myths, vitamins and cheese do not have particular therapeutic benefits for PCP intoxication.

94. **(C)** This patient is suffering from major depression with psychotic features. Psychosis cannot be treated with antidepressant medication alone, because psychosis should be treated with an antipsychotic such as risperidone. Depression should be treated with an antidepressant such as sertraline. Lithium and synthroid can both effectively augment antidepressants such as paroxetine. Lorazepam, a benzodiazepine, may help with anxiety, but will not be effective against psychosis or depression. Similarly, a combination of lorazepam and clozapine, an atypical antipsychotic, will not treat the depression.

95. **(I)** PCP, AKA angel dust, intoxication produces these symptoms as well as hyperthermia, depersonalization, and hallucinations in auditory, tactile, and visual modalities.

96. **(E)** These symptoms may begin within a day for severe alcoholics in withdrawal, and they can progress to DTs by 3 days. DTs are associated with a risk of lethal autonomic collapse.

97. **(C)** These symptoms tend to be mild and last 1–2 days post last use in a regular cocaine user. Occasionally, the depression can be great enough to raise the risk of self-injurious behavior or suicide attempts.

98. **(G)** Heroin withdrawal peaks at about 72 hours post last use in dependent users. It is experienced with many flu-like symptoms and gastrointestinal complaints, such as cramping, nausea, and diarrhea. The appearance of piloerection in the syndrome gave rise to the slang term *cold turkey* to describe the action of total cessation of use of the drug. Cannabis intoxication (A) heightens sensitivity to external stimuli and impairs motor skills. Cocaine intoxication (B) is marked by elated mood, hallucinations, and agitation. Alcohol intoxication (D) involves characteristic behavioral changes, as well as slurred speech, ataxia, and other

neurologic findings. It can progress to coma if severe. Heroin intoxication **(F)** is marked by an altered mood, psychomotor retardation, and drowsiness. The syndromes of MDMA **(H)** and methamphetamine **(J)** intoxication are similar to those of cocaine intoxication. MDMA users typically report an increased "sense of closeness" with other people. Intoxication by inhalants **(K)** (volatile substances such as gasoline fumes) is marked by disorientation and fear and is short-lived. Nicotine intoxication **(L)** is not a category of the DSM-IV-TR. Nitrous oxide intoxication **(M)** produces euphoria and light-headedness and usually subsides within hours without treatment. Withdrawal from psilocybin **(N)**, a hallucinogen derived from mushrooms, is not well-described.

99. **(B)** Clozapine causes agranulocytosis in about 1% of patients. For this reason, weekly blood counts are measured for the first 6 months of treatment, then every 2 weeks thereafter.

100. **(G)** Lithium is associated with clinical hypothyroidism in about 5% of patients, most commonly women. Thyroid supplementation may be added to counter this side effect. Up to 30% of patients may show elevated thyroid-stimulating hormone levels.

Bibliography

American Medical Association. *Code of Medical Ethics: Current Opinions and Annotations 2004–2005.* Chicago, IL: American Medical Association; 2004.

American Psychiatric Association. *Diagnostic and Statistical Manual of Mental Disorders.* 4th ed. Text Revision. Washington, DC: American Psychiatric Press; 2000.

American Psychiatric Association. *DSM-IV-TR Casebook.* Washington, DC: American Psychiatric Press; 2002.

Arana GW, Rosenbaum JF. *Handbook of Psychiatric Drug Therapy.* 4th ed. Boston, MA: Little, Brown & Company; 2000.

Becker AE, Grinspoon SK, Klibanski A, et al. Current concepts: eating disorders. *N Engl J Med.* 1999;340:1092–1098.

Benedetti F, Sforzini L, Colombo C, et al. Low dose clozapine in acute and continuation treatment of severe borderline personality disorder. *J Clin Psychiatry.* 1998;59:103–107.

Check JR. Munchausen syndrome by proxy: an atypical form of child abuse. *J Practical Psychiatry Behavl Health.* 1998;4:340–345.

Conley RR. Optimizing treatment with clozapine. *J Clin Psychiatry.* 1998;59:S44–S48.

Fogel B, Schiffer R, Rao S, eds. *Neuropsychiatry: A Comprehensive Textbook.* Baltimore, MD: Williams & Wilkins; 2003.

Friedman M. Current and future drug treatment for post-traumatic stress disorder. *Psychiatr Ann.* 1998;28:461.

Hyman S, Nestler E. *The Molecular Foundations of Psychiatry.* Washington, DC: American Psychiatric Press; 1993.

Kane JM, Jeste DV, Barnes TRE, et al. *Tardive Dyskinesia: A Task Force Report of the American Psychiatric Association.* Washington, DC: American Psychiatric Association; 1992.

Kaplan HI, Sadock BJ, eds. *Comprehensive Textbook of Psychiatry.* 7th ed. Baltimore, MD: Williams & Wilkins; 2000.

Katona CLE, Robertson MM. *Psychiatry at a Glance.* Cambridge, MA: Blackwell Science; 2000.

Levenson JL. Neuroleptic malignant syndrome. *Am J Psychiatry.* 1985;142:1137–1145.

Lewis M. *Child & Adolescent Psychiatry: A Comprehensive Textbook.* 3rd ed. Baltimore, MD: Williams & Wilkins; 2002.

Lezak MD. *Neuropsychological Assessment.* New York, NY: Oxford University Press; 1995.

Lindenmayer JP, Czobor P, Volavka J, et al. Changes in glucose and cholesterol levels in patients with schizophrenia treated with typical or atypical antipsychotics. *Am J Psychiatry.* 2003;160:290–296.

Lishman WA. *Organic Psychiatry: The Psychological Consequences of Cerebral Disorder.* Malden, MA: Blackwell Science; 1998.

Lowinson J, Ruiz P, Millman R, Langrod J, eds. *Substance Abuse.* 4th ed. Baltimore, MD: Williams & Wilkins; 2004.

O'Malley S, Jaffe AJ, Chang G, et al. Six-month follow-up of naltrexone and psychotherapy for alcohol dependence. *Arch Gen Psychiatry.* 1996;53:217–224.

Ollendick TH, Hersen M, eds. *Handbook of Child Psychopathology.* 3rd ed. New York, NY: Plenum Press; 1998.

Preskorn SH. Clinically relevant pharmacology of selective serotonin reuptake inhibitors. *Clin Pharmacokinet.* 1997;32:S1–S21.

Price L, Heninger G. Lithium in the treatment of mood disorders. *N Engl J Med.* 1994;331:591–598.

Sadock BJ, Sadock VA. *Kaplan and Sadock's Synopsis of Psychiatry:Behavioral Sciences, Clinical Psychiatry.* 9th ed. Baltimore, MD: Williams & Wilkins; 2002.

Schatzberg A, Cole J, DeBattista C, eds. *Manual of Clinical Psychopharmacology.* 3rd ed. Washington, DC: American Psychiatric Press; 1997.

Schatzberg A, Nemeroff C. *Textbook of Psychopharmacology.* 2nd ed. Washington, DC: American Psychiatric Press; 2003.

Stahl S. *Essential Psychopharmacology.* 2nd ed. Cambridge, UK: Cambridge University Press; 2000.

Sternbach H. The serotonin syndrome. *Am J Psychiatry.* 1991;148:705–713.

Tasman A, Kay J, Lieberman J, eds. *Psychiatry.* Hoboken, NJ: John Wiley & Sons; 2003.

Yudofsky SC, Hales RD, eds. *Textbook of Neuropsychiatry and Clinical Neurosciences.* 4th ed. Washington, DC: American Psychiatric Press; 2002.

Index